Springer Proceedings in Mathematics & Statistics

Volume 398

This book series features volumes composed of selected contributions from workshops and conferences in all areas of current research in mathematics and statistics, including data science, operations research and optimization. In addition to an overall evaluation of the interest, scientific quality, and timeliness of each proposal at the hands of the publisher, individual contributions are all refereed to the high quality standards of leading journals in the field. Thus, this series provides the research community with well-edited, authoritative reports on developments in the most exciting areas of mathematical and statistical research today.

Regina Bispo · Lígia Henriques-Rodrigues ·
Russell Alpizar-Jara · Miguel de Carvalho
Editors

Recent Developments in Statistics and Data Science

SPE2021, Évora, Portugal, October 13–16

Springer

Editors
Regina Bispo
NOVA School of Science
and Technology
Caparica, Portugal

Russell Alpizar-Jara
University of Évora
Évora, Portugal

Lígia Henriques-Rodrigues
University of Évora
Évora, Portugal

Miguel de Carvalho
University of Edinburgh
Edinburgh, UK

ISSN 2194-1009 ISSN 2194-1017 (electronic)
Springer Proceedings in Mathematics & Statistics
ISBN 978-3-031-12765-6 ISBN 978-3-031-12766-3 (eBook)
https://doi.org/10.1007/978-3-031-12766-3

Mathematics Subject Classification: 62-06, 62P10, 62P25, 62R07

This Springer imprint is published by the registered company Springer Nature Switzerland AG
The registered company address is: Gewerbestrasse 11, 6330 Cham, Switzerland

Organization

SPE 2021 was organized by the University of Évora and by the Portuguese Statistical Society (SPE).

Executive Commitee

Russell Alpizar-Jara (President), University of Évora (PT)
Dulce Gomes, University of Évora (PT)
Lígia Henriques-Rodrigues, University of Évora (PT)
Patrícia A. Filipe, ISCTE, University Institute of Lisbon (PT)

Scientific Committee

Miguel de Carvalho (President), University of Edinburgh (UK)
Fátima Ferreira, University of Trás-os-monte e Alto Douro (PT)
João Andrade e Silva, University of Lisbon (PT)
Luís Meira-Machado, University of Minho (PT)
Marco Costa, University of Aveiro (PT)
Maria Eduarda Silva, University of Oporto (PT)
Marílía Antunes, University of Lisbon (PT)
Paula Brito, University of Oporto (PT)
Regina Bispo, Nova University of Lisbon (PT)
Rosário Oliveira, University of Lisbon (PT)
Russell Alpizar-Jara, University of Évora (PT)

Partners and Sponsoring Institutions

International Statistical Associations:

- Bernoulli Society
- Brazilian Statistical Association
- CWS (Caucus for Women in Statistics)
- FENStatS (Federation of the European National Statistical Societies)
- ISBA (International Society for Bayesian Analysis)
- RBras (Brazilian Region International Biometric Society)
- SGaPEIO (Sociedade Galega para a promoción da Estatística e da Investigación de Operacions)

National Statistical Associations:

- CLAD (Portuguese Association for Classification and Data Analysis)

Industry and Official Statistics:

- GADES (Data Analysis Solutions)
- INE (Statistics Portugal)
- PSE—Your Data Specialists
- PORDATA—Estatísticas sobre Portugal e Europa

Referees for Proceedings

Ana Freitas
Andy Lynch
Carlos A. Braumann
Clara Cordeiro
Dulce Gomes
Filipe Marques
Inês Sousa
Isabel Pereira
Jessica Silva Lomba
Kamil Turkman
Lisete Sousa
Luís Machado
M. Filomena Teodoro
Manuela Neves
Marco Costa
Maria Antónia Turkman
Maria de Fátima Ferreira
Maria Ivette Gomes
Maria Polidoro

Marília Antunes
Maurizio Sanarico
Nuno Sepúlveda
Patrícia de Zea Bermudez
Patrícia Filipe
Paula Brito
Paulo C. Rodrigues
Paulo M. M. Rodrigues
Pedro Campos
Raquel Menezes
Rita Sousa
Soraia Pereira
Tiago Marques
Vanda Lourenço

Welcome Message from the Editors

XXV Congresso
Sociedade Portuguesa
de Estatística
2021 Évora

Dear authors, referees, and readers of

Recent Developments in Statistics and Data Science,

It is a great pleasure to welcome you to the proceedings of the XXV Congress of the Portuguese Statistical Society—**SPE 2021**—held during 13–16 October 2021 at Évora, Portugal. This was the first-time, ever, online SPE conference, and it gathered more than 200 delegates from all over the world.

The meeting was hosted by University of Évora, Portugal, in collaboration with the Portuguese Statistical Society, and we had a fantastic program including 4 plenary lectures, 31 sessions, and 22 posters. A variety of societies had virtual rooms at SPE 2021 including *Bernoulli Society, Brazilian Statistical Association, Caucus for Women in Statistics*, and the *International Society for Bayesian Analysis*—just to name a few. Institutional members of the Portuguese Statistical Society were also represented (e.g. Statistics Portugal, Banco de Portugal, PORDATA). For more details on the meeting please, see *www.spe2021.uevora.pt/en/*.

Recent Developments in Statistics and Data Science highlights some selected contributions that were presented at SPE 2021. This volume covers a broad range of topics lying at the interface between Statistics and Data Science, such as applied statistics, computational statistics, extremes and outliers, medical statistics, modeling time series and stochastic processes, and data visualization, among others.

And speaking of visualization, Fig. 1 depicts a word cloud of all the titles and abstracts in this volume. While this chart is not a substitute for a table of contents, it does not summarize the order by which the articles appear in this issue! it offers a visual roadmap of what is to be found ahead. Given the broad scope of topics covered, we have opted for clustering articles according to the similarity of topics.

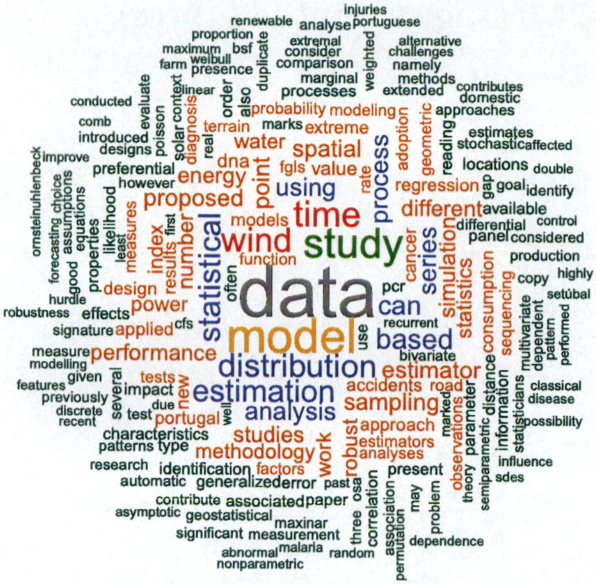

Fig. 1 Word cloud summarizing all titles, keywords, and abstracts of contributions included in this issue

And, as the tag cloud in Fig. 1 reveals, *data* are the common denominator across most contributions.

We are indebted to many people. First, we would like to thank the authors for their contributions and to everyone involved in the peer-review process who did a superb job on meeting tight deadlines in a thoughtful manner. They all worked hard so that the community keeps breaking new ground, and should be proud of their achievements. We are also indebted to Springer for their excellent collaboration on the production of this issue, and to the Scientific Committee and keynote speakers for their contributions to the meeting. Last but not the least, our words of thanks go to the organizers of SPE 2021 for their outstanding work, and to the community of the Portuguese Statistical Society for their continuous, and yet unbounded! support.

March 2022

Regina Bispo
Lígia Henriques-Rodrigues
Russell Alpizar-Jara
Miguel de Carvalho

Contents

How to Increase the Visibility of Statisticians in the Modern World of Dataism?

Nuno Sepúlveda

Abstract In the view of the historian Yuval Noah Harari, current human thought can be characterized by a deep belief in data, whether big or small, as the main vehicle to understand and control the world. This belief is referred to as Dataism. Notwithstanding their key role as guarantors of high-quality statistical exercises and data curators, statisticians typically remain in the shadow of big decisions in multi-disciplinary and highly collaborative environments. This situation can be overcome by operating a change in the mindset of statisticians from *shoe clerks* to *statistical leaders*. Under the assumption that a statistician has already achieved a certain level of statistical proficiency, this paper aims to discuss useful skills, such as active listening, networking, and effective communication, which can foster statistical leadership and increase recognition and merit by non-statisticians inside and outside academia.

Keywords Impact · Interpersonal skills · Leadership · Statistical career

1 Introduction

We are living in a world in which data are an integral part of our daily experience as human beings. Take the example of our little good friend smartphone, which can collect data on the number of daily steps. With these data, we can judge whether we should be more active and, if so, we can get other data-collection apps to help us tracing that increase in activity. Data and the respective collection are so engrained in our lives that the famous historian Yuval Noah Harari writes in his best-selling book *Homo Deus: a Brief History of Tomorrow* about Dataism, a kind of new religion deeply rooted on the general belief that data and its flow are all that matters to understand and hold control of the world [1]. This religion made us to invest in

N. Sepúlveda (✉)
Faculty of Mathematics and Information Science, Warsaw University of Technology, Warsaw, Poland
e-mail: N.Sepulveda@mini.pw.edu.pl

CEAUL - Centro de Estatística e Aplicações da Universidade de Lisboa, Lisbon, Portugal

R. Bispo et al. (eds.), *Recent Developments in Statistics and Data Science*,
Springer Proceedings in Mathematics & Statistics 398,
https://doi.org/10.1007/978-3-031-12766-3_1

innovative technologies in data acquisition, storage, and management [2]. As a result, current data can be big, huge, humungous!

In this brave new world of big data, our privacy, autonomy, and individuality are often given away to ensure our essential role as data providers. At the same time, such a profound and often blind belief on Dataism makes us all too vulnerable to unscrupulous politicians who use fake news or incomplete data to convince us to join their malicious cause. In this scenario, we statisticians can be seen as whistleblowers of data abuses, rationale and neutral players that can denounce disinformation, misinformation, or statistical malpractices [3]. A kind of justice league members of this data world. But is anyone out there who is willing to listen to us given that even the use of our *friend* p-value in Science is under debate and controversy [4]?

Unfortunately, the deep faith in Dataism did not make statisticians more visible in the society over the years. In fact, this reduced visibility can be traced back to the time of the great statisticians of the past. In 1938, Fisher [5] famously wrote in his usual cut-throat style that:

> To consult the statistician after an experiment finished is often merely to ask him to conduct a postmortem examination. He can perhaps say what the experiment died of.

This sentence is an open criticism to the still-prevailing attitude of seeking a statistician as a last resort. It also subtlety hints that statisticians are somehow invisible to their peers from the non-statistical world. In the past, statisticians were hidden disciples of Mathematics and now are simply *data crunchers* or *p-value providers*. To make things worse, statisticians are currently in direct competition with data scientists, bioinformaticians, and mathematical modellers in terms of their contribution to multidisciplinary, and above all, cutting-edge research. The fundamental question that we all statisticians face at the moment is then how to increase our visibility and value in this wondrous world of big data.

A first answer to this question can be found in the thought-provoking article entitled *The role of the Statistician: scientist or shoe clerk* by Irving Bross [6]. This author discusses the immediate and the long-term implications of a statistician adopting a posture similar of a shoe clerk whose primary objective is to please current and future customers. On the one hand, a shoe-clerk attitude has the advantage of neutrality and minimal hassle in moments of tension amongst team's members. It has also the advantage of fattening the resumé of applied statisticians (including the author of this paper) with a large number of middle-author publications; the underlying idea seems to be: minimal effort, maximum outcome, and a big boost of the ego. This advantage is in agreement with an increased number of middle authors in biomedical research [7], but it remains to be uncovered what is the contribution of statisticians to this trend. On the other hand, the hard truth is that, in the long-term, statisticians who solely act as shoe clerks will always be treated like one. Ultimately, the cordial, complacent but often neglecting treatment by their non-statistical peers suggests a certain *be a lamb* stereotype for the statistician as a professional. Finally, the quality of the statistical product itself could be also compromised, because it is intrinsically difficult for shoe-clerk-type statisticians to go against their customers who are typically in a standpoint of *I know what I want or need for my data* at the start of a collaboration.

More recently, Gibson [8] intertwines the concepts of visibility and the value of a statistician with leadership skills; however, the use of the word *value* has the unnecessary connotation that a statistician like a commodity can be sold up or down in the stock (or job) market. According to this author, the visibility of a statistician can be increased by creating a new culture around statistical leadership. This culture requires the acquisition of specific skills and the mindset of a leader, which will be discussed in Sect. 2. Such skills can be learned, practised, and improved. However, there is a limited number of universities offering courses on these leadership skills.

In this scenario, this paper is a collection of ideas and concepts scattered around the literature about leadership; a more personal account of this topic can be found elsewhere [9]. It is particularly directed to all the statisticians who wish to embrace a joyful journey towards a more impactful, fulfilling, and meaningful collaborations. Statistical leadership is above all a personal choice and not an authority, rank, or position. As such, it is accessible to everyone.

2 Statistical Leadership and Its Key Competences

According to Gibson [8], statistical leadership can be broadly defined as the use of influence without authority to guide the design, strategy, and decisions of a multidisciplinary team. The same author outlines three competences or soft skills essential for successful statistical leadership: (i) active listening; (ii) networking; and (iii) effective communication. These skills are not new and can be found in the popular book entitled *12 Rules for Life: Antidote to Chaos* by the clinical psychologist Jordan Peterson [10], but formulated as follows:

- Active listening: *Assume that the person you are listening to might know something you don't*;
- Networking: *Make friends with people who want the best for you*;
- Effective communication: *Be precise in your speech.*

A brief discussion on these skills will be presented in the next three subsections.

2.1 Active Listening

It is universally regarded that Nelson Mandela (1918–2013) was a great leader. He was the elected president in the first free democratic elections in South Africa after the end of the apartheid. One of the remarkable Mandela's leadership skills was his power of listening and using it for strategic and reflective questioning [11]. This power was developed by witnessing community meetings with his father who was the chief of his tribe [12]. He learned that everyone was seated in a circle and his father was always the last one to speak. The amazing capacity of listening to everyone before speaking and, more importantly, before any rushed judgement deeply resides the transformative power of active listening.

At the surface, one might think that active listening is just giving free and undivided attention to the speaker. However, it is more than that [13]. It involves (Table 1):

1. adopting an appropriate body language while listening;
2. reflecting in what is being heard;
3. understanding the consequences and implications of the information received.

As a consequence, active listening is able to generate mutual understanding, commitment between parties, and the joyful and fulfilling sensation that each side was heard. Ultimately, active listening builds trust and respect, which are necessary to maintain harmonious and sustainable collaborative environments.

We statisticians like medical doctors, nurses, and other professionals alike are required to develop such a listening skill due to our line of work. Unfortunately, this skill is taken for granted, because it is supposedly to be natural to have it. In the truth of the matter, it is not easy to master it without any effort and even more so in the modern world of constant distractions by smartphones, social media, amongst other factors. As suggested in the Introduction, this skill can be learned, trained, and improved. In the book entitled *How to be heard: Secrets for Powerful Speaking and Listening*, Julian Treasure [14] suggests simple exercises to improve one's listening capacities such as:

1. enjoy the sound of silence (or simply enjoy the song of Simon and Garfunkel or the cover by the Disturbed);
2. listen to mundane sounds like a bus passing by or a working dishwasher;
3. try to identify how many different sounds can be heard in a bar;
4. changing listening positions such as passive versus active or critical versus empathic;
5. follow RASA (Receive, Appreciate, Summary, and Ask) in a conversation.

The crisis in listening is so severe nowadays that the same author in his 2011 Ted Talk about this topic gathered more than 10 million views on YouTube since then [15]. Hence, it is time to sharpen our hearing and try to listening better.

2.2 *Networking*

Current scientific agenda aims to provide answers to complex societal problems, such as the impact of climate change in the world, the prediction of a new pandemic, or the reduction of social inequality. The complexity of these problems motivates the creation of large research teams, research consortia, or networks, in which people with different expertise converge. In this regard, statisticians are sought as strategic partners of these enterprises, because they can help with the design of a project and

Table 1 Active listening skills according to Robertson [13]

Attentive body language
Posture and gestures showing involvement and engagement
Appropriate body movement
Appropriate facial expressions
Appropriate eye contact
Non-distracting environment
Following skills
Interested *door openers*
Minimal verbal encouragers
Infrequent, timely and considered questions
Attentive silences
Reflective skills
Paraphrase (check periodically that you've understood)
Reflect back feelings and content
Summarize the major issues

deliver advanced statistical analysis that is typically out of reach of non-statistically-trained researchers. However, working in such multidisciplinary environments can be challenging and overwhelming for statisticians, because they need to interact with other researchers often enough to negotiate different strategic decisions for the course of a project. The development of networking skills is then necessary.

These skills consist in developing an interpersonal intuition on how different members of a research team fit together in order to understand team dependencies, responsibilities, and dynamics. For example, in a large epidemiological study, statisticians are typically asked to join forces with epidemiologists, mathematical modellers, and bioethical experts. Statisticians can increase visibility by talking to each of these colleagues in order to decide on the best study design. In a sentence, higher visibility comes when a statistician is a team player and sets the team's goal as his/her top priority.

Networking skills are also mandatory for choosing collaborators wisely. Like ice-creams, collaborators come in different flavours and, therefore, statisticians who intend to be treated as equal should create a network of collaborators who share the same principles, attitudes, and ambitions. When it comes to evaluating the success of a given collaboration, statisticians should weight the immediate research output (i.e., a high-impact paper or a funded project) against the sense of mutual respect, harmony, and sustainability in the long term. One cannot forget that, given the high demand for statistical services in academia and elsewhere, statisticians have all the autonomy and power to choose and embrace only durable and harmonious collaborations with their non-statistical peers.

The important question is then to know how to improve networking skills. Besides taking formal training, statisticians can also join a professional society such as the

Portuguese Statistical Society in Portugal, the Royal Statistical Society in the United Kingdom (UK), or the International Biometrical Society. Active citizenship in these societies allows statisticians to find and connect easily with other professionals with the same research interests. Alternatively, statisticians can make an effort to seek networking opportunities outside the field of Statistics. For example, being a member of COST actions funded by the European Union is a unique opportunity for statisticians to increase their network of collaborators across Europe. In the UK, the Academy of Medical Sciences and the Royal Society offer specific funding for creating new networks between UK-based and overseas researchers.

2.3 *Effective Communication*

The primary objective of any act of verbal communication is to create understanding from what is being said and heard. The same objective is also expected when communication takes the form of the written word. Effective communication goes beyond this basic objective by aiming to create impact, to generate action, or to motivate change.

In the case of applied statisticians, effective communication is likely to come in the shape of presenting or writing the results of a statistical analysis to a non-specialized audience. In this scenario, impactful communication should not be understood as the delivery of catchy and simple soundbites or keywords, or just speaking to the audience's emotions, or even more so sacrificing technical accuracy and rigour. Impact should be seen in a broader sense in which the target audience understands the results and the respective implications clearly. Impactful communication also sets the scene for statisticians to manage expectations and negotiations that might occur during the lifetime of a project or collaboration. Unsurprisingly, there is no magical solution for effective and impactful communication. However, some of the tips below are extremely useful for a scientist in general to learn, practice, and improve.

In the current work and scientific culture of frequent meetings and conferences, effective and impactful verbal communication is intimately related to delivering a good talk or presentation. In this regard, the TED curator Chris Anderson provides a set of tricks for public speaking [16]. According to this author, delivering a decent talk is at the reach of everyone's hand. Delivering a talk in the format of a story is always a very compelling way to fuel people's imagination. Stories are also easy to follow and natural for all of us given that we learn life through stories since childhood. Simplify the message and never underestimate the power of rehearsing are two other tips for effective talks. The Indian Yoga's master Sadhguru [17] also provides a very useful advice for speaking in general:

> *See if you can articulate the same things that you are saying with half the number of words. Suddenly you will become extremely conscious of everything.*

When preparing slides supporting a presentation, the humorous and bold David Phillips [18] advises five tips *to avoid death by powerpoint*:

1. one message per slide to increase focus of the audience and avoid distraction amongst competing content;
2. avoid the use of text to reduce the mental strain of listening and reading simultaneously;
3. increase the size of key objects to maximize their readability and interpretability by the audience;
4. use contrast of colours to guide people's attention;
5. use a maximum of 6 objects per slide to minimize the time for the audience to grasp what is on each slide.

From the above five tips, avoiding text should be the mantra for any public speaker including a statistician. In fact, slides with insane amounts of text might be one of the deadliest sins in public speaking. It can give the impression that the text is not there for the audience to read, but for the speaker not forget what to say. As a consequence, one might feel that the speaker is neither prepared, nor confident, nor comfortable in his/her shoes. While lack of preparation suggests some sort of disrespect for the audience, lack of confidence might generate empathy to some listeners; after all, we all have been out there, exposed in front of the audience with sharp eyes, but it ultimately generates pity rather impact. Reducing the amount of text has the benefit of creating the right motivation for a speaker to be brief and simple, and to rehearse the presentation. We should never forget that the speaker and what he/she is saying are the main focus of a talk. By logic, if the speaker wishes the audience to read from slides, why is he/she there?

For effective writing in scientific papers and reports, Ehrenberg [19] suggests the following guidelines:

1. to start at the end (or focus on findings first);
2. be prepared to revise;
3. cut down the long words;
4. be brief;
5. think of the reader.

Presenting and discussing the results first is the writing format that some scientific journals such as the Nature-branded and PLoS journals are adopting nowadays; the Materials & Methods section where statisticians feel more comfortable, is typically placed at the end of the paper or, in some extreme cases, buried in an online supplementary material. This writing format might be challenging for statisticians given their natural inclination and enthusiasm for methodological issues. However, at the same time, this inclination and enthusiasm should not be totally silenced, because providing detailed information about the statistical methodology is a moral and ethical obligation that promotes scientific replication and reproducibility [3].

To be prepared to revise is the joyful art for some or the painstaking task for others of making tweaks and adjustments to the text for better readability. This task is intimately related to be brief and cut down unnecessary jargon which is typically encapsulated in long words. It takes an underestimated number of iterations, specially, by students and early-career statisticians. The revision of a paper written in English might be challenging for non-native speakers. In this case, one should operate in a benevolent regime of *practice makes perfect*; that and a lot of patience. Finally, thinking of the reader helps deciding the level of (statistical) detail that statisticians can dive in a report or paper.

If one seeks to master the art of effective (oral) communication to inspire others, Simon Sinek [20] proposes a simple but useful concept: the golden circle (Fig. 1). The way that we communicate on the daily basis is by progressing from *what*, *how*, and *why*. For example, if one aims to present the content of this paper in a conference, the traditional way to start the presentation could be the following:

> Today I will share with you some tips that I have learned about statistical leadership. These tips are related to active listening, networking, and effective communication. I will first define what they mean and then tell you how you can improve them. I hope all of these tips are useful for you and your future career.

This is the natural way of communicating for most of us, because we start from the most precise to the most vague piece of information. That is, (almost) everyone knows what he/she is supposed to do, some really know how to do it, but only a few know the reason for what they are doing. This way of communication is not necessarily ineffective per se, but fails to deliver impact to the audience; we listen to the same communication format over and over again and, therefore, boredom might set in with these repetitions.

According to Simon Sinek, simply reversing the order of the information given generates more impact on the listener. Let's come back to the above example. After some tweaking, one could alternatively start the presentation like this:

> Big data are the brave new world. However, we statisticians remain hidden in the shadow of this world of wonder. We are simply seen as data crunchers or p-value providers. We

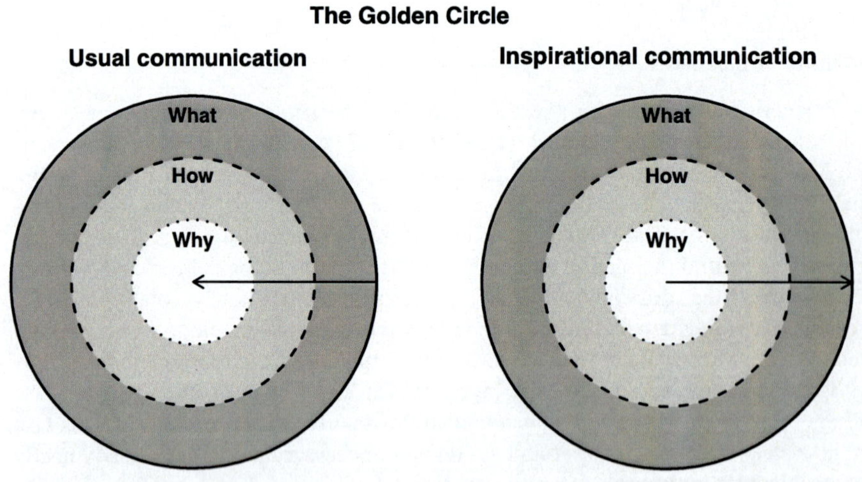

Fig. 1 The golden circle of communication by Simon Sinek [20]: usual communication travels from what, how, and why, while inspirational communication does the opposite

> should change this narrow view of our profession. How to operate this change? By thinking of statistical leadership and how we can develop it. Today I will give you some tips about active listening, networking, and effective communication, which we can use routinely in our profession. In the end, if we are little ambassadors of statistical leadership, everyone wins.

The clear articulation of *why* talks to our emotions and, as we all know it, they are capable to convince us to do wonderful things. However, for this communication approach to work, there is the challenge of knowing the reason of what we are doing. In this regard, the philosophical discussion about the role of a statistician, the duality between a scientist and shoe clerk as smartly put it by Bross [6], helps to solve this challenge. If a statistician acts like a shoe clerk, it is difficult to inspire anyone by simply pleasing the customer, getting a salary at the end of the month, or climbing up the academic ladder. In contrast, if a statistician considers him/herself as a scientist first of all, it is much easier to find a purpose for being part of a given project. After all, a scientist is a curious person about the world and an eternal chaser of the truth.

3 Increasing Visibility in Academia

In theory, the academic recognition and visibility of a statistician should be in a direct correlation with the publication record and the amount of funding awarded. Hence, any attempt to increase the number of publications and funding awarded are straightforward steps towards a higher recognition and visibility of statisticians in academia. In practice, there are other factors that one must consider.

Firstly, increasing the number of publications might require to extend the number of collaborators and projects involved. Managing different collaborators and projects might imply to become a *slave* of them. This can dramatically reduce the time dedicated to pursuit personal research interests. Therefore, applied statisticians should find their optimal balance between their own projects and statistical consultancy activities.

Secondly, funding opportunities for the development of statistical methodologies are scarce and, when available, are often shared with mathematical modellers, mathematicians, bioinformaticians, and data scientists. Given this scenario and the multidisciplinary nature of the statistical exercise, applied statisticians could try to widen their research interests beyond statistical methodology; genetics and climate changes are just two examples of scientific areas where a deep knowledge of statistics and statistical modelling is a requirement. Such a widening of the research agenda increases the chance of getting a project funded and provides an opportunity for statisticians to lead a project. Leading a project increases the visibility of the respective leader irrespective of the scientific area. In this regard, we should follow the footsteps of the great statisticians of the past who made remarkable contributions outside the field of Statistics: Ronald Fisher-population and quantitative genetics; Karl Pearson-biometrics; Egon Pearson and Walter Shewhart-quality control; Francis Galton-psychometrics; amongst others.

There are also less conventional ways that statisticians can use to increase their visibility in academia. Statisticians can find inspiration in a recent review of global travelling and infectious diseases using James Bond's movies as case studies [21]. At the time of writing, this review gathered almost 3,500 likes and 2,000 mentions on Twitter. The infamous Christmas edition of the prestigious British Medical Journal also offers the publication of formal and rigorous scientific enquiries to quirky, light-hearted, or funny biomedical questions, including the estimation of teaspoons disappearance from shared kitchens in a research institute [22], risk estimation of neck and head injuries in heavy metal lovers [23], or the reporting of side-effects in sword-swallowing [24]. A final example comes from James Carlisle who gained the nickname of *data detective* [25]. This Englishman is a trained anesthesiologist but spends his part-time screening the biomedical literature for unusual statistical consistency, data fabrication, and statistical anomalies [26, 27]. Of course, his hobby does not make him particular popular amongst the targets of his investigations [28]. However, his sleuth efforts were not left unnoticed by the research community and hopefully, they served the purpose of raising awareness on the statistical problems in the existing literature while promoting better science and better use of statistical methodology.

4 Increasing Visibility in Society

Imagination, creativity, and personal motivation are the only limits that can hold someone's back in the track of increased visibility in society. For example, statisticians can embrace the technological revolution in mass communication provided by the internet. Social media platforms such as Facebook or Twitter offer quick and cheap ways to disseminate research findings amongst collaborators, colleagues, family, and friends. These platforms also provide an informal forum of discussion between researchers and the general public who ultimately fund research through taxes. The production of podcasts dedicated to disseminate scientific ideas are also gaining popularity in different corners of science [29]. In this regard, the podcast called *The Effective Statistician* by Alexander Schacht [30] helps statisticians to improve efficiency at the workplace, to think more strategically about their career, and to appreciate leadership and negotiation skills.

An interesting opportunity to increase visibility amongst the youngsters is provided by the journal *Frontiers for Young Minds*. The journal publishes conceptual papers to be read by the young ones. The peer-review process is conducted by a young reviewer, but under the guidance of a professional scientist. The *modus operandi* of the journal offers the chance of disseminating statistical ideas and promoting their use amongst the young readers, as the case of Sendef and Robbins [31], who explored the concepts of population, statistics, and probability. The review was done by Joseph of 12 years of age with the help of Jonathan Montaño from the New Mexico State University.

5 Concluding Remarks

This paper discusses some useful skills with the potential of increasing the visibility and the potential of a statistician at the individual level. These skills require permanent and, if needed, formal training. Unfortunately, traditional statistical courses are mainly focused on the hardcore technical skills even if a successful statistician is required to master interpersonal skills given the translational nature of the statistical exercise. Therefore, there is a mismatch between the formal training of Statistics at the university and the prerequisites for a successful career in academia and elsewhere, namely, in the long-term. It is then advised for future or even established statisticians to seek opportunities for improving their interpersonal skills. The acquisition and practising of these skills will make them more prepared, more comfortable, and more confidence to go beyond the "shoe-clerk"-type mindset.

The underlying assumption of this discussion is that a statistician reached a certain *badge* of statistical proficiency when it is reasonable to think of leadership and visibility. This badge does not necessarily mean a world-class recognition of someone's achievements in terms of statistical methodology and modelling. It only means a level of understanding of what a statistical analysis is and what it entails. In other words, statistical leadership and visibility come naturally when a statistician understands not only the methodology, but also the *big picture* beyond the remit of a given statistical analysis. In this scenario, early-career statisticians would find themselves less inclined to invest time in developing leadership skills and taking the necessary steps towards a more impactful career. This comes more naturally to mid-career statisticians who were already involved in enough collaborations and projects, and therefore, have a better idea of the pros and cons of the statistical profession. However, it is important to emphasize again that leadership and visibility are personal choices and, as such, every one of us should make an introspective exercise at least once in a lifetime to answer the question whether statistical leadership is a sufficiently appealing or attractive journey to take. At the end of the day, a career of any professional should be joyful.

Statisticians with the intention to increase their (professional) influence should be aware of two possible psychological roadblocks. The first one is that leadership and increased visibility should be perceived as journeys rather than goals. These journeys require a great amount of patience, persistence, and resilience. These personal capacities typically clash with current culture of instant gratification and constant pursuit for impact. Anxiety might come along the way. If such happens, statisticians should make a step back and revaluate their situation. The second roadblock is the so-called impostor phenomenon. In this phenomenon, people express self-doubt on their accomplishments and skills, despite factual evidence or other people indicating otherwise. People who suffer from this phenomenon believe that their success is due to some kind of luck or error, and they live in constant fear of being unmasked as unintelligent or less capable. These impostor feelings can diminish career planning, career prospective, and the motivation to lead [32]. Therefore, it is possible that future highly visible statistical leaders should feel something similar. In that case, statisticians should embrace these feelings as a motivation and an opportunity for self-improvement and not for self-doubt.

The final remark is to make a clear distinction amongst individual, organizational, and policy levels of statistical leadership and visibility, as discussed by Gibson [8]. In this scenario, the present paper mainly focused the discussion at the individual level. This level relates to small research groups and day-to-day interactions between a statistician and his/her colleagues or collaborators. Statistical visibility and leadership at the organizational level is related to the situation where the influence of a (senior) statistician or a group of them aims to be felt at the level of a given institution, such as company or research consortium. This influence can take the form of trying to change a given statistical practice amongst all members of the same institution. In turn, statistical leadership and visibility at the policy level is operated by statisticians who sit at technical advisory committees representing different stakeholders. For example, statisticians together with epidemiologists, medical doctors, nurses, and other health staff might be put together to discuss with the national health authorities whether an existing policy needs to be change or whether a new policy needs to be created at the light of new data. An interesting example of statistical leadership at this level is the discussion around the salt consumption and health held by the Institute of Medicine (currently, named National Academy of Medicine) from the USA provided by Nancy Cook [33]. Another example is given by the statistician Mike Campbell who works on the NICE appraisal committee in the UK [34]; NICE is the agency that decides which new therapies should be allowed in the British National Health System. These two levels of statistical leadership are more challenging than the individual one, and require a deeper discussion of other skills (e.g., negotiation, conflict management, and mediation skills) that are beyond the scope of this paper. A more extensive discussion about these two levels of statistical leadership can be found in Gibson [8].

Acknowledgements The author would like to thank João Malato (Instituto de Medicina Molecular, Lisbon, Portugal), Emanuele Giorgi (Lancaster University, Lancaster, UK), Francisco Westermeier (FH Joanneum University of Applied Sciences, Graz, Austria) and Alexander Schacht (The Effective Statistician, Germany) for proof-reading the manuscript and providing insightful comments and suggestions. The author acknowledges funding from the Fundação para a Ciência e Tecnologia, Portugal (ref. UIDB/00006/2020), and the Polish National Agency for Academic Exchange, Poland (ref. PPN/ULM/2020/1/00069/U/00001).

References

1. Harari, Y.N.: Homo Deus: A Brief History of Tomorrow. Vintage, London, London (2017)
2. Leonelli, S.: Data-from objects to assets. Nature **574**, 317–320 (2019)
3. Stark, P.B., Saltelli, A.: Cargo-cult statistics and scientific crisis. Significance **15**, 40–43 (2018)
4. Wasserstein, R.L., Lazar, N.A.: The ASA statement on p-values: context, process, and purpose. Am. Stat. **70**, 129–133 (2016)
5. Fisher, R.A.: Presidential address (1933–1960). Sankhya: The Indian J. Stat. **4**(1), 14–17 (1938)
6. Bross, I.D.J.: The role of the statistician: scientist or shoe clerk. Am. Stat. **28**, 126–127 (1974)
7. Mongeon, P., Smith, E., Joyal, B., Lariviére, V.: The rise of the middle author: Investigating collaboration and division of labor in biomedical research using partial alphabetical authorship. PLoS One **12**, e0184601 (2017)
8. Gibson, E.W.: Leadership in statistics: increasing our value and visibility. Am. Stat. **73**, 109–116 (2018)
9. Sepúlveda, N.: Ser ou não ser um líder (estatístico)?. In: Boletim SPE Primavera, pp. 39–48, SPE Editions (2022)
10. Peterson, J.B.: 12 Rules for Life: An Antidote to Chaos. Penguin Allen Lane, London (2021)
11. Bunkers, S.S.: The power and possibility in listening. Nurs. Sci. Q. **23**, 22–27 (2009)
12. Mandela, N.R.: Long Walk to Freedom. Hachette Book Group, New York (1994)
13. Robertson, K.: Active listening: More than just paying attention. Aust. Family Phys. **34**, 1053–1055 (2005)
14. Treasure, J.: How to be Heard: Secrets for Powerful Speaking and Listening. Mango Publishing Group, Coral Gable (2017)
15. Treasure, J.: 5 ways to listen better. https://www.ted.com/talks/julian_treasure_5_ways
16. Anderson, C.: TED Talks: The Official TED Guide to Public Speaking. Houghton Mifflin Harcourt, Boston (2016)
17. Sadhguru: The importance of silence
18. Phillips, D.J.P.: How to avoid death by powerpoint. https://www.youtube.com/watch?v=KpMbR7WCLXI
19. Ehrenberg, A.S.C.: Writing technical papers or reports. Am. Stat. **36**, 326–329 (1982)
20. Sinek, S.: Start with Why: How Great Leaders Inspire Everyone to Take Action. Portfolio, London (2009)
21. Graumans, W., Stone, W.J., Bousema, T.: No time to die: An in-depth analysis of James Bond's exposure to infectious agents. Travel Med. Infect. Dis. **44**, 102175 (2021)
22. Lim, M.S.C., Hellard, M.E., Aitken, C.K.: The case of the disappearing teaspoons: longitudinal cohort study of the displacement of teaspoons in an australian research institute. BMJ **331**, 1498–1500 (2005)
23. Patton, D., McIntosh, A.: Head and neck injury risks in heavy metal: head bangers stuck between rock and a hard bass. BMJ **337**, a2825–a2825 (2008)
24. Witcombe, B., Meyer, D.: Sword swallowing and its side effects. BMJ **333**, 1285–1287 (2006)
25. Adam, D.: How a data detective exposed suspicious medical trials. Nature **571**, 462–464 (2019)
26. Carlisle, J.B.: The analysis of 168 randomised controlled trials to test data integrity. Anaesthesia **67**, 521–537 (2012)
27. Carlisle, J.B.: Data fabrication and other reasons for non-random sampling in 5087 randomised, controlled trials in anaesthetic and general medical journals. Anaesthesia **72**, 944–952 (2017)
28. Fujii, Y.: The analysis of 168 randomised controlled trials to test data integrity. Anaesthesia **67**, 669–670 (2012)
29. Kwok, R.: How to make your podcast stand out in a crowded market. Nature **565**, 387–389 (2019)
30. Schacht, A.: The effective statistician podcast. http://theeffectivestatistician.com/podcast/
31. Sendef, J., Robbins, A.: How scientists use statistics, samples, and probability to answer research questions. Front. Young Minds **7**, 118 (2019)
32. Neureiter, M., Traut-Mattausch, E.: An inner barrier to career development: preconditions of the impostor phenomenon and consequences for career development. Front. Psychol. **7** (2016)

33. Cook, N.R.: Salt: how much less should we eat for health?: understanding the recent IOM report. Significance **10**, 6–10 (2013)
34. Campbell, M.: A statistician on a NICE committee. Significance **7**, 81–84 (2010)

A Robust Hurdle Poisson Model in the Estimation of the Extremal Index

Manuela Souto de Miranda, M. Cristina Miranda, and M. Ivette Gomes

Abstract In statistical extreme value theory, the occurrence of clusters of exceedances above a high threshold is related to the extremal index (*EI*), when that parameter exists. In such cases, the *EI* represents the reciprocal of the mean cluster dimension in the limit distribution. The set of observed cluster sizes may contain too many zeroes, depending on the scheme used in the identification of the clusters and posterior estimation process, as it happens with the Blocks estimator. We consider the estimation of the mean cluster size by modelling the clusters dimension with a hurdle zero truncated Poisson regression model. The goal is to find a robust estimator with a good performance along increasing quantiles and computationally user friendly. The paper highlights the importance of the last question also, since many statisticians use or do not use some methods, depending on the free software devoted to the method and respective confidence in their optimization procedures and results. A simulation study explores and compares different proposals.

Keywords Blocks estimator · Extremal index · Hurdle model · Robustness

M. Souto de Miranda (✉)
CIDMA, University of Aveiro, Aveiro, Portugal
e-mail: manuela.souto@ua.pt

M. C. Miranda
ISCA and CIDMA, University of Aveiro, Aveiro, Portugal
e-mail: cristina.miranda@ua.pt

CEAUL, University of Lisbon, Cidade Universitária, Campo Grande, Portugal

M. I. Gomes
Faculty of Science of Lisbon (FCUL/DEIO) and CEAUL, University of Lisbon, Cidade Universitária, Campo Grande, Portugal
e-mail: ivette.gomes@fc.ul.pt

R. Bispo et al. (eds.), *Recent Developments in Statistics and Data Science*,
Springer Proceedings in Mathematics & Statistics 398,
https://doi.org/10.1007/978-3-031-12766-3_2

1 The Extremal Index

1.1 Motivation

There is a great interest in modelling extreme values, particularly when they represent the exceedance of high thresholds. The theory is extensively developed for extremes in the independence framework. Nevertheless, many phenomena are more realistically modelled by the occurrence of clusters of extreme values than assuming a scenery of isolated independent ones. That is the case with heat or cold waves, extremely rainy days, price crashes in the stock market and so on. The duration of those phenomena can be traduced by a counting process that represents the cluster size, whose mean is related to the *EI*, when it exists. Thus, the *EI* estimation procedure deserves a great practical interest. But it is not enough to look for a method with good mathematical properties from a classical point of view. The procedure must be robust, in the sense that gives good estimates in the assumed model and, simultaneously, it is not very sensitive to small deviations from the model assumptions, for instance, gross error values or even the functional form of the cluster size distribution. Robust estimation theory has been widely investigated for location and regression models, particularly with continuous distributions. With respect to counting processes, the research is still very active nowadays.

Another important point of view is the existence of computation facilities that allow easy access to the *EI* estimates, either in individual case studies or in simulations. Computational techniques cover two main fields: the numerical questions, since many estimators depend on complex optimization problems that become more evident in simulation environments; and open access software tools, like the *R* platform with its packages, which are already programmed in a devoted way and well tested by investigators. It is also desirable that software is user friendly, so that it can be used by statisticians in general. Those aspects are essential to the success of the *EI* estimation process (and others), mainly outside the more popular Gaussian and independence scenarios.

1.2 Theoretical Introduction

Assume a strictly stationary sequence of random variables $\{X_n\}_{n\geq 1}$, from a *cumulative distribution function* (*CDF*) denoted by F, under general asymptotic and long-range dependence restrictions, like the long-range dependence condition **D** (see [1]) and the local dependence condition **D**” (see [2]). Let $\{X_{i:n}\}_{n\geq 1}$, $1 \leq i \leq n$, denote the associated sequence of ascending order statistics.

The stationary sequence $\{X_n\}_{n\geq 1}$ is said to have an *EI*, θ, with $(0 < \theta \leq 1)$, if for all $\tau > 0$, we can find a sequence of levels $u_n = u_n(\tau)$ such that, with $\{Y_n\}_{n\geq 1}$ the associated *independent, identically distributed* (*i.i.d.*) sequence (*i.e.*, an *i.i.d.* sequence from the same CDF F),

$$P\left(Y_{n:n} \le u_n\right) = F^n(u_n) \underset{n\to\infty}{\longrightarrow} e^{-\tau}$$

and

$$P\left(X_{n:n} \le u_n\right) \underset{n\to\infty}{\longrightarrow} \exp^{-\theta\tau}.$$

Since $0 < \theta \le 1$, there is thus a *'shrinkage'* of the values in the limit *CDF*, but after linearly normalized, $X_{n:n}$ has still an *extreme value* (*EV*) distribution, with a *CDF* with a functional form of the type

$$\mathrm{EV}_\xi(x) = \begin{cases} \exp\{-(1+\xi x)^{-1/\xi}\},\ 1+\xi x > 0, & \text{if } \xi \ne 0 \\ \exp(-\exp(-x)),\ x \in R, & \text{if } \xi = 0. \end{cases} \quad (1)$$

Under the two mixing conditions **D** and **D''**, the *EI* can also be defined as:

$$\theta = \frac{1}{\text{limiting mean size of clusters}} = \lim_{n\to\infty} P(X_2 \le u_n | X_1 > u_n),$$

with

$$u_n: \quad F(u_n) = 1 - \tau/n + o(1/n), \quad \text{as } n \to \infty, \text{ with } \tau > 0, \text{ fixed.} \quad (2)$$

The m-dependent (m-dep) processes are used here for illustration. It is known that for these processes the *EI* is given by $\theta = 1/m$. They may be based on *i.i.d.* Fréchet (ξ) random variables Y_i, $i \ge 1$, from a *CDF* $\Phi_\xi^{1/m}$, with $\Phi_\xi(x) = \exp\left(-x^{-1/\xi}\right)$, $x \ge 0$, the standard Fréchet *CDF*. They are then built upon the relation $X_i = \max_{i\le j\le i+m-1} Y_j$, $i \ge 1$. An illustration of clustering of high values with an asymptotic mean size equal to m, is presented in Fig. 1 as illustrated in [12].

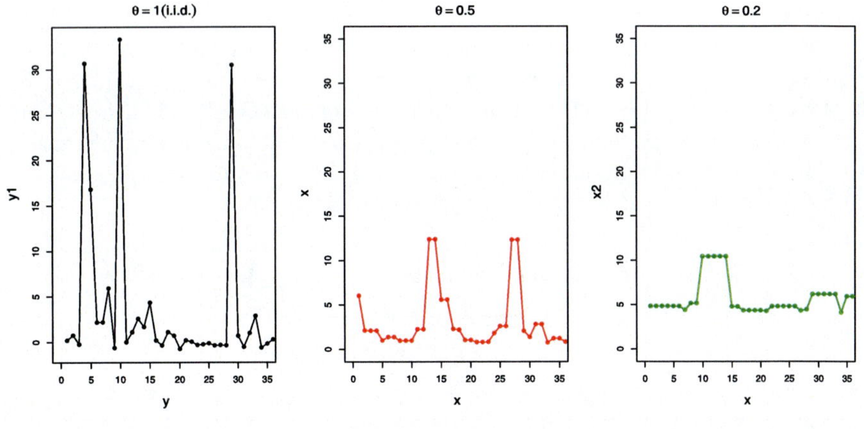

Fig. 1 Sample paths of an *i.i.d.* (left), 2-dep (center) and 5-dep (right) processes from the same underlying Fréchet ($\Phi_{\xi=1}$), but with *EI*s, respectively, equal to 1, 0.5 and 0.2 [12]

When $\theta = 1$ it corresponds to the occurrence of independent extreme values. As θ decreases to zero, m-dependence has an increasing m and leads to a number of sequential extreme values forming clusters that tend to have greater size. Thus we are more concerned with the estimation of low θ values (high dependence).

1.3 EI Estimators

Since the last 80s, several authors have proposed different *EI* estimators. The most distinguishable feature is the scheme used in the clusters of exceedances identification. The Blocks estimator is the most known, in spite of still existent current doubts about optimizing the number of blocks to be considered; the problem is investigated, e.g., in [3]. The Blocks estimator was initially suggested by [4], and it has been improved in different versions, like the equivalent weighted version in [5], or the sliding blocks versions as studied in [6]. Inference questions about the limiting cluster size distribution are studied in [7]. Basically, the Blocks estimator start by identifying a cluster when it occurs an observation higher than a pre-fixed threshold. The dimension of the cluster is the number of observations in the block above that fixed threshold. Notice that, dealing with extremely high observations, the great majority of the blocks do not contain clusters. The Blocks estimator corresponds to the inverse of the mean cluster size estimate.

With more detail, the sample is divided into k blocks of equal range. The total number of exceedances above a fixed high threshold is counted *per* each block. Those blocks that do not contain exceedances are ignored. Then,

$$\widehat{\theta_B} = (N_n/Z_n)^{-1} = Z_n/N_n,$$

where N_n is the number of exceedances and Z_n is the number of blocks that contain at least one exceedance.

There are other type of estimators, like the Runs estimator (see [8]), the Nandagopalan estimator, those based in the inter-exceedance times, e.g., [5], or the k-gaps estimator (see [9] or [10]). In the paper of Gomes and Guillou [11], the authors present a review of the topic. The present paper is devoted to the Blocks estimator, continuing and improving the previous work [12]. For computational purpose, the authors used the equivalent form suggested by Robert in [7]:

$$\widehat{\theta_B} = -\frac{\log\left(\frac{1}{k}\sum_{i=1}^{k} I\left(M_{(i-1)r,ir} \leq u_n\right)\right)}{\frac{1}{k}\sum_{i=1}^{rk} I(X_i > u_n)}, \tag{3}$$

with $M_{s,r} = \max_{s<i\leq r} X_i$, for $0 \leq s < r$. The estimator $\widehat{\theta}_{\text{B}}$ is a consistent and asymptotically normal EI-estimator.

1.4 Scope of the Article

The main goal is to find the best robust version of the EI-estimator in (3), in the sense of an estimator with a good performance under model assumptions, but that it does not breakdown in the neighbourhoods of the model, namely in the presence of atypical observations or of small deviations from the assumed model. In Section 2, a Hurdle model for fitting the clusters dimension asymptotic distribution is proposed. In Section 3, a robust estimation of the model in the framework of the generalized linear model is considered. The last two sections, Section 4 and 5, include a simulation study and the analysis of results.

2 The Hurdle Model

2.1 Why the Hurdle Poisson Model?

Since the Blocks estimator counts the number of extreme values above a fixed threshold, there exist a lot of blocks with no exceedances, i.e., with zero observations of exceedances. Among the most known counting models prepared for dealing with an excess of zeroes (see [13]), we considered mixed models with two components, and we decided that the hurdle model with a zero truncated distribution was the best choice. Actually, a possible candidate model would be a Zero Inflated Model. But that one would assume that the zeroes could be generated by both components of the model. In the opposite, the hurdle model with a zero truncated distribution admits that all the zeroes must be generated by a single component of the model, while the strictly positive counts are in the second component. Observations belonging to the zero truncated component occur conditionally based on a Bernoulli distribution. Therewith, it is necessary to assume a discrete distribution for the cluster dimension.

In the limit distribution, it was proven in [14] that under a broad condition, the number of exceedances N_n converges to a compound Poisson process with multiplicities equal to the dimension of the clusters. Moreover, clusters' size distribution is given by

$$\pi_n(j) = \mathbb{P}\left[\sum_{i=1}^{r_n} \mathbb{I}_{(X_i>u_n)} = j | M_{r_n} > u_n\right], \quad j = 1, 2, \ldots$$

where $\mathbb{I}$ stands for the indicator function. If the limit exists when $n \to \infty$, the distribution of the clusters' size associated with the compound Poisson process is $\pi = \lim_{n\to\infty} \pi_n$.

In general, π is not known. Some authors assume a Poisson distribution. Taking into account that the Poisson distribution should not fit with the excess of zeroes, we will consider that the limit distribution of the strictly positive cluster dimension belongs to the neighbourhood of a *Zero Truncated Poisson* (*ZTP*) model. Observations belonging to the *ZTP* component occur conditionally based on a Bernoulli distribution.

The hurdle *ZTP* model can be characterized by

$$\mathbb{P}[Y_i = y_i] = \begin{cases} 1 - p(x_i), & y_i = 0, \\ p(x_i)\frac{\exp[-\lambda(\mu_i)][\lambda(\mu_i)]^{y_i}}{y_i![1-\exp[\lambda(\mu_i)]]}, & y_i = 1, 2, \ldots, \end{cases} \tag{4}$$

where Y_i represent the countings y_i, $x_i \in \mathbb{R}$, $\mu_i \in \mathbb{R}$. The corresponding expectation is

$$\mathbb{E}[Y_i|x_i] = \mu_i = \frac{\lambda_i}{1 - \exp(-\lambda_i)}. \tag{5}$$

Thus, once the parameter λ_i of the complete Poisson distribution is estimated it is easy to obtain the estimated expected value of the *ZTP*.

There are other advantages in treating the hurdle *ZTP* in the *General Linear Model* (*GLM*) framework: besides treating the mean as the constant term of the Poisson regression (after inverting the link function), the *GLM* estimation is intensively studied, particularly, whenever dealing with robust estimation.

3 Robust Estimation of the Hurdle Model

Let us consider the generalization of (4) to the case of covariates $\mathbf{x}_i \in \mathbb{R}^p$, with $\boldsymbol{\mu}_i \in \mathbb{R}^{\tilde{p}}$, with p and $\tilde{p}$ not necessarily the same:

$$\mathbb{P}[Y_i = y_i] = \begin{cases} 1 - p(\mathbf{x}_i), & y_i = 0, \\ p(\mathbf{x}_i)\frac{\exp[-\lambda(\boldsymbol{\mu}_i)][\lambda(\boldsymbol{\mu}_i)]^{y_i}}{y_i![1-\exp[\lambda(\boldsymbol{\mu}_i)]]}, & y_i = 1, 2, \ldots. \end{cases}$$

Each component of the model can be interpreted as a *GLM*, namely, the Bernoulli component as a logistic regression with link function

$$logit[p(\boldsymbol{x}_i)] = \log\left[\frac{p(\boldsymbol{x}_i)}{1 - p(\boldsymbol{x}_i)}\right] = \boldsymbol{x}_i^T\boldsymbol{\alpha}, \quad (\boldsymbol{\alpha} \in \mathbb{R}^p)$$

and the second component as a log-linear regression conditional to $p(\boldsymbol{x}_i)$, with link function

$$\log[\lambda(\boldsymbol{\mu}_i)] = \boldsymbol{\mu}_i^T \boldsymbol{\gamma} \quad (\boldsymbol{\gamma} \in \mathbb{R}^{\tilde{p}}).$$

The log-likelihood function of the model is presented in Cantoni and Zedini [15]:

$$l(\boldsymbol{\alpha}, \boldsymbol{\gamma}; y) = \sum_{y_i=0} \log\left(\frac{1}{1+\exp(\boldsymbol{x}_i^T\boldsymbol{\alpha})}\right) + \sum_{y_i>0} \log\left(\frac{\boldsymbol{x}_i^T\boldsymbol{\alpha}}{1+\exp(\boldsymbol{x}_i^T\boldsymbol{\alpha})}\right) +$$
$$+ \sum_{y_i>0} \left(y_i(\boldsymbol{\mu}_i^T\boldsymbol{\gamma}) - \exp(\boldsymbol{\mu}_i^T\boldsymbol{\gamma}) - \log\left(1-\exp(-\exp(\boldsymbol{\mu}_i^T\boldsymbol{\gamma}))\right)\right) - \log(y_i!).$$

The expression above can be written as a sum of the type

$$l(\boldsymbol{\alpha}, \boldsymbol{\gamma}; y) = l_1(\boldsymbol{\alpha}; y) + l_2(\boldsymbol{\gamma}; y),$$

where l_1 does not depend on $\boldsymbol{\gamma}$ and l_2 does not depend on $\boldsymbol{\alpha}$. So, maximization of $l(\boldsymbol{\alpha}, \boldsymbol{\gamma}; y)$ in order to each parameter is independent from the other. That means that parameters $\boldsymbol{\alpha}$ and $\boldsymbol{\gamma}$ of the *GLM* are orthogonal. Thus, the estimation of both components of the model can be independent. In the same paper, the authors present also the variance and the deviance functions computed originally in [16], where the *ZTP* was treated as a *GLM* for the first time. One of the advantages in considering the *GLM* framework is that the expected value of the complete Poisson is the constant term of the previous log regression with a Poisson error term. Besides, since our main goal is to get a robust estimate of the expectation of the *ZTP*, we are only interested in estimating the second component of the model.

Robust regression estimators for the *GLM* are already available for some distributions, namely for the complete Poisson or the Bernoulli distributions. The estimators are included in free software like *R*, particularly, in the *robustbase* package. They have already been deeply studied, used and tested by the community, thus avoiding numerical questions with optimization problems. Taking into account the relation (5) between expectations of the Poisson and the *ZTP*, we begin by looking for the robust fit of the complete Poisson parameter, using just the strictly positive observations in the estimation process. The zeroes are ignored, as it is usual with non-observed values in a sample, in spite of belonging to distribution support. With that procedure we hope to find the λ_i estimates that better fit the strictly positive cluster size, independently of the zeroes frequency. Once we have a good estimate for the Poisson parameter, the mean cluster size estimate considering the *ZTP* is obtained directly from (5).

The *R* package *robustbase* includes the *glmrob* function, which collects the most recognized or computationally disposable robust counterparts to the common *GLM* estimators. For the Poisson distribution, there are implemented two main families of robust estimators (particularly, M-estimators): MT-type estimators and Mallows's or Huber-type estimators. MT-estimators are based on a stabilizing variance transformation proposed in [17]; in the *glmrob* function, those estimators correspond to the option *method*="MT". They can be computationally more time consuming, depending on the initial value used in the algorithm and they did not produce the best results according to the authors previous studies. Mallows's or Huber estimators correspond to the option *method*="Mqle", as suggested in [18] and [15], but they are computed using a pure influence algorithm, with the possibility of several choices through the *glmrob.control* function. For the *GLM* with different covariates, they have the following form:

$$\sum_{i=1}^{n} \psi(y_i, \boldsymbol{\mu}_i) = \sum_{i=1}^{n} \left[\psi_c(r_i)\omega(\boldsymbol{x}_i)\frac{1}{\sqrt{\nu_{\mu_i}}}\boldsymbol{\mu}_i)_i^T - a(\boldsymbol{\beta}) \right] = \mathbf{0},$$

where ψ_c is the Huber function with tuning constant c; $r_i = (y_i - \mu_i)/\sqrt{\nu_{\mu_i}}$ are the Pearson residuals; $\nu_{\mu_i} = \mathbb{V}[Y_i|\boldsymbol{x}_i]$; $\omega(\boldsymbol{x}_i)$ are weights that control $\boldsymbol{x}_i$; $\boldsymbol{\mu}_i = \mathbb{E}[Y_i|\boldsymbol{x}_i]$; and $a(\boldsymbol{\beta})$ assures Fisher consistency (see Cantoni and Zedini [15]). Since our goal is to estimate just the constant term of the *GLM*, we have $\omega(\boldsymbol{x}_i) = 1, \forall i$. The tuning constant is recommended by [15] as $c \in (1.2, 1.8)$. We obtained better results with $c = 1.6$, but the value of c determines the efficiency of the estimator and that issue has not been theoretically investigated by the authors. From previous simulation studies, Mallows's type estimators seem to be preferable.

The result obtained by the *GLM* model, let it be denoted by $\hat{\lambda}^\star$, is the estimate of the *GLM* constant term. Inversion of the link function gives the estimate for the expected value of the Poisson, $\tilde{\lambda} = \exp(\hat{\lambda}^\star)$.

The relation (5) between the expected values of the *ZTP* and the Poisson, i.e.,

$$\hat{\lambda}_{ZTP} = \frac{\tilde{\lambda}}{1 - \exp(-\tilde{\lambda})},$$

gives the estimate of the mean cluster dimension (assuming a *ZTP*). Finally, the *EI* estimate is

$$\hat{\theta}_{Rob.ZTP} = 1/\hat{\lambda}_{ZTP}. \tag{6}$$

4 Simulation Study

The present simulation study aims to find the best robust alternative as a robust version of the Blocks *EI* estimator. The evaluation of the performance of the robust version when compared with other *EI* estimators, in the same dependence structure, takes into account the results of the methods in both cases: "clean" samples, in the sense that they are generated according with model assumptions; but the results must be satisfactory also when the samples are contaminated. By contaminated samples, we mean that the sample may contain atypical values according to the assumed model, or that the real distribution lies in some neighbourhoods of the assumed model. A robust estimator should not break down under those conditions.

The evaluation criteria were the following:

- For each sample, the performance was evaluated for high percentiles (30 levels from 80% to 99%).
- Estimators are compared in terms of bias, through the mean estimates of the *EI*; and in terms of variability, which is evaluated through the root mean square error.
- Stability along the percentiles also matters. That is analyzed by graphical comparisons.
- Computational facilities and reliability of estimates along repetitive simulations. The authors consider that the development of free packages that are simple to use is essential for the application of the methods in a real environment.

4.1 Simulated Scenarios

The generated samples must contain extreme values, higher than fixed thresholds, particularly, in scenarios of distributions defined by (1). Thus, observations were generated according to a unit Fréchet distribution. In what concerns the dependence structure, the work was focused in low values of θ, since $0 < \theta < 1$ when the extreme values present dependence and $\theta = 1$ corresponds to the independent case. Herein, we present results for m-dependent processes with $\theta = 0.2$, but similar results were obtained for other values of m. In the case of m-dependent processes, it is possible to compute explicitly the *EI* value, which is $\theta = 1/m$. Thus, 5-dependent processes allow to investigate a scenery quite away from independence.

Each generated sample has a dimension $n = 2000$. The number of blocks is prefixed and it is an issue still under current research (see [3]). We choose $b = 100$ blocks, in accordance with other similar simulation studies. Finally, the number of replicates is 500. Those conditions are related to the "clean" samples.

For producing contaminated samples, notice that the introduction of contamination should be not in the observed values from the Fréchet processes, but necessarily in the size of the clusters of exceedances. That goal was achieved with the following procedure: the samples were partially randomly generated in such a manner that, in every sample, at least one cluster of exceedances should contain an atypical dimension. Thus, the 25 central observations in each sample were replaced by the maxima observed in the block where they were registered.

To access robust properties, every procedure and criterion was repeated using both clean and contaminated samples.

Table 1 *R* packages and functions used for obtaining estimates by different methods

estim.	Function	*Package*	Method
$\hat{\theta}_B$	Programmed		
$\hat{\theta}_W$	Programmed		
$\hat{\theta}_{Runs}$	extremalindex	*extRemes*	
$\hat{\theta}_{Int}$	ext.index	*mev*	Intervals
$\hat{\theta}_{Rob}$	glmrob	*robustbase*	Mqle
$\hat{\theta}_{MT}$	glmrob	*robustbase*	MT
$\hat{\theta}_{Gaps}$	iwls	*exdex*	
$\hat{\theta}_N$	spm	*exdex*	
$\hat{\theta}_{BB}$	spm	*exdex*	

4.2 Software Tools

All the computations were performed with *R* software, since it has free access and many already tested packages, namely, devoted to robustness and extreme value distributions. We used self-programmed software in some cases.

In past studies about the same topic the authors noticed that was not possible to compare results using some *EI* estimators, namely, the k-gaps estimator $\hat{\theta}_{Gaps}$, the semiparametric maxima Northrop $\hat{\theta}_N$ estimator or the MT-estimator $\hat{\theta}_{MT}$. Then, they produced the estimates just with specific samples, but they presented serious problems in the simulation of many samples, probably due to numerical lack of convergence.

Nowadays those problems seem to have been solved with important computational improvements. The package *exedex* can compute $\hat{\theta}_{Gaps}$, Northrop estimator $\hat{\theta}_N$ and also a similar estimator proposed by Berghaus and Büche (see [19]), here denoted by $\hat{\theta}_{BB}$. Unfortunately that package does not allow visual comparisons of the two last estimators with the rest, quantile by quantile. So, they appear in Table 1 (respecting to the non-sliding block version), but they do not appear in the following graphical evaluations. We just present numerical comparisons of their estimates with $\hat{\theta}_{Rob.ZTP}$ global results.

In spite of the referred great improvements in the computational tools, there are some difficulties not yet solved.

5 Analysis of Results

Remember that $\hat{\theta}_{Rob.ZTP}$ represents the robust version of the *EI* estimator computed by the Mallows's type estimator. Next figures represent the curves of the estimates of θ obtained by different methodologies. The empirical quantiles are chosen as pre-fixed thresholds, in the abscissa axis. The results are shown for 30 quantiles of the

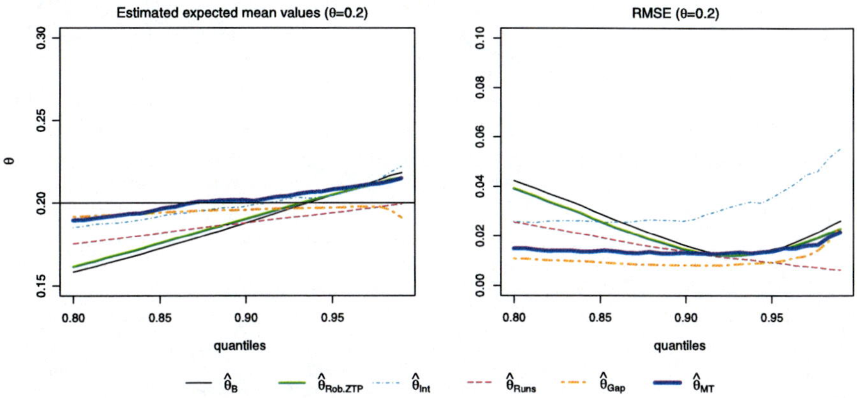

Fig. 2 Estimated means (left) and estimated root mean square errors (right) by different methods with "clean" samples and $\theta = 0.2$

empirical distribution from 0.80 until 0.99. Almost all the methods and packages provide estimates according with that choice of thresholds.

We start by comparing robust versions of Blocks estimator with other *EI* estimators, in the "clean" samples scenery, with $\theta = 0.2$. Figure 2 shows the results.

In what concerns bias (in the left of Fig. 2) it is possible to see that the robust version $\hat{\theta}_{Rob.ZTP}$ and the Blocks estimator have a similar behaviour under "clean" samples, with increasing bias when the quantiles increase; in terms of root mean square error, $\hat{\theta}_{Rob.ZTP}$ shows a slightly reduction on variability. Comparing with the robust alternative $\hat{\theta}_{MT}$, the latter performs better when there is no contamination. Notice that under the simulated condition $\hat{\theta}_{Gap}$ has the best performance—minimum values and stability for almost all the quantiles.

The conclusions are not the same when we consider the contaminated scenery, as in Fig. 3.

$\hat{\theta}_{Rob.ZTP}$ estimates show a bias reduction when compared with original version of Blocks estimates, but only until somewhere between the 85% and 90% quantiles; and the advantage in terms of variability is lost from (about) the same threshold. Analyzing the estimates, the comparative results with the other robust estimator, $\hat{\theta}_{MT}$, is even more disappointing. We must conclude that under this type of contamination there is not a great improvement in *EI* estimation through $\hat{\theta}_{Rob.ZTP}$, which was our initial choice in the sequence of previous work. Nevertheless, the performance of the $\hat{\theta}_{Gap}$ estimator is remarkable, both with or without contamination. Actually, without contamination, that estimator seems to present (in general) the smaller bias and the smaller root mean square error, being also quite stable along the increasing quantiles; with contaminated samples (in general) $\hat{\theta}_{Gap}$ is preferable.

The authors think that the improvement on the $\hat{\theta}_{Gap}$ estimates is due to the computational evolution. In spite of working with the same samples, previous simulations were difficult and worse than the present ones, perhaps due to divergence problems

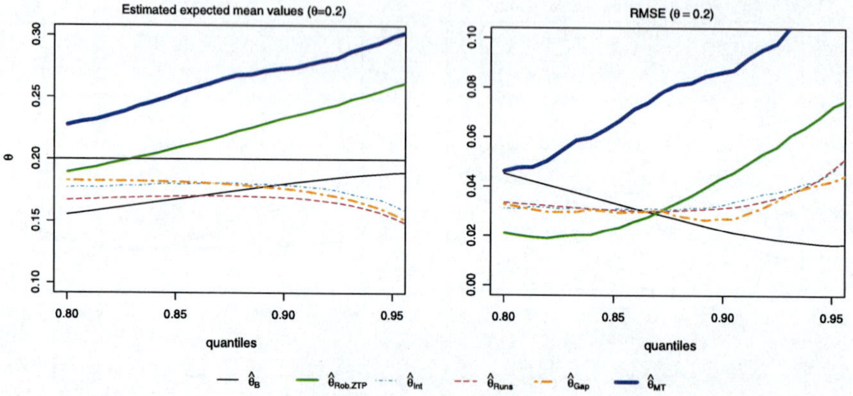

Fig. 3 Estimated means (left) and estimated root mean square errors (right) by different methods with contaminated samples and $\theta = 0.2$

Table 2 Comparison of $\hat{\theta}_N$ and $\hat{\theta}_{BB}$ estimates with global results of $\hat{\theta}_{Rob.ZTP}$ and $\hat{\theta}_{Gap}$ estimates (bold digits for smaller cases)

	Clean samples		Contaminated samples	
	Est. bias	RMSE	Est.absol.bias	RMSE
$\hat{\theta}_N$	0.0079	0.0368	**0.0010**	0.0498
$\hat{\theta}_{BB}$	0.0176	0.0393	0.0101	0.0505
$\hat{\theta}_{Rob.ZTP}$	0.0112	0.0213	0.0112	0.0486
$\hat{\theta}_{Gap}$	**0.0049**	**0.0102**	0.0395	**0.0446**

in the numerical optimization. The present use of the *R* package *exdex* (with the original settings), which was not disposable when we did the previous similar study, led to completely different conclusions.

The analysis of the results under the simulated conditions highlights the importance of the associated computational methods in the evaluation of the estimators and their comparisons. With the package *exdex* is possible to analyze the estimates obtained with the Northrop and the Berghaus and Büche estimators, respectively, $\hat{\theta}_N$ and $\hat{\theta}_{BB}$. As mentioned before, the results are presented in a different format, so we did not compare them in the same type of graphical representation. The package includes a sliding blocks version for each of those estimators, but we dealt just with disjoint blocks, in coherence with Blocks estimator versions. Thus, we present the next table for comparing their estimates with $\hat{\theta}_{Rob.ZTP}$ global results and with $\hat{\theta}_{Gap}$, since apparently, it provided the best results.

Observing Table 2 we see that with clean samples there are no great differences, like those pointed in the graphics. Both in what respects to estimated bias or estimated root mean square error, $\hat{\theta}_{Gap}$ had the best performance. When there is contamination, the robust Mallows type estimator is overpassed by the Northrop estimator, the last one being almost unbiased. The estimated root mean square error is very similar for all the estimators considered in the table and slightly better for the k-gaps estimator. Concluding, with the introduced contamination, $\hat{\theta}_N$ is the best in terms of bias, while $\hat{\theta}_{Gap}$ is the best in terms of root mean square error.

6 Final Comments

The dimension of clusters of exceedances distribution was modelled with a Hurdle model with a zero truncated Poisson. We have improved past computations of the robust Mallows type version of the Blocks estimators (see [12]), but that did not improve the comparative results. Some estimators that could not be compared in previous simulations (due to frequent optimization problems) are now available with good estimates, using the present version of *exdex R* package (see [20]). That points out the importance of free access, good and user friendly software. According to the simulated scenarios and the studied type of contamination, we can conclude that: unfortunately the M-estimators proposed showed lower performance than expected (particularly the MT-estimator); The k-Gap estimator seems to be the best, considering either "clean" or contaminated samples, and for different criteria, followed by Northrop estimator. Future research is needed to study robust estimators under other simulated dependence structures and contaminations.

Acknowledgements This work was partially supported by Fundação para a Ciência e a Tecnologia (FCT), through projects UIDB/MAT/0006/2020 (CEA/UL) and UIDP/04106/2020 (CIDMA).

References

1. Leadbetter, M.R., Nandagopalan, S.: On Exceedance Point Processes for Stationary Sequences Under Mild Oscillation Restrictions, pp. 69–80. Springer, New York, NY (1989)
2. Leadbetter, L.G., M. R. Rootzén, H.: Extremes and Related Properties of Random Sequences and Processes. Springer, New-York (1983)
3. Ferreira, H., Ferreira, M.: Estimating the extremal index through local dependence. Annales de l'Institut Henri Poincaré-Probabilités et Statistiques **54**, 587–605 (2018)
4. Hsing, T.: On tail estimation using dependent data. Ann. Stat. **19**, 1547–1569 (1991)
5. Ferro, C.A.T., Segers, J.: Inference for clusters of extreme values. J. R. Stat. Soc. Ser. B **65**(2), 545–556 (2003)
6. Northrop, P.J.: An efficient semiparametric maxima estimator of the extremal index. Extremes **18**, 585–603 (2015)
7. Robert, C.Y.: Inference for the limiting cluster size distribution of extreme values. Ann. Stat. **37**, 271–310 (2009)
8. Hsing, T.: Extremal index estimation for a weakly dependent stationary sequence. Ann. Stat. **21**, 2043–2071 (1993)
9. Süveges, M.: Likelihood estimation of the extremal index. Extremes **10**(1–2), 41–55 (2007)
10. Süveges, M., Davison, A.C.: Model misspecification in peaks over threshold analysis. Ann. Appl. Stat. **4**(1), 203–221 (2010)

11. Gomes, M.I., Guillou, A.: Extreme value theory and statistics of univariate extremes: a review. Int. Stat. Rev. **83**(2), 263–292 (2015)
12. Gomes, M.I., Miranda, M., Souto de Miranda, M.: A note on robust estimation of the extremal index. Springer Proc. Math. Stat. **339**, 213–225 (2020)
13. Heritier, S., Cantoni, E., Samuel, C.: Robust Methods in Biostatistics. Wiley (2009)
14. Hsing, H.J., T. Leadbetter, M.R.: On the excedance of point process for a stationary sequence. Prob. Theory Related Fields **78**, 97–112 (1988)
15. Cantoni, E., Ronchetti, E.: Robust inference for generalized linear models. J. Am. Stat. Assoc. **96**, 1022–1030 (2011)
16. Barry, S.C., Welsh, A.H.: Generalized additive modelling and zero inflated count data. Ecol. Model. **157**, 179–188 (2002)
17. Valdora, M., Yohai, V.: Robust estimators for generalized linear models. J. Stat. Plann. Inference **146**, 31–48 (2014)
18. Cantoni, E., Ronchetti, E.: A robust approach for skewed and heavy-tailed outcomes in the analysis of health care expenditures. J. Health Econ. **25**(2), 198–213 (2006)
19. Berghaus, B., Bücher, A.: Weak convergence of a pseudo maximum likelihood estimator for the extremal index. Ann. Stat. **46**, 2307–2335 (Oct 2018)
20. Northrop, P.: Introducing `exdex`: Estimation of the Extremal Index (2019). https://cran.r-project.org/web/packages/exdex/vignettes/exdex-vignette.html

Computational Study of the Adaptive Estimation of the Extreme Value Index with Probability Weighted Moments

Frederico Caeiro and M. Ivette Gomes

Abstract In statistics of extremes, the estimation of the extreme value index (EVI) is an important and central topic of research. We consider the probability weighted moment estimator of the EVI, based on the largest observations. Due to the specificity of the properties of the estimator, a direct estimation of the threshold is not straightforward. In this work, we consider an adaptive choice of the number of order statistics based on the double bootstrap methodology. Computational and empirical properties of the methodology are here provided.

Keywords Bootstrap · Extreme value index · Heavy tails · Probability weighted moment · Semi-parametric estimation

1 Introduction and Scope of the Article

Let $(X_1, \ldots, X_n)$ denote a random sample of size n from a population with unknown *cumulative distribution function* (CDF) $F(x) = \mathbb{P}(X \leq x)$ and consider the associated sample of ascending *order statistics* (OSs) $(X_{1:n} := \min_{1 \leq i \leq n} X_i \leq \cdots \leq X_{n:n} := \max_{1 \leq i \leq n} X_i)$. Further assume that for large values of x, $F(x)$ is a Pareto-type model, i.e., a model with a regular varying right tail with a negative index of regular variation equal to $-1/\xi$ $(\xi > 0)$. Consequently,

$$\overline{F}(x) := 1 - F(x) = \mathbb{P}(X > x) = x^{-1/\xi} L(x), \quad \text{as } x \to \infty, \tag{1}$$

F. Caeiro (✉)
NOVA School of Science and Technology (FCT NOVA) and CMA, NOVA University of Lisbon, Campus de Caparica, Lisbon, Portugal
e-mail: fac@fct.unl.pt

M. I. Gomes
Faculty of Science of Lisbon (FCUL/DEIO) and CEAUL, University of Lisbon, Cidade Universitária, Campo Grande, Portugal
e-mail: ivette.gomes@fc.ul.pt

R. Bispo et al. (eds.), *Recent Developments in Statistics and Data Science*, Springer Proceedings in Mathematics & Statistics 398,
https://doi.org/10.1007/978-3-031-12766-3_3

with $L(\cdot)$ a slowly varying function, i.e.

$$\lim_{t\to\infty} \frac{L(tx)}{L(t)} = 1, \quad \forall\, x > 0.$$

Models satisfying the condition (1) are in the domain of attraction for maxima of a non-degenerate distribution. This means that there exist normalizing constants $a_n > 0$ and $b_n \in \mathbb{R}$ such that

$$\lim_{n\to\infty} \mathbb{P}\left(\frac{X_{n:n} - b_n}{a_n} \le x\right) = \lim_{n\to\infty} F^n\left(a_n x + b_n\right) = G(x), \tag{2}$$

with $G(\cdot)$ a non-degenerate CDF. With the appropriate choice of the normalizing constants in (2), and under a general framework, G is the general *extreme value* (EV) distribution,

$$G(x) \equiv \mathrm{EV}_\xi(x) := \begin{cases} \exp\left(-(1+\xi x)^{-1/\xi}\right), \ 1+\xi x > 0, & \text{if } \xi \neq 0, \\ \exp(-\exp(-x)), \ x \in \mathbb{R}, & \text{if } \xi = 0, \end{cases} \tag{3}$$

given here in the von Mises-Jenkinson form (see [1, 2]). Whenever such a non-degenerate limit exists, we write $F \in \mathcal{D_M}(EV_\xi)$, and the real parameter ξ is the *extreme value index* (EVI).

As already mentioned, we shall deal with Pareto right-tails, i.e. heavy right-tails or equivalently a model with a positive EVI. Then, the right-tail function is of regular variation with an index of regular variation equal to $-1/\xi$, i.e.

$$F \in \mathcal{D_M}(EV_\xi)_{\xi>0} \iff \overline{F} := 1 - F \in RV_{-1/\xi}, \tag{4}$$

where the notation RV_α stands for the class of *regularly varying* functions at infinity with an *index of regular variation* equal to α, i.e. positive measurable functions g such that $\lim_{t\to\infty} g(tx)/g(t) = x^\alpha$, for all $x > 0$. With the notation

$$U(t) := F^{\leftarrow}(1 - 1/t),\ t \ge 1, \quad F^{\leftarrow}(y) := \inf\{x : F(x) \ge y\}, \tag{5}$$

condition (4) is equivalent to $U \in RV_\xi$. Pareto-type models are extremely important in practice due to the frequency and magnitude of extreme values and inference on extreme and large events is usually performed on the basis of the $k+1$ largest order statistics in the sample, as sketched in Fig. 1.

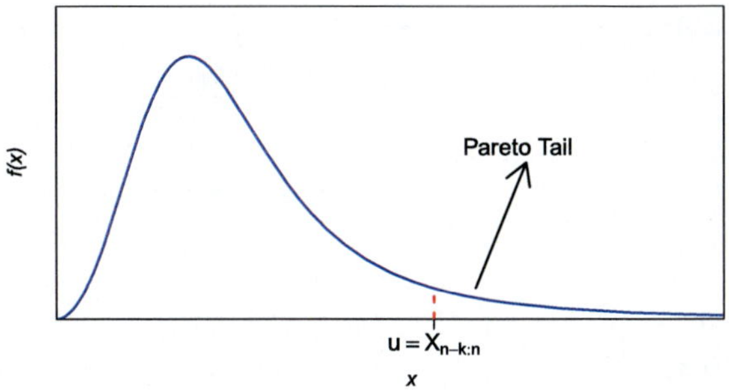

Fig. 1 A Pareto right-tail probability density function

1.1 EVI-Estimators Under Consideration

One of the first classes of semi-parametric estimators of a positive EVI was the class of Hill (H) estimators introduced in [3] and given by

$$\hat{\xi}^{\mathrm{H}}_{k,n} := \frac{1}{k}\sum_{i=1}^{k}\{\ln X_{n-i+1:n} - \ln X_{n-k:n}\}\,,\ k = 1, 2, \ldots, n-1. \tag{6}$$

This estimator can be highly sensitive to the choice of k, especially in the presence of a substantial bias. As an alternative, we shall also consider the *Pareto probability weighted moments* (PPWM) EVI-estimators, introduced in [4]. They are consistent for $0 < \xi < 1$, compare favourably with the Hill estimator, and are given by

$$\hat{\xi}^{\mathrm{PPWM}}_{k,n} := 1 - \frac{\hat{a}_1(k)}{\hat{a}_0(k) - \hat{a}_1(k)}, \tag{7}$$

with

$$\hat{a}_0(k) := \frac{1}{k}\sum_{i=1}^{k} X_{n-i+1:n} \quad \text{and} \quad \hat{a}_1(k) := \frac{1}{k}\sum_{i=1}^{k}\frac{i}{k}\, X_{n-i+1:n}.$$

For other alternative estimators of the EVI see Refs. [5–7], among others. Consistency of the EVI-estimators in (6) and (7) is achieved if $X_{n-k:n}$ is an *intermediate* OS, i.e. if

$$k = k_n \to \infty \quad \text{and} \quad k/n \to 0, \quad \text{as} \quad n \to \infty.$$

In order to derive the asymptotic normality of these EVI-estimators, it is often assumed the validity of a second-order condition, like

$$\lim_{t\to\infty}\frac{\ln U(tx) - \ln U(t) - \xi \ln x}{A(t)} = \begin{cases} \frac{x^{\rho}-1}{\rho}, & \text{if } \rho < 0,\\ \ln x, & \text{if } \rho = 0,\end{cases} \tag{8}$$

Table 1 Asymptotic variance and bias' rulers of H and PPWM EVI–estimators

	H ($\xi > 0$)	PPWM ($0 < \xi < 1/2$)
$\sigma_\bullet^2$	ξ^2	$\xi^2 \frac{(1-\xi)(2-\xi)^2}{(1-2\xi)(3-2\xi)}$
$b_\bullet$	$\frac{1}{1-\rho}$	$\frac{(1-\xi)(2-\xi)}{(1-\xi-\rho)(2-\xi-\rho)}$

where $U(\cdot)$ is defined in (5) and $|A| \in RV_\rho$, $\rho \leq 0$. Under such a second-order framework, if $\sqrt{k}A(n/k) \to \lambda_A$, finite, as $n \to \infty$, these EVI-estimators are asymptotically normal. Denoting $\hat{\xi}^\bullet_{k,n}$, any of the estimators above, we have, with $Z_k^\bullet$ an asymptotically standard normal random variable and for adequate $(b_\bullet, \sigma_\bullet) \in (\mathbb{R}, \mathbb{R}^+)$,

$$\hat{\xi}^\bullet_{k,n} \stackrel{d}{=} \xi + \frac{\sigma_\bullet Z_k^\bullet}{\sqrt{k}} + b_\bullet\, A(n/k)(1 + o_{\mathbb{P}}(1)), \quad \text{as} \quad n \to \infty, \tag{9}$$

with $b_\bullet$ the asymptotic bias, and $\sigma_\bullet^2$ the asymptotic standard deviation of the approximation, given in Table 1.

Under the above second-order framework, in (8), but with $\rho < 0$, let us use the parametrization

$$A(t) = \xi\beta t^\rho, \quad \text{with } \beta \neq 0 \text{ and } \rho < 0,$$

where β and ρ are generalized scale and shape second-order parameters, which need to be adequately estimated on the basis of the available sample. Let us denote the optimal level by

$$\tilde{k}_0^\bullet(n) := \arg\min_k \text{MSE}(\hat{\xi}^\bullet_{k,n}),$$

with MSE standing for *mean squared error*. With $\mathbb{E}$ denoting the mean value operator and AMSE standing for *asymptotic* MSE, a possible substitute for $\text{MSE}(\hat{\xi}^\bullet_{k,n})$ is

$$\text{AMSE}(\hat{\xi}^\bullet_{k,n}) := \mathbb{E}\left(\frac{\sigma_\bullet}{\sqrt{k}} Z_k^\bullet + b_\bullet A(n/k)\right)^2 = \frac{\sigma_\bullet^2}{k} + b_\bullet^2\, \xi^2\, \beta^2 \left(\frac{n}{k}\right)^{2\rho},$$

cf. Eq. (9). Then, with the notation $k_0^\bullet(n) := \arg\min_k \text{AMSE}\big(\hat{\xi}^\bullet_{k,n}\big)$, we get

$$k_0^\bullet(n) = \left(\frac{\sigma_\bullet^2\, n^{-2\rho}}{(-2\rho)\, b_\bullet^2\, \xi^2 \beta^2}\right)^{1/(1-2\rho)} = \tilde{k}_0^\bullet(n)(1 + o(1)). \tag{10}$$

For the Hill estimator in (6), and as can be seen in Table 1, we have $(b_{\rm H}, \sigma_{\rm H}) = (1/(1-\rho), \xi)$. Consequently, with $(\hat{\beta}, \hat{\rho})$ a consistent estimator of (β, ρ) and $[x]$ denoting the integer part of x, we have an asymptotic justification for the estimator

$$\hat{k}_0^{\mathrm{H}} := \left[\left(\frac{(1-\hat{\rho})^2 n^{-2\hat{\rho}}}{(-2\hat{\rho}\hat{\beta}^2)} \right)^{1/(1-2\hat{\rho})} \right] + 1.$$

The same does not happen with the PPWM EVI-estimators, due to the fact that σ_{PPWM}, b_{PPWM} and consequently k_0^{PPWM} depend on the value of ξ (see Table 1, again). It is thus sensible to use the bootstrap methodology for the adaptive choice of the threshold associated to the PPWM EVI-estimation.

1.2 Scope of the Article

The main goal is the adaptive estimation of the EVI. For that purpose, the choice of the threshold is crucial and we study computationally a recent bootstrap algorithm. After a review, in Sect. 2, of the role of the bootstrap methodology in the estimation of optimal sample fractions, we provide an algorithm for the adaptive estimation through the Hill and the PPWM EVI-estimators. In Sect. 3 we provide results from a Monte Carlo simulation study. In Sect. 4, as an illustration, we apply such methodology to a data set in the field of insurance. Section 5 concludes the paper.

2 Adaptive EVI-Estimation and the Bootstrap Methodology

Similarly to what has been done in Gomes and Oliveira [8], for the H estimator, and in Gomes et al. [9], for adaptive reduced-bias estimation, we can use the algorithm in Caeiro et al. [10] (see also [4]), considering the auxiliary statistic,

$$T^{\bullet}_{k,n} := \hat{\xi}^{\bullet}_{[k/2],n} - \hat{\xi}^{\bullet}_{k,n}, \quad k = 2, \ldots, n-1, \tag{11}$$

which converges to the known value zero, and double-bootstrap it adequately, in order to estimate $k_0^{\bullet}(n)$, through a bootstrap estimate $\hat{k}_0^{\bullet,*}$. Indeed, again under the second-order framework, in (8), we get, for the auxiliary statistic $T^{\bullet}_{k,n}$, in (11), the asymptotic distributional representation,

$$T^{\bullet}_{k,n} \stackrel{d}{=} \frac{\sigma_{\bullet}\, Q^{\bullet}_k}{\sqrt{k}} + b_{\bullet}(2^{\rho}-1)\, A(n/k) + o_{\mathbb{P}}(A(n/k)),$$

with $Q^{\bullet}_k$ asymptotically standard normal, and $(b_{\bullet}, \sigma_{\bullet})$ given in Table 1. The AMSE of $T^{\bullet}_{k,n}$ is thus minimal at a level $k^{\bullet}_{0|T}(n)$ such that $\sqrt{k}\, A(n/k) \to \lambda'_{A} \neq 0$, i.e. a level of the type of the one in (10), with $b_{\bullet}$ replaced by $b_{\bullet}(2^{\rho}-1)$, and we consequently have

$$k_0^{\bullet}(n) = k^{\bullet}_{0|T}(n)\, (1-2^{\rho})^{\frac{2}{1-2\rho}}\, (1+o(1)).$$

2.1 The Bootstrap Methodology in Action

Given the sample $\underline{X}_n = (X_1, \ldots, X_n)$ from an unknown model F, consider for any $n_1 = O(n^{1-\epsilon})$, with $0 < \epsilon < 1$, the bootstrap sample $\underline{X}^*_{n_1} = (X^*_1, \ldots, X^*_{n_1})$, from the model $F^*_n(x) = \frac{1}{n}\sum_{i=1}^n I_{\{X_i \le x\}}$, the empirical CDF associated with the original sample $\underline{X}_n$. We choose the resample size n_1 to be less than the original sample size to avoid underestimation of the bias (see Hall [11]). Next, associate to that bootstrap sample the corresponding bootstrap auxiliary statistic, denoted $T^{\bullet,*}_{k_1,n_1}$, $1 < k_1 < n_1$. Then, with the notation

$$k^{\bullet,*}_{0|T}(n_1) = \arg\min_{k_1} \mathrm{AMSE}\big(T^{\bullet,*}_{k_1,n_1}\big),$$

we have that

$$\frac{k^{\bullet,*}_{0|T}(n_1)}{k^{\bullet,*}_{0|T}(n)} = (n_1/n)^{-\frac{2\rho}{1-2\rho}}(1 + o(1)).$$

Consequently, for another sample size $n_2 = n_1^2/n$,

$$\frac{\big(k^{\bullet,*}_{0|T}(n_1)\big)^2}{k^{\bullet,*}_{0|T}(n_2)} = k^{\bullet}_{0|T}(n)(1 + o(1)), \quad \text{as } n \to \infty.$$

We are now able to estimate $k^{\bullet}_0(n)$, on the basis of any estimate $\hat{\rho}$ of ρ. With $\hat{k}^{\bullet,*}_{0|T}$ denoting the sample counterpart of $k^{\bullet,*}_{0|T}$, $\hat{\rho}$ the ρ-estimate and taking into account (10), we can build the k_0-estimate,

$$\hat{k}^{\bullet,*}_0 \equiv \hat{k}^{\bullet,*}_0(n; n_1) := \min\left(n - 1, \left[\frac{\big(1 - 2^{\hat{\rho}}\big)^{\frac{2}{1-2\hat{\rho}}}\big(\hat{k}^{\bullet,*}_{0|T}(n_1)\big)^2}{\hat{k}^{\bullet,*}_{0|T}([n_1^2/n] + 1)}\right] + 1\right), \tag{12}$$

and the ξ-estimate

$$\hat{\xi}^{\bullet,*} \equiv \hat{\xi}^{\bullet,*}(n; n_1) := \hat{\xi}_{\hat{k}^{\bullet,*}_{0|T}(n;n_1),n}. \tag{13}$$

A few questions, some of them with answers outside the scope of this paper, may be raised: How does the bootstrap method work for small or moderate sample sizes? Is the method strongly dependent on the choice of n_1? What is the type of the sample path of the EVI-estimator, as a function of n_1? What is the sensitivity of the bootstrap method with respect to the choice of the ρ-estimate? Although aware of the theoretical need to have $n_1 = o(n)$, what happens if we choose $n_1 = n$?

2.2 An Algorithm for the Adaptive EVI-Estimation

The estimates $(\hat{\beta}, \hat{\rho})$, of the vector (β, ρ) of second-order parameters, are the ones already used in previous papers:

1. Given a sample $(x_1, \ldots, x_n)$, consider the observed values of the ρ-estimators $\hat{\rho}_\tau(k)$, introduced and studied in Fraga Alves et al.[12], for tuning parameters $\tau = 0$ and $\tau = 1$.
2. Select $\{\hat{\rho}_\tau(k)\}_{k\in\mathcal{K}}$, with $\mathcal{K} = ([n^{0.995}],\ [n^{0.999}])$, and compute their median, denoted by η_τ, $\tau = 0, 1$.
3. Next compute $I_\tau := \sum_{k\in\mathcal{K}} \left(\hat{\rho}_\tau(k) - \eta_\tau\right)^2$, $\tau = 0, 1$, and choose the *tuning parameter* $\tau^* = 0$ if $I_0 \le I_1$; otherwise, choose $\tau^* = 1$.
4. Work with $\hat{\rho} \equiv \hat{\rho}_{\tau^*} = \hat{\rho}_{\tau^*}(k_1)$ and $\hat{\beta} \equiv \hat{\beta}_{\tau^*} := \hat{\beta}_{\hat{\rho}_{\tau^*}}(k_1)$, $k_1 = [n^{0.999}]$ and $\hat{\beta}_{\hat{\rho}}(k)$ given in Gomes and Martins [13].

Now, and with $\hat{\xi}^{\rm H}_{k,n}$ and $\hat{\xi}^{\rm PPWM}_{k,n}$ respectively defined in (6) and (7), the algorithm goes on with the following steps:

5. Compute $\hat{\xi}^{\bullet}_{k,n}$, $k = 1, \ldots, n-1$, $\bullet =$ H and/or PPWM.
6. Next, consider a sub-sample size $n_1 = o(n)$, and $n_2 = [n_1^2/n] + 1$.
7. For l from 1 until B, generate independently B bootstrap samples $(x_1^*, \ldots, x_{n_2}^*)$ and $(x_1^*, \ldots, x_{n_2}^*, x_{n_2+1}^*, \ldots, x_{n_1}^*)$, of sizes n_2 and n_1, respectively, from the empirical CDF, $F_n^*(x) = \frac{1}{n}\sum_{i=1}^{n} I_{\{X_i \le x\}}$, associated with the observed sample $(x_1, \ldots, x_n)$.
8. Denoting by $T^{\bullet,*}_{k,n}$ the bootstrap counterpart of $T^{\bullet}_{k,n}$, defined in (11), obtain $(t^{\bullet,*}_{k,n_1,l},\ t^{\bullet,*}_{k,n_2,l})$, $1 \le l \le B$, the observed values of the statistic $T^{\bullet,*}_{k,n_i}$, $i = 1, 2$. For $k = 2, \ldots, n_i - 1$, compute

$$\mathrm{MSE}^{\bullet,*}(n_i, k) = \frac{1}{B}\sum_{l=1}^{B} \left(t^{\bullet,*}_{k,n_i,l}\right)^2,$$

and obtain

$$\hat{k}^{\bullet,*}_{0|T}(n_i) := \arg\min_{1<k<n_i} \mathrm{MSE}^{\bullet,*}(n_i, k), \quad i = 1, 2.$$

9. Compute the threshold estimate $\hat{k}^{\bullet,*}_0$, in (12).
10. Finally obtain

$$\hat{\xi}^{\bullet,*} \equiv \hat{\xi}^{\bullet,*}(n; n_1) = \hat{\xi}_{\hat{k}^{\bullet,*}_{0|T}(n;n_1),n},$$

already provided in (13).

Such an algorithm needs to be computationally validated, a topic we deal with in the next section. Further, note that bootstrap *confidence intervals* (CIs) are easily associated with the estimates presented through the replication of this algorithm r times.

3 A Small-Scale Simulation Study

In this section, we have implemented a multi-sample Monte Carlo simulation experiment of size 1000, to obtain the distributional behaviour of the EVI adaptive bootstrap estimates $\hat{\xi}^{H,*}$ and $\hat{\xi}^{PPWM,*}$ in (6) and (7), respectively. We have considered a re-sample of size $n_1 = [n^{0.955}]$ for samples of size $n = 100, 200, 500, 750, 1000, 2000$ and 5000 from the following models:

- the Fréchet model, with d.f.

$$F(x) = \exp(-x^{-1/\xi}), \quad x > 0, \quad \xi > 0,$$

  with $\xi = 0.25$ ($\rho = -1$);
- the Burr model, with d.f.

$$F(x) = 1 - (1 + x^{-\rho/\xi})^{1/\rho}, \quad x > 0,$$

  with $(\xi, \rho) = (0.25, -0.75)$;
- the Half-t_4 model, i.e., the absolute value of a Student's t with $\nu = 4$ degrees of freedom ($\xi = 0.25$, $\rho = -0.5$).

In Table 2 we present, for the above mentioned models, the multi-sample simulated (mean) double bootstrap optimal sample fraction (OSF), the mean (E) and median (med) of the EVI-estimates and the simulated RMSE for both EVI-estimators, as a function of the sample size n. The less biased EVI-estimate and the smallest RMSE is presented in **bold**. Although both estimators over-estimate the EVI, the consideration of the PPWM EVI-estimator leads to a less biased EVI-estimate, as expected. The PPWM estimation can also lead to a smaller RMSE, for models with $|\rho| < 1$.

4 A Case Study

Here, the performance of the adaptive double bootstrap procedure is illustrated through the analysis of a real dataset. The analysis was made in R software with the computer code developed in Caeiro and Gomes [14]. We used the dataset AutoClaims from a motor insurance portfolio. The data is available in the R package `insuranceData` [15]. The variable of interest is the amount paid on a closed claim, in dollars. There are $n = 6773$ claims available. Since large claims are a topic of great concern in the Insurance Industry, accurate modelling of the right tail of the underlying distribution is extremely important. The Histogram and the Pareto Quantile-Quantile (QQ) Plot, in Fig. 2, are compatible with a Pareto-type underlying distribution.

In Fig. 3, we present the EVI-estimates provided by the Hill and the PPWM EVI-estimators in (6) and (7), respectively. Both estimators are upward biased for large k.

Table 2 Simulated OSF, EVI-estimates (provided by the mean and median) and RMSE estimates obtained through the Hill and PPWM estimators and the double bootstrap methodology

	Hill				PPWM			
n	OSF	$E(\hat{\xi}^*)$	$med(\hat{\xi}^*)$	$RMSE(\hat{\xi}^*)$	OSF	$E(\hat{\xi}^*)$	$med(\hat{\xi}^*)$	$RMSE(\hat{\xi}^*)$
	Fréchet with $\xi = 0.25$ ($\rho = -1$)							
100	0.3458	0.2665	0.2716	**0.0706**	0.3677	**0.2446**	**0.2533**	0.0728
200	0.3246	0.2675	0.2701	**0.0561**	0.3453	**0.2503**	**0.2559**	0.0573
500	0.2750	0.2656	0.2674	**0.0390**	0.3101	**0.2544**	**0.2587**	0.0395
750	0.2567	0.2646	0.2680	**0.0322**	0.2826	**0.2532**	**0.2571**	0.0353
1000	0.2420	0.2630	0.2640	**0.0282**	0.2632	**0.2528**	**0.2566**	0.0332
2000	0.2027	0.2614	0.2628	**0.0217**	0.2269	**0.2538**	**0.2569**	0.0244
5000	0.1602	0.2588	0.2601	**0.0163**	0.1832	**0.2539**	**0.2562**	0.0177
	Burr with $\xi = 0.25$, $\rho = -0.75$							
100	0.1756	0.2963	0.3020	0.1390	0.1676	**0.2611**	**0.2737**	**0.0969**
200	0.1503	0.2913	0.2988	0.0931	0.1389	**0.2614**	**0.2702**	**0.0761**
500	0.1202	0.2885	0.2927	0.0612	0.1133	**0.2614**	**0.2686**	**0.0590**
750	0.1021	0.2836	0.2882	0.0525	0.0979	**0.2602**	**0.2660**	**0.0500**
1000	0.0974	0.2833	0.2854	0.0503	0.0912	**0.2604**	**0.2654**	**0.0464**
2000	0.0768	0.2780	0.2813	0.0391	0.0733	**0.2595**	**0.2639**	**0.0372**
5000	0.0550	0.2703	0.2724	**0.0292**	0.0570	**0.2577**	**0.2623**	0.0306
	Half-t_4 ($\xi = 0.25$, $\rho = -0.5$)							
100	0.0986	0.3492	0.3520	0.2877	0.0951	**0.2922**	**0.3025**	**0.1318**
200	0.0843	0.3391	0.3463	0.1907	0.0761	**0.2887**	**0.3012**	**0.1105**
500	0.0628	0.3382	0.3371	0.2858	0.0562	**0.2862**	**0.2960**	**0.0874**
750	0.0550	0.3279	0.3361	0.1037	0.0492	**0.2849**	**0.2934**	**0.0794**
1000	0.0500	0.3243	0.3300	0.0973	0.0436	**0.2807**	**0.2906**	**0.0736**
2000	0.0392	0.3133	0.3179	0.0799	0.0340	**0.2755**	**0.2839**	**0.0618**
5000	0.0268	0.2993	0.3030	0.0604	0.0244	**0.2715**	**0.2786**	**0.0498**

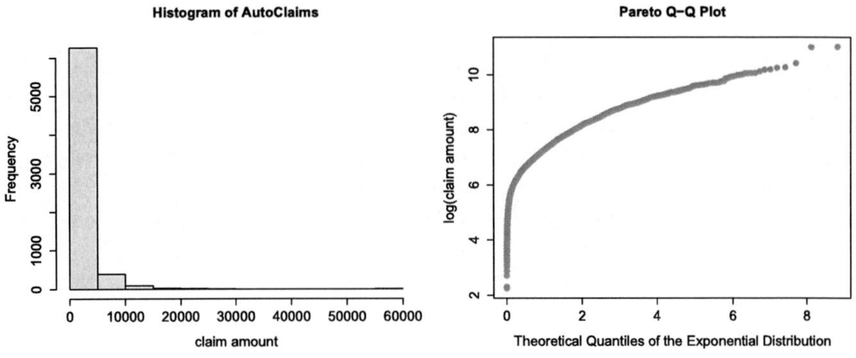

Fig. 2 Histogram and Pareto QQ plot for the AutoClaims dataset

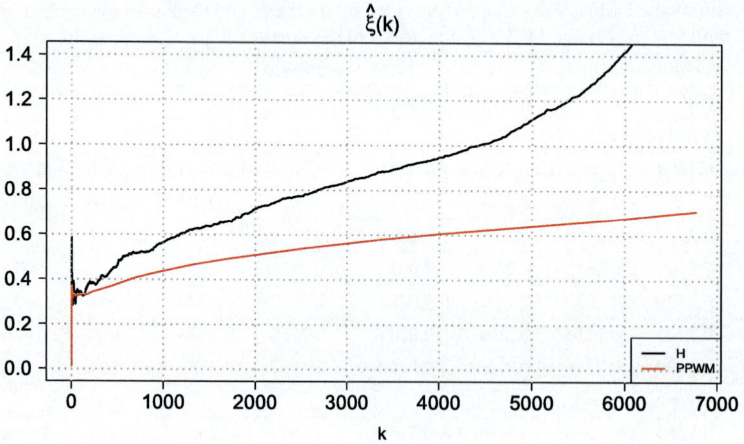

Fig. 3 Estimates of the EVI for the AutoClaims dataset

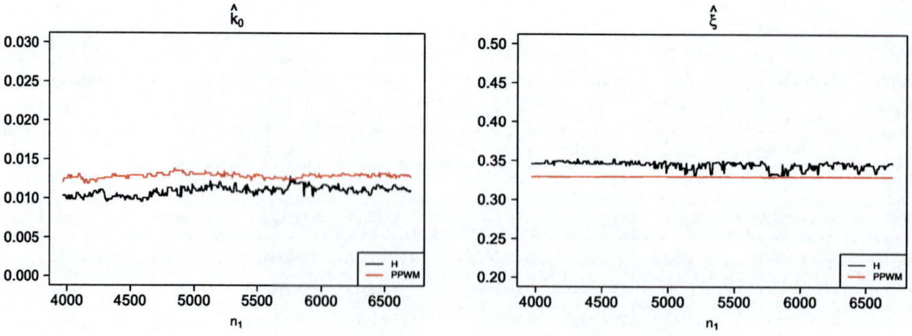

Fig. 4 Estimates of the OSF's $\hat{k}_0^{\bullet,*}/n$ (*left*) and the bootstrap adaptive extreme value index estimates $\hat{\xi}^{\bullet,*}$ (*right*), as functions of the sub-sample size n_1, for the amount paid on a closed claim

In Fig. 4, as a function of the sub-sample size n_1, ranging from $n_1 = 3990$ until $n_1 = 6700$, we picture, at the left, the estimates $\hat{k}_0^{\bullet,*}(n_1)/n$ of the optimal sample fraction, $k_0^{\bullet}/n$, for the adaptive double bootstrap estimation of ξ through the H and the PPWM estimators. Associated bootstrap EVI-estimates are pictured at the right. Contrarily to the bootstrap Hill, the bootstrap PPWM EVI-estimates are quite stable as a function of the sub-sample size n_1 (see Fig. 4, right).

For a re-sample size $n_1 = [n^{0.955}] = 4554$, and $B = 250$ bootstrap generations, we were led to $\hat{k}_0^{H,*} = 67$ and to $\hat{\xi}^{H,*} = 0.3463$. This same algorithm applied to the PPWM estimator provide the bootstrap estimates $\hat{k}_0^{PPWM,*} = 88$ and $\hat{\xi}^{PPWM,*} = 0.3301$.

5 Conclusions

In this paper we addressed the adaptive estimation of the EVI with the double bootstrap methodology associated to the Hill and the PPWM estimators. The presented simulation study shows that the adaptive PPWM EVI-estimator is usually less biased and provides a similar or a smaller RMSE than the adaptive Hill EVI-estimator. Moreover, the efficiency of the adaptive PPWM estimator relatively to the adaptive Hill estimator seems to improve as the asymptotic bias of estimators increases (as ρ increases). Further research concerning the sensitivity of the method on the choice of n_1 will be addressed in the future.

Acknowledgements Research partially supported by National Funds through **FCT**—Fundação para a Ciência e a Tecnologia, projects UIDB/00006/2020 and UIDP/00006/2020 (CEA/UL) and UIDB/00297/2020 and UIDP/00297/2020 (CMA/UNL).

References

1. Jenkinson, A.F.: The frequency distribution of the annual maximum (or minimum) values of meteorological elements. Q. J. R. Meteorol. Soc. **81**, 158–171 (1955)
2. Von Mises, R.: La distribution de la plus grande de *n* valuers. Rev. Math. Union Interbalcanique **1**, 141–160 (1936)
3. Hill, B.M.: A simple general approach to inference about the tail of a distribution. Ann. Stat. **3**(5), 1163–1174 (1975)
4. Caeiro, F., Gomes, M.I.: Semi-parametric tail inference through probability-weighted moments. J. Stat. Plann. Inference **141**(2), 937–950 (2011)
5. Beirlant, J., Herrmann, K., Teugels, J.: Estimation of the extreme value index. In: Extreme Events in Finance, pp. 97–115. Wiley (2016)
6. Fedotenkov, I.: A review of more than one hundred Pareto-tail index estimators. Statistica (Bologna) **80**(3), 245–299 (2020)
7. Beirlant, J., Caeiro, F., Gomes, M.I.: An overview and open research topics in statistics of univariate extremes. Revstat-Stat. J. **10**(1), 1–31 (2012)
8. Gomes, M.I., Oliveira, O.: The bootstrap methodology in statistics of extremes–choice of the optimal sample fraction. Extremes **4**(4), 331–358 (2001)
9. Gomes, M.I., Mendonça, S., Pestana, D.: Adaptive reduced-bias tail index and var estimation via the bootstrap methodology. Commun. Stat.-Theory and Methods **40**(16), 2946–2968 (2011)
10. Caeiro, F., Gomes, M.I., Vandewalle, B.: Semi-parametric probability-weighted moments estimation revisited. Methodol. Comput. Appl. Probab. **16**(1), 1–29 (2014)
11. Hall, P.: Using the bootstrap to estimate mean squared error and select smoothing parameter in nonparametric problems. J. Multivar. Anal. **32**(2), 177–203 (1990)
12. Fraga Alves, M.I., Gomes, M.I., De Haan, L.: A new class of semi-parametric estimators of the second order parameter. Portugaliae Math. **60**(2), 193–213 (2003)
13. Gomes, M.I., Martins, M.J.: Asymptotically unbiased estimators of the tail index based on external estimation of the second order parameter. Extremes **5**(1), 5–31 (2002)
14. Caeiro, F., Gomes, M.: Threshold selection in extreme value analysis. In: Extreme Value Modeling and Risk Analysis. Chapman and Hall/CRC, Boca Raton, FL
15. Wolny-Dominiak, A., Trzesiok, M.: `insuranceData`: A collection of insurance datasets useful in risk classification in non-life insurance (2014). R package version 1.0

Estimation of the Weibull Tail Coefficient Through the Power Mean-of-Order-p

Frederico Caeiro, M. Ivette Gomes, and Lígia Henriques-Rodrigues

Abstract The *Weibull tail coefficient* (WTC) is the parameter θ in a right-tail function of the type $\overline{F} := 1 - F$, such that $H := -\ln \overline{F}$ is a *regularly varying* function at infinity with an index of regular variation equal to $\theta \in \mathbb{R}^+$. In a context of extreme value theory for maxima, it is possible to prove that we have an *extreme value index* (EVI) $\xi = 0$, but usually a very slow rate of convergence. Most of the recent WTC-estimators are proportional to the class of Hill EVI-estimators, the average of the log-excesses associated with the k upper order statistics, $1 \le k < n$. The interesting performance of EVI-estimators based on generalized means leads us to base the WTC-estimation on the power *mean-of-order-p* (MO_p) EVI-estimators. Consistency of the WTC-estimators is discussed and their performance, for finite samples, is illustrated through a small-scale Monte Carlo simulation study.

Keywords Power mean-of-order-p · Semi-parametric estimation · Statistics of extremes · Weibull tail coefficient

F. Caeiro (✉)
NOVA School of Science and Technology (FCT NOVA) and CMA, NOVA University of Lisbon, Campus de Caparica, Lisbon, Portugal
e-mail: fac@fct.unl.pt

M. I. Gomes
Faculty of Science of Lisbon (FCUL/DEIO) and CEAUL, University of Lisbon, Cidade Universitária, Campo Grande, Lisbon, Portugal
e-mail: ivette.gomes@fc.ul.pt

L. Henriques-Rodrigues
School of Science and Technology (ECT-UE) and CIMA, University of Évora, Évora, Portugal
e-mail: ligiahr@uevora.pt

R. Bispo et al. (eds.), *Recent Developments in Statistics and Data Science*, Springer Proceedings in Mathematics & Statistics 398,
https://doi.org/10.1007/978-3-031-12766-3_4

1 A Brief Introduction

Extreme value theory (EVT) and *statistics of extremes* help us to control potentially disastrous events, of high relevance to society and with a high social impact. Domains of application of EVT are quite diverse. We mention *biostatistics, finance, insurance, structural engineering* and also *environment, hydrology, meteorology* and *seismology*. Earthquakes, fires, floods and other extreme events have provided impetus for several recent re-developments of *extreme value analysis* (EVA), of *statistics of univariate extremes* (SUE) and also multivariate and spatial extremes.

By the late seventies, it was common to work in the field of parametric statistics of extremes, essentially through the use of the limiting models for extremes. The developments of the asymptotic EVT led researchers to work under semi-parametric and non-parametric frameworks. Nowadays, with the increase in computational resources, the parametric modelling gained a new dynamism with the use of Bayesian and spatial techniques.

Apart from the estimation of the *extreme value index* (EVI), one of the primary parameters in EVA, the reliable estimation of other important parameters of rare events, like the *Weibull tail coefficient* (WTC), the shape parameter in a Weibull-type right-tail, will be among the topics to be addressed. Among a large variety of Weibull-type right-tails, we mention the Exponential, the Gamma, the Logistic and the Normal tails. They thus form an important and large subgroup of light and exponential right-tailed distributions of a Gumbel type, being of high interest in hydrology, meteorology, environmental and actuarial science, among other areas of application. As mentioned above, we shall emphasize the use of generalized means (GMs) in the WTC-estimation.

2 A Brief Motivation for the Need of EVT

To motivate the interest for this area, and despite the great variety of disasters that have happened recently, we merely mention the historical floods in the North Sea, on February 1, 1953. According to Encyclopaedia Britannica [1], this was the worst storm recorded in the North Sea with extensive floodings in several North sea countries that caused 2551 deaths and vast destruction.

As a way of preventing future floods, the Dutch government created the Delta project, to determine the height of the dikes and dams so that the probability of flooding in a future year would be extremely small [1]. And EVT was used as a tool to reliably answer this question.

When dealing with extreme or rare events, we are interested in working with maximum or minimum values and we want to characterize the tails' behaviour. For this, we need to use asymptotic methods, being necessary to make a compromise since there are generally not many observations in the tails of the distributions and extrapolation upwards or downwards of the observed sample is required.

EVT is a Statistics' branch that provides the probabilistic tools to fully characterize and understand extreme and rare events. Even when dealing with 'big data', the tails are scarce, and just as mentioned above it is often required an estimation beyond the sample extremes. The answer to the question, '*Is there a hidden pattern underlying this type of extreme events?*', is positive, being next partially and briefly provided.

3 A Brief Touch on Asymptotical EVT

Some of the key tools that have led to the way statistical EVT has been exploding in these last decades are the following ones: 1 – The key result obtained by Fréchet [2], on the functional equation of stability for maxima, which led him to the now rightly called Fréchet law; 2 – Such a functional equation was later solved, still with some restrictions, by Fisher and Tippett [3], who derived the possible non-degenerate limiting laws of the linearly normalized sample maxima,

$$\frac{X_{n:n} - b_n}{a_n}, \quad a_n > 0,\ b_n \in \mathbb{R}, \quad X_{n:n} := \max(X_1, \ldots, X_n), \tag{1}$$

associated with an *independent and identically distributed* (IID) random sample, $\underline{X}_n := (X_1, \ldots, X_n)$ from a *cumulative distribution function* (CDF) F.
They then arrived at the *extreme value* (EV) CDFs,

$$\text{Type I}: \quad \Lambda(x) = \mathrm{e}^{-\mathrm{e}^{-x}},\ x \in \mathbb{R} \qquad [Gumbel], \tag{2}$$

$$\text{Type II}: \ \Phi_\alpha(x) = \mathrm{e}^{-x^{-\alpha}},\ x > 0,\ \alpha > 0\ [Fr\acute{e}chet], \tag{3}$$

$$\text{Type III}: \Psi_\alpha(x) = \mathrm{e}^{-(-x)^\alpha},\ x < 0,\ \alpha > 0\ [Max - Weibull]; \tag{4}$$

3 – Such a result was initially formalized by Gnedenko [4], used by Gumbel [5], for applications of EVT in engineering and hydrology, and finally formalized by de Haan [6].

SUE is thus mainly based on the aforementioned EV models, also called *max-stable* laws, related to the non-degenerate limiting behaviour of the sequence of linearly normalized maximum values, as in (1). SUE deals thus essentially with the above-mentioned EV CDFs, in (2), (3) and (4), which can be encompassed in the *general extreme value* (GEV) CDF,

$$G_\xi(x) \equiv \mathrm{GEV}_\xi(x) = \begin{cases} \mathrm{e}^{-(1+\xi x)^{-1/\xi}},\ 1 + \xi x \geq 0, & \text{if } \xi \neq 0, \\ \mathrm{e}^{-\mathrm{e}^{-x}},\ x \in \mathbb{R}, & \text{if } \xi = 0, \end{cases} \tag{5}$$

with ξ the so-called EVI, the primary parameter in SUE. But SUE is also based on asymptotic results related to the non-degenerate limiting behaviour of a set of upper *order statistics* (OSs), either individually or jointly (Weissman [7, 8]; Pickands [9]; Gomes [10–12]; Smith [13]), or of excesses over high thresholds (Davison [14];

Smith [15]; Davison and Smith [16]), linked to *generalized Pareto* CDFs ($\mathrm{GP}_\xi(\cdot) = 1 + \ln\ \mathrm{GEV}_\xi(\cdot)$). And the fact that $\min(X_1, \ldots, X_n) = -\max(-X_1, \ldots, -X_n)$ enables the derivation of analogous results for minima and lower OSs.

The aforementioned main theoretical result on the non-degenerate limiting behaviour of the linearly normalized maximum in (1) is commonly known as the Fisher–Tippett–Gnedenko's theorem, also called *extremal types theorem* (ETT), and has a role similar to the *central limit theorem* (CLT) for averages (or sums). The CDF F is then said to belong to the *max-domain of attraction* (MDA) of GEV_ξ, and we write $F \in \mathcal{D}_\mathcal{M}\left(\mathrm{GEV}_\xi\right)$. The EVI measures the heaviness of the *right-tail function* (RTF), $\overline{F}(x) := 1 - F(x)$. The heavier the right-tail, the larger ξ is.

Statistical applications of EVT have given emphasis to the relaxation of the independence condition and homoscedasticity, to the consideration of multidimensional and spatial frameworks and from a theoretical point of view, to a deeper and deeper use of regular variation and point processes.

4 Semi-parametric Estimation in SUE

The crucial parameter in SUE is the already defined EVI, denoted by ξ ($\in \mathbb{R}$). For dependent samples, we also have the extremal index, related to the mean size of clusters of extreme events. Under a semi-parametric framework, there is no fitting of an adequate parametric model. It is only assumed that $F \in \mathcal{D}_\mathcal{M}(\mathrm{GEV}_\xi)$, with $\mathrm{GEV}_\xi(\cdot)$ given in (5), ξ being the unique primary parameter of extreme events to be initially estimated, on the basis of a few upper observations, and according to an adequate methodology.

It is then common to consider the k upper observations above the random threshold $X_{n-k:n}$, i.e. $X_{n:n} \ge \cdots \ge X_{n-k+1:n}$. Such a threshold needs to be an upper intermediate OS, i.e.

$$k = k_n \to \infty, \quad k \in [1, n), \quad k = o(n) \quad \text{as } n \to \infty. \tag{6}$$

Let $F^{\leftarrow}$ denote the generalized inverse function associated with the underlying CDF, F. Let U be the associated *reciprocal tail quantile function*:

$$U(t) := F^{\leftarrow}(1 - 1/t), \quad t \in [1, \infty]. \tag{7}$$

The model F is commonly said to have a heavy right-tail if and only if there exists a positive real ξ such that

$$\overline{F} = 1 - F \in RV_{-1/\xi} \ \text{ if and only if } \ U \in RV_\xi, \tag{8}$$

with $U(\cdot)$ defined in (7) and where the notation RV_β stands for the class of regularly varying functions at infinity with an index of regular variation equal to β, i.e. positive measurable functions $g(\cdot)$ such that $\lim_{t\to\infty} g(tx)/g(t) = x^\beta$, for all $x > 0$.

Since risks are more dangerous when we deal with a heavy RTF, we often consider heavy-tailed models, i.e. Pareto-type underlying CDFs, with a positive EVI, working thus in

$$\mathcal{D_M}^+ := \mathcal{D_M}\left(\text{GEV}_{\xi>0}\right), \tag{9}$$

or equivalently, models F such that (8) holds.

4.1 A Class of GM EVI-Estimators

Among the large variety of EVI-estimators, we mention the Hill (H) estimators [17]. The H EVI-estimators are the average of the log-excesses, $V_{ik} := \ln X_{n-i+1:n} - \ln X_{n-k:n}$, $1 \le i \le k < n$, i.e.

$$\text{H}_{k,n} \equiv \text{H}(k) \equiv \text{H}(k; \underline{X}_n) := \frac{1}{k}\sum_{i=1}^{k} V_{ik}, \qquad 1 \le k < n. \tag{10}$$

We further mention one of the competitive generalizations of $\text{H}(k)$, recently introduced in the literature, and based on a simple GM.

First, note that we can write

$$\text{H}(k) = \sum_{i=1}^{k} \ln\left(\frac{X_{n-i+1:n}}{X_{n-k:n}}\right)^{1/k} = \ln\left(\prod_{i=1}^{k}\frac{X_{n-i+1:n}}{X_{n-k:n}}\right)^{1/k}.$$

The H EVI-estimator in (10) is thus the logarithm of the *geometric mean* (or *power mean-of-order*-0) of

$$U_{ik} := \frac{X_{n-i+1:n}}{X_{n-k:n}}, \quad 1 \le i \le k < n. \tag{11}$$

Almost simultaneously, Brilhante et al. [18], Paulauskas and Vaičiulis [19] and Beran et al. [20] (see also [21]) considered as basic statistics, the power mean-of-order-p (MO_p) of U_{ik}, $1 \le i \le k$, in (11), for $p \ge 0$. More generally, Caeiro et al. [22] considered the same statistics for any $p \in \mathbb{R}$, i.e.

$$\text{M}_p(k) = \begin{cases} \left(\frac{1}{k}\sum_{i=1}^{k} U_{ik}^p\right)^{1/p}, & \text{if } p \neq 0, \\ \left(\prod_{i=1}^{k} U_{ik}\right)^{1/k}, & \text{if } p = 0, \end{cases}$$

and the associated class of MO_p EVI-estimators:

$$\mathrm{H}_{k,n,p} \equiv \mathrm{H}_p(k) = \mathrm{H}_p(k; \underline{X}_n) := \begin{cases} \left(1 - \mathrm{M}_p^{-p}(k)\right)/p, \text{ if } p < 1/\xi,\ p \neq 0, \\ \ln \mathrm{M}_0(k) = \mathrm{H}(k), \ \text{ if } p = 0. \end{cases} \tag{12}$$

The use of the extra tuning parameter $p \in \mathbb{R}$ and the MO_p methodology can thus provide a much more adequate EVI-estimation. Asymptotic normality is achieved for $p \leq 1/(2\xi)$. But, on the basis of Gomes et al. [23] (see also [24]), we can now go up to $p = 1/\xi$, getting then a sum-stable behaviour, with an index of sum-stability $\alpha = 1/(p\xi)$. And for $p = 1/\xi$, we get, for $\mathrm{H}_p(k) - \xi$, a deterministic dominant component, of the order of $1/\ln k$.

4.2 Semi-parametric Estimation of the WTC

The WTC is the parameter θ in an RTF of the type

$$\overline{F}(x) = 1 - F(x) =: e^{-H(x)}, \quad H \in RV_{1/\theta},\ \theta \in \mathbb{R}^+. \tag{13}$$

Equivalently to (13), we can say that

$$U(e^t) = H^{\leftarrow}(t) \in RV_\theta \iff U(t) =: (\ln t)^\theta L(\ln t), \tag{14}$$

with $L \in RV_0$, a slowly varying function.

In a context of EVT for maxima, it is possible to prove that we have an EVI $\xi = 0$, but usually a very slow rate of convergence. We are working with those tails, like the Normal RTF, in the MDA of Gumbel's law $\Lambda(\cdot)$, in (2), which can exhibit a penultimate (or pre-asymptotic) behaviour, a concept introduced in the aforementioned seminal paper by Fisher and Tippett, [3]. Such RTFs, despite double-exponential, look more similar either to

- Max-Weibull, $\Psi_\alpha(x) = \exp(-(-x)^\alpha)$, $x < 0$ ($\xi = -1/\alpha < 0$)
- or to Fréchet, $\Phi_\alpha(x) = \exp(-x^{-\alpha})$, $x > 0$ ($\xi = 1/\alpha > 0$)

right-tails, according to $\theta < 1$ or $\theta > 1$, respectively. Details on penultimate behaviour can be found in Gomes [10, 25] and Gomes and de Haan [26], among others.

Here, we merely mention the most relevant WTC-estimators in Gardes and Girard [27], which are given by

$$\widehat{\theta}^{\mathrm{H}}_{k,n} := \frac{\ln(n/k)}{k} \sum_{i=1}^{k} V_{ik} = \ln(n/k)\mathrm{H}_{k,n}, \tag{15}$$

with $\mathrm{H}_{k,n}$ the already defined H EVI-estimators, in (10). More generally than $\widehat{\theta}^{\mathrm{H}}_{k,n}$, we now suggest the consideration of MO$_p$ WTC-estimators, based on the aforementioned GM EVI-estimators, in (12), i.e.

$$\widehat{\theta}^{\mathrm{MO}_p}_{k,n} := \ln(n/k)\mathrm{H}_{k,n,p}. \tag{16}$$

And recently, Lehmer's mean-of-order-p EVI-estimators (Penalva et al. [28–30]) have revealed even a higher efficiency, but have not yet been considered for the WTC-estimation.

4.3 Consistency of the WTC-Estimators

To achieve the consistency of the new class of WTC-estimators, we just need to consider $p \neq 0$, in (16), since the case $p = 0$ that corresponds to the class $\widehat{\theta}^{\mathrm{H}}_{k,n}$, in (15), was already studied in Gardes and Girard [27]. We start by observing that, for any $p \neq 0$, and with $U(\cdot)$ defined in (7),

$$\left(\frac{U(tx)}{U(t)}\right)^p = \left(1 + \frac{\ln x}{\ln t}\right)^{p\theta} \left(\frac{L(\ln t + \ln x)}{L(\ln t)}\right)^p.$$

Since $L(\cdot)$, defined in (14), is in RV_0, and applying a first-order Taylor expansion to the first term, we can write

$$\left(\frac{U(tx)}{U(t)}\right)^p \sim 1 + p\,\theta\,\frac{\ln x}{\ln t}.$$

Let $Y_{1:n}, Y_{2:n}, \ldots, Y_{n:n}$ denote the OSs associated with a random sample of n independent standard Pareto random variables with CDF $F_Y(y) = 1 - 1/y$, $y \geq 1$. Then $X_{i:n} \stackrel{d}{=} U(Y_{i:n})$, $1 \leq i \leq n$ and $Y_{n-i+1:n}/Y_{n-k:n} \stackrel{d}{=} Y_{k-i+1:k}$. In this case, the following distributional representation holds, with U_{ik} defined in (11),

$$\begin{aligned} U_{ik}^p &\stackrel{d}{=} \left(\frac{U(Y_{n-i+1:n})}{U(Y_{n-k:n})}\right)^p \\ &\stackrel{d}{=} \left(\frac{U(Y_{n-k:n}Y_{k-i+1:k})}{U(Y_{n-k:n})}\right)^p \sim 1 + \frac{p\,\theta \ln Y_{k-i+1:k}}{\ln(n/k)}. \end{aligned}$$

Since $E_i = \ln Y_i$ are IID exponentially random variables with mean value 1 and $E_{n-k:n} \sim \ln(n/k) \to \infty$, for intermediate sequences of OSs satisfying (6), we then get

$$\frac{1}{k}\sum_{i=1}^{k} U_{ik}^p \stackrel{d}{=} 1 + \frac{p\,\theta}{\ln(n/k)}(1 + o_{\mathbb{P}}(1)), \quad p \neq 0,$$

with $o_{\mathbb{P}}(1)$ uniform in i, $1 \leq i \leq k$ (see [22]). From (12) and (16), the consistency of the MO_p WTC-estimators in (16) follows, in the whole $\mathcal{D}_{\mathcal{M}}{}^{+}$, in (9), provided that (6) holds.

5 Finite Sample Behaviour with Simulated Data

In this section, we evaluate the finite sample performance of the class of estimators $\widehat{\theta}_{k,n}^{\mathrm{MO}_p}$, in (16), through a Monte Carlo simulation study. The values for the tuning parameter p were selected from a preliminary simulation study. The value $p = 0$ was always used, since it provides the estimator in (15). The value $p = 1$ was also used as an example of a positive tuning parameter. We have considered the following typical distributions within the class of Weibull-type models: the Gamma distribution with a shape parameter equal to 0.75 ($\theta = 1$) and the Half-Normal model ($\theta = 0.5$). In Figs. 1 and 2, we present, at the left, the simulated mean value and, at the right, the corresponding simulated *root mean squared error* (RMSE), as a function of k, provided by the aforementioned class of WTC-estimators and 20,000 samples of size $n = 1000$. The horizontal solid line, at the left plot, indicates the true WTC value. Similar patterns were obtained for other simulated models and sample sizes.

In Table 1, we present the simulated values of the RMSE at the simulated optimal level, for samples of sizes 100, 200, 500, 1000, 2000 and 5000. For each model and sample size, the smallest RMSE is written in **bold**. The smallest RMSE is always achieved by $\widehat{\theta}_{k,n}^{\mathrm{MO}_p} := \ln(n/k)\mathrm{H}_{k,n,p}$, in (16), with $p < 0$. Moreover, the optimal p decreases, as the sample size n increases. For large sample sizes, the choices -3 and -1.5 seem to provide an overall good performance for the Gamma and Half-Normal models, respectively.

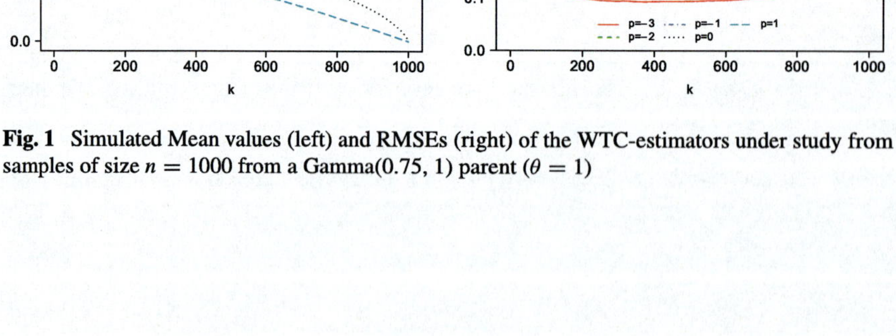

Fig. 1 Simulated Mean values (left) and RMSEs (right) of the WTC-estimators under study from samples of size $n = 1000$ from a Gamma(0.75, 1) parent ($\theta = 1$)

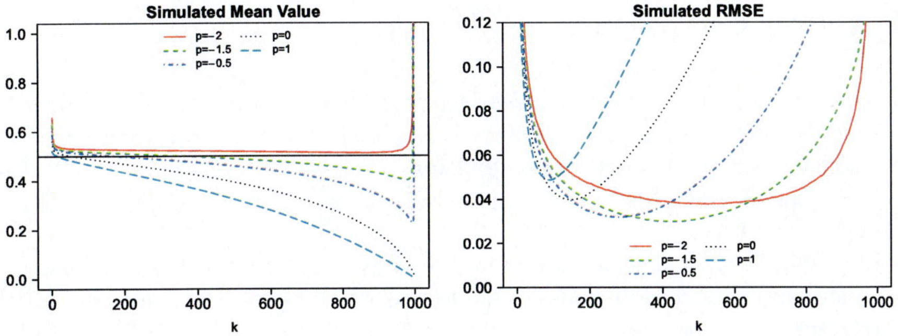

Fig. 2 Simulated Mean values (left) and RMSEs (right) of the WTC-estimators under study from samples of size $n = 1000$ from a Half-Normal parent ($\theta = 0.5$)

Table 1 Simulated RMSE at the simulated optimal level

Sample size:	100	200	500	1000	2000	5000
	Gamma(0.75, 1)					
$p = -3$	0.2808	0.1868	**0.1206**	**0.0942**	**0.0781**	**0.0653**
$p = -2$	0.2311	**0.1768**	0.1369	0.1173	0.1023	0.0867
$p = -1$	**0.2302**	0.1948	0.1619	0.1413	0.1248	0.1068
$p = 0$	0.2547	0.2242	0.1880	0.1651	0.1478	0.1273
$p = 1$	0.2910	0.2573	0.2180	0.1936	0.1738	0.1494
	Half-Normal					
$p = -2$	0.1191	0.0814	0.0512	0.0377	0.0280	0.0195
$p = -1.5$	0.0985	0.0678	**0.0419**	**0.0300**	**0.0215**	**0.0137**
$p = -1$	0.0878	**0.0637**	0.0430	0.0320	0.0237	0.0157
$p = 0$	**0.0873**	0.0694	0.0507	0.0398	0.0311	0.0220
$p = 1$	0.0961	0.0792	0.0605	0.0489	0.0396	0.0295

A few general comments:

- For all simulated parents, we could always find a value of p (negative, contrary to what happens with the MO_p EVI-estimation), such that, for adequate k-values, there is a reduction in RMSE, as well as in bias, and for such a value of p, the MO_p often strongly beats the $H \equiv MO_0$ WTC-estimators.
- Algorithmic details on the choice of tuning parameters under play are still under progress, but can be easily devised, similar to what has been done for an EVI-estimation in Caeiro and Gomes [31] and Gomes et al. [32], where R-scripts are provided.

6 Overall Conclusions

- Risk analyses related to extreme events are challenging and require the combined expertise of statisticians and domain experts in climatology, hydrology, finance, insurance, medicine, sports and other fields.
- In our opinion, even SUE is still a quite lively topic of research, of high relevance in risk modelling.
- Important developments have appeared recently in the area of *spatial extremes*, where *parametric models*, both asymptotic and pre-asymptotic, became again quite relevant.
- And in a semi-parametric framework, topics like *threshold selection* and the PORT methodology, with PORT standing for *peaks over random thresholds*, a terminology coined in Araújo Santos et al. [33], are still quite challenging.
- The lack of efficiency of the MO_p WTC-estimators for $p > 0$, and of the MO_p EVI-estimators for $p < 0$, together with the results in Stehlík et al. [34], related to the robustness of the MO_{-1} EVI-estimators, deserves a further discussion of the topic 'robustness versus efficiency'.
- Related statistical research with critical risk assessment applications can be found in several books, like Embrechts et al. [35], Beirlant et al. [36], Gomes et al. [37] and Dey and Yan [38], among others. For recent overviews on SUE and its possible application in risk modelling, see Davison and Huser [39] and Gomes and Guillou [40].
- We have here considered the univariate case only, but EVT is of high relevance both in the multivariate and in the spatial setup, whenever dealing with the modelling of extreme events or equivalently the modelling of risk.
- A comparative study with other WTC-estimators, like the ones in Diebolt et al. [41], Gardes and Girard [42, 43], Goegebeur et al. [44], Gong and Ling [45] and Kpanzou et al. [46], among others, is expected to be developed in the near future.
- In a way similar to what has been done in Worms and Worms [47], the new estimator can be developed for censored data.
- Also corresponding estimators of extreme quantiles can be developed either for complete or censored (mild/heavy) settings.

Acknowledgements The research was partially supported by National Funds through FCT—Fundação para a Ciência e a Tecnologia (Portuguese Foundation for Science and Technology) through projects UIDB/00297/2020 (CMA/UNL), UIDB/00006/2020 (CEA/UL) and UIDB/04674/2020 (CIMA).

References

1. Encyclopaedia Britannica.: The Editors of Encyclopaedia Britannica, North Sea flood. Encyclopaedia Britannica (2022). https://www.britannica.com/event/North-Sea-flood. https://doi.org/10.57805/revstat.v4i3.37
2. Fréchet, M.: Sur la loi de probabilité de l'écart maximum. Annales de la Société Polonaise de Mathematique **6**, 93–116 (1927)
3. Fisher, R.A., Tippett, L.H.C.: Limiting forms of the frequency distributions of the largest or smallest member of a sample. Proc. Camb. Philos. Soc. **24**, 180–190 (1928). https://doi.org/10.1017/S0305004100015681
4. Gnedenko, B.V.: Sur la distribution limite du terme maximum d'une série aléatoire. Ann. Math. **44**, 423–453 (1943). https://doi.org/10.2307/1968974
5. Gumbel, E.J.: Statistics of Extremes. Columbia University Press, NY (1958). https://doi.org/10.7312/gumb92958
6. Haan, L. de: On Regular Variation and its Application to the Weak Convergence of Sample Extremes. Mathematical Centre Tract 32, Amsterdam (1970)
7. Weissman, I.: Multivariate extremal processes generated by independent non-identically distributed random variables. J. Appl. Probab. **12**, 477–487 (1975). https://doi.org/10.2307/3212862
8. Weissman, I.: Estimation of parameters and large quantiles based on the k largest observations. J. Amer. Stat. Assoc. **73**, 812–815 (1978). https://doi.org/10.2307/2286285
9. Pickands III, J.: Statistical inference using extreme order statistics. Ann. Stat. **3**, 119–131 (1975). https://doi.org/10.1214/aos/1176343003
10. Gomes, M.I.: Some Probabilistic and Statistical Problems in Extreme Value Theory. Ph.D. Thesis, The University of Sheffield (1978)
11. Gomes, M.I.: An i-dimensional limiting distribution function of largest values and its relevance to the statistical theory of extremes. In: Taillie, C., et al. (eds.) Statistical Distributions in Scientific Work, vol. 6, pp. 389–410. D. Reidel, Dordrecht (1981)
12. Gomes, M.I.: Statistical theory of extremes–comparison of two approaches. Stat. Decis. **2**, 33–37 (1985)
13. Smith, R.L.: Extreme value theory based on the r largest annual events. J. Hydrol. **86**, 27–43 (1986). https://doi.org/10.1016/0022-1694(86)90004-1
14. Davison, A.C.: Modeling excesses over high threshold with an application. In: Tiago de Oliveira, J. (eds.) Statistical Extremes and Applications, pp.461–482. D. Reidel, Dordrecht (1984). https://doi.org/10.1007/978-94-017-3069-3_34
15. Smith, R.L.: Threshold methods for sample extremes. In: Tiago de Oliveira, J. (ed.) Statistical Extremes and Applications, pp. 621–638. D. Reidel, Dordrect (1984). https://doi.org/10.1007/978-94-017-3069-3_48
16. Davison, A.C., Smith, R.L.: Models for exceedances over high thresholds. J. R. Stat. Soc. B Stat. Meth. **52**, 393–442 (1990). http://www.jstor.org/stable/2345667
17. Hill, B.M.: A simple general approach to inference about the tail of a distribution. Ann. Stat. **3**, 1163–1174 (1975). https://doi.org/10.1214/aos/1176343247
18. Brilhante, M.F., Gomes, M.I., Pestana, D.: A simple generalisation of the Hill estimator. Comput. Statist. Data Anal. **57**(1), 518–535 (2013). https://doi.org/10.1016/j.csda.2012.07.019
19. Paulauskas, V., Vaičiulis, M.: On the improvement of Hill and some other estimators. Lith. Math. J. **53**, 336–355 (2013). https://doi.org/10.1007/s10986-013-9212-x
20. Beran, J., Schell, D., Stehlík, M.: The harmonic moment tail index estimator: asymptotic distribution and robustness. Ann. Inst. Statist. Math. **66**, 193–220 (2014). https://doi.org/10.1007/s10463-013-0412-2
21. Segers, J.: Residual estimators. J. Stat. Plann. Infer. **98**(1–2), 15–27 (2001). https://doi.org/10.1016/s0378-3758(00)00321-9
22. Caeiro, F., Gomes, M.I., Beirlant, J., de Wet, T.: Mean-of-order p reduced-bias extreme value index estimation under a third-order framework. Extremes **19**(4), 561–589 (2016). https://doi.org/10.1007/s10687-016-0261-5

23. Gomes, M.I., Henriques-Rodrigues, L., Pestana D.: Non-regular Frameworks and the Mean-of-order p Extreme Value Index Estimation. J. Stat. Theory Practice **16**(37) (2022). https://doi.org/10.1007/s42519-022-00264-w
24. Gomes, M.I., Henriques-Rodrigues, L., Pestana, D.: Estimação de um índice de valores extremos positivo através de médias generalizadas e em ambiente de não-regularidade. In: Milheiro, P. et al. (eds.) Estatística: Desafios Transversais às Ciências com Dados – Atas do XXIV Congresso da Sociedade Portuguesa de Estatística, Edições SPE, pp. 213–226 (2021)
25. Gomes, M.I.: Penultimate behaviour of the extremes. In: Galambos, J., Lechner, J., Simiu, E. (eds.) Extreme Value Theory and Applications, pp. 403–418. Kluwer Academic Publishers (1994). https://doi.org/10.1007/978-1-4613-3638-9
26. Gomes, M.I., de Haan, L.: Approximation by penultimate extreme value distributions. Extremes **2**(1), 71–85 (1999). https://doi.org/10.1023/A:1009920327187
27. Gardes, L., Girard, S.: Comparison of Weibull tail-coefficient estimators. Revstat.—Stat. J. **4**, 163–188 (2006). https://doi.org/10.57805/revstat.v4i2.34
28. Penalva, H., Caeiro, F., Gomes, M.I., Neves, M.M.: An Efficient Naive Generalization of the Hill Estimator-Discrepancy between Asymptotic and Finite Sample Behaviour. Notas e Comunicações CEAUL 02/2016 (2016). http://ceaul.org/wp-content/uploads/2018/10/NotaseCom-2.pdf
29. Penalva, H., Gomes, M.I., Caeiro, C., Neves, M.M.: A couple of non reduced bias generalized means in extreme value theory: an asymptotic comparison. Revstat.—Stat. J. **18**(3), 281–298 (2020). https://doi.org/10.57805/revstat.v18i3.301
30. Penalva, H., Gomes, M.I., Caeiro, C., Neves, M.M.: Lehmer's mean-of-order-p extreme value index estimation: a simulation study and applications. J. Appl. Stat. **47**, 13–15, 2825–2845 (2020). https://doi.org/10.1080/02664763.2019.1694871
31. Caeiro, F., Gomes, M.I.: Threshold selection in extreme value analysis. In: Dey Yan (eds.) Extreme Value Modeling and Risk Analysis: Methods and Applications (Chap. 4), pp. 69–87. Chapman-Hall/CRC (2015). https://doi.org/10.1201/b19721-5
32. Gomes, M.I., Caeiro, F., Henriques-Rodrigues, L., Manjunath, B.G.: Bootstrap methods in statistics of extremes. In: Longin, F. (ed.) Handbook of Extreme Value Theory and Its Applications to Finance and Insurance (Chap. 6), pp. 117–138 . Wiley (2016). https://doi.org/10.1002/9781118650318.ch6
33. Araújo Santos, P., Fraga Alves, M.I., Gomes, M.I.: Peaks over random threshold methodology for tail index and high quantile estimation. Revstat.—Statist. J. **4**(3), 227–247 (2006). https://doi.org/10.57805/revstat.v4i3.37
34. Stehlík, M., Potocký, R., Waldl, H., Fabián Z.: On the favourable estimation of fitting heavy tailed data. Comput. Stat. **25**, 485–503 (2010). https://doi.org/10.1007/s00180-010-0189-1
35. Embrechts, P., Klüppelberg, C., Mikosch, T.: Modelling Extremal Events for Insurance and Finance. Springer, Berlin (1997). https://link.springer.com/book/10.1007/978-3-642-33483-2
36. Beirlant, J., Goegebeur, Y., Segers, J., Teugels, J.: Statistics of Extremes: Theory and Applications. Wiley, England (2004). https://onlinelibrary.wiley.com/doi/book/10.1002/0470012382
37. Gomes, M.I., Fraga Alves, M.I., Neves, C.: Análise de Valores Extremos: uma Introdução. Edições S.P.E. and I.N.E. (2013). ISBN: 978-972-8890-30-8
38. Dey, D.K., Yan, J.: Extreme Value Modeling and Risk Analysis: Methods and Applications. Chapman and Hall/CRC (2015). https://doi.org/10.1201/b19721
39. Davison, A.C., Huser, R.: Statistics of extremes. Ann. Rev. Stat. Appl. **2**(1), 203–235 (2015). https://doi.org/10.1146/annurev-statistics-010814-020133
40. Gomes, M.I., Guillou, A.: Extreme value theory and statistics of univariate extremes: a review. Intern. Stat. Rev. **83**(2), 263–292 (2015). https://doi.org/10.1111/insr.12058
41. Diebolt, J., Gardes, L., Girard, S., Guillou, A.: Bias-reduced extreme quantile estimators of Weibull tail distributions. J. Stat. Plan. Infer. **138**, 1389–1401 (2008). https://doi.org/10.1016/j.jspi.2007.04.025
42. Gardes, L., Girard, S.: Estimation of the Weibull tail-coefficient with linear combination of upper order statistics. J. Stat. Plan. Infer. **138**, 1416–1427 (2008). https://doi.org/10.1016/j.jspi.2007.04.026f

43. Gardes, L., Girard, S.: On the estimation of the functional Weibull tail-coefficient. J. Multivar. Anal. **146**(C), 29–45 (2016). https://doi.org/10.1016/j.jmva.2015.05.007
44. Goegebeur, Y., Beirlant, J., de Wet T.: Generalized kernel estimators for the Weibull-tail coefficient. Commun. Stat. Theory Methods **39**, 3695–3716 (2010). https://doi.org/10.1080/03610920903324882
45. Gong, C., Ling, C.: Robust estimations for the tail index of Weibull-type distribution. Risks **6**, 119 (2018). https://doi.org/10.3390/risks6040119
46. Kpanzou T.A., Gamado K.M., Hounnon H.: A Beran-inspired estimator for the Weibull-type tail coefficient. J. Stat. Theory Pract. **13** (2019). https://doi.org/10.1007/s42519-018-0013-8
47. Worms, J., Worms, R.: Estimation of extremes for Weibull-tail distributions in the presence of random censoring. Extremes **22**, 667–704 (2019). https://doi.org/10.1007/s10687-019-00354-2

On the Maximum of a Bivariate Max-INAR(1) Process

Sandra Dias and Maria da Graça Temido

Abstract In this paper, we introduce a $\mathbb{Z}_+^2$-valued strictly stationary bivariate max-INAR(1) model, which is an extension of the univariate max-INAR(1) model, introduced and studied in [1]. We consider that the marginals have a double geometric distribution in the sense of Marshall and Olkin [2]. As a consequence, we deduce that the innovations have a tail equivalent to a bivariate geometric distribution. By proving that the restriction dependence conditions introduced in [3] hold, we establish asymptotic lower and upper bounds for the distribution function of the double maxima.

Keywords Bivariate geometric distribution · Extreme value theory · Max-stability · Max-INAR(1) process

1 Introduction

The study of time series for count data has attracted the interest of many authors in the last three decades. Understanding the discreteness of the data, that are common in practice, strongly impacts a wide variety of fields, particularly engineering, marketing, finance and health science.

The literature on univariate time series for counts is largely developed, whereas the research of multivariate time series models is progressing more slowly and is not so detailed.

In the successful attempt to establish a parallel with the moving average or autoregressive classic models, the very well-known Binomial thinning operator is introduced by Steutel and van Harn [4]. Assuming that X is a non-negative integer-valued

S. Dias (✉)
CEMAT, Department of Mathematics, University of Trás-os-Montes e Alto Douro, Vila Real, Portugal
e-mail: sdias@utad.pt

M. da Graça Temido
University of Coimbra, Department of Mathematics, FSTUC, CMUC, Coimbra, Portugal

R. Bispo et al. (eds.), *Recent Developments in Statistics and Data Science*, Springer Proceedings in Mathematics & Statistics 398,
https://doi.org/10.1007/978-3-031-12766-3_5

random variable and $\alpha \in]0, 1[$, this operator, when applied to (α, X), gives

$$\alpha \circ X = \sum_{s=1}^{X} B_s(\alpha) ,$$

where $\{B_s(\alpha)\}$ is a sequence of independent and identically distributed (i.i.d.) random variables with Bernoulli distribution satisfying $P(B_s(\alpha) = 1) = \alpha$ and independent of X. This interesting counterpart of the usual multiplication allowed the flowering of such models, which started with the so-called integer autoregressive model (INAR), introduced by MacKenzie [5] and Al-Osh and Alzaid [6]. Interesting results of bivariate count models can be found in Pedeli and Karlis [7], who discuss the bivariate INAR(1) model with negative binomial innovations, and in [8] for the parameter inference context.

Despite the wide variety of results that seems to cover a significant number of practical situations, many discrete models used in the above-mentioned fields remain to be studied with respect to their extreme values. In part, this is due to the fact that many integer-valued distributions do not belong to the domain of attraction of any extreme-value distribution. Anderson [9] gave an important contribution to overtaking this limitation by obtaining upper and lower bounds for the limiting distribution of the maximum of i.i.d. sequences with marginal discrete distributions exhibiting an exponentially decaying tail. Indeed, Anderson [9] proved that an integer-valued distribution function (d.f.) F, with infinite right endpoint, satisfies

$$\lim_{n\to\infty} \frac{1 - F(n-1)}{1 - F(n)} = r,\ r \in]1, +\infty[, \tag{1}$$

if and only if

$$\begin{cases} \limsup\limits_{n\to\infty} F^n(x + b_n) \le \exp(-r^{-x}) \\ \liminf\limits_{n\to\infty} F^n(x + b_n) \ge \exp(-r^{-(x-1)}) \end{cases}$$

for any real x and b_n suitably chosen. In the literature on extremes, the class of distributions satisfying (1) is usually called Anderson's class. A simple example of a d.f. in this class is the Negative Binomial.

When the univariate approach is considered, one can find in the literature of extremes the study of the extremal behaviour of integer-valued autoregressive models as well as moving average models in a few number of papers. Among these, we cite [1, 10–14]. In these works, dealing with the stationary or non-stationary process, with distributions in Anderson's class and satisfying Leadbeter's dependence restrictions (or some natural extensions), the limiting extremal behaviour is obtained.

In what concerns the multivariate case, little has been done so far with respect to extreme values of integer-valued data. Hüsler et al. [15] establishes asymptotics for the distribution of the maximum term of stationary sequences $\{(X_n, Y_n)\}$, where the marginals are defined by non-negative integer-valued moving average sequences of the general form

$$(X_n, Y_n) = \left(\sum_{i=-\infty}^{+\infty} \alpha_i \circ V_{n-i}, \sum_{i=-\infty}^{+\infty} \beta_i \circ W_{n-i} \right),$$

with i.i.d. innovation sequence $\{(V_n, W_n)\}$ and $\alpha_i, \beta_i \in]0, 1[$. Assuming also that $\alpha \circ V$ and $\beta \circ W$ are independent given (V, W), it is established that, for all $(x, y) \in \mathbb{R}^2$, it holds

$$\begin{cases} \limsup_{n\to\infty} P(M_n^{(1)} \le u_n, M_n^{(2)} \le v_n) \le \exp\{-r_1^{-x} - r_2^{-y}\} \\ \liminf_{n\to\infty} P(M_n^{(1)} \le u_n, M_n^{(2)} \le v_n) \ge \exp\{-r_1^{-x+1} - r_2^{-y+1}\} \end{cases},$$

where $r_1 > 1$ and $r_2 > 1$ are parameters of the model.

Due to the aim of this paper, we pay special attention to [1], where the univariate max-INAR(1) model is introduced and studied. Given an innovation sequence $\{Z_n\}$ of i.i.d. random variables, the max-INAR(1) stationary process is defined in [1] by

$$X_n = \max\{\alpha \circ X_{n-1}, Z_n\},$$

with $\alpha \in]0, 1[$ and $\{Z_n\}$ independent of X_1. Considering that the marginal d.f. F of $\{X_n\}$ belongs to Anderson's class and proving that Leadbeter's dependence restrictions $D(u_n)$ and $D'(u_n)$ hold, for a suitable sequence of normalizations $\{u_n\}$ with $u_n := u_n(x)$, these authors have established the following bounds:

$$\begin{cases} \limsup_{n\to\infty} P(M_n \le u_n) \le \exp\{-r^{-x}\} \\ \liminf_{n\to\infty} P(M_n \le u_n) \ge \exp\{-r^{-(x-1)}\} \end{cases} \tag{2}$$

for any real x. Another approach with F in the domain of attraction of the Fréchet d.f. is also considered in [1].

In this work, we extend the univariate max-INAR model, proposed and studied in [1], to a bivariate one, considering that the marginal stationary distribution is the bivariate geometric distribution introduced in [2]. The details follow.

We introduce the bivariate max-INAR(1) process

$$(X_n, Y_n) = (\max\{\alpha \circ X_{n-1}, Z_n\}, \max\{\beta \circ Y_{n-1}, W_n\}), \tag{3}$$

where $\alpha \in]0, 1[$ and $\{(Z_n, W_n)\}$ is a sequence of i.i.d. bivariate random variables which are independent of (X_1, Y_1).

We first prove that the process is strictly stationary. Also, for suitable normalizations $\{u_n\}$ and $\{v_n\}$, we prove that the process $\{(X_n, Y_n)\}$ satisfies the long-range condition $D(u_n, v_n)$ and the local dependence condition $D'(u_n, v_n)$ introduced in [3]. Consequently, for the normalized double maxima, the expected extension of (2) is obtained.

2 Stationarity of the Process

The multivariate distribution of any vector of the process $\{(X_n, Y_n)\}$ can be obtained from the following lemma.

Lemma 1 *The probability function of* $(X_1, Y_1, X_2, Y_2, ..., X_n, Y_n)$ *is given by*

$$\begin{aligned} &P(X_1 = x_1, Y_1 = y_1, X_2 = x_2, Y_2 = y_2, ..., X_n = x_n, Y_n = y_n) \\ &= P(X_1 = x_1, Y_1 = y_1) \prod_{i=2}^{n} \big[F_{Z,W}(x_i, y_i) F_{\alpha \circ x_{i-1}, \beta \circ y_{i-1}}(x_i, y_i) \\ &\quad - F_{Z,W}(x_i - 1, y_i) F_{\alpha \circ x_{i-1}, \beta \circ y_{i-1}}(x_i - 1, y_i) \\ &\quad - F_{Z,W}(x_i, y_i - 1) F_{\alpha \circ x_{i-1}, \beta \circ y_{i-1}}(x_i, y_i - 1) \\ &\quad + F_{Z,W}(x_i - 1, y_i - 1) F_{\alpha \circ x_{i-1}, \beta \circ y_{i-1}}(x_i - 1, y_i - 1) \big] , \end{aligned}$$

where $F_{\alpha \circ u, \beta \circ t}(k, \ell) = P(\alpha \circ X \leq k, \beta \circ Y \leq \ell | X = u, Y = t)$ *and* $F_{Z,W}$ *represents the d.f. of* (Z, W).

Proof For any $n \geq 2$, the conditional d.f. of the process is given by

$$\begin{aligned} P(X_n \leq k_1, Y_n \leq \ell | X_{n-1} = u, Y_{n-1} = t) &= P(Z_n \leq k_1, W_n \leq \ell) \times \\ &\times P(\alpha \circ X_{n-1} \leq k, \beta \circ Y_{n-1} \leq \ell | X_{n-1} = u, Y_{n-1} = t) \\ &= F_{Z,W}(k, \ell) F_{\alpha \circ u, \beta \circ t}(k, \ell) . \end{aligned}$$

Therefore, we can write the conditional probability function as follows:

$$\begin{aligned} &P(X_n = k, Y_n = \ell | X_{n-1} = u, Y_{n-1} = t) \\ &= P(X_n \leq k, Y_n \leq \ell | X_{n-1} = u, Y_{n-1} = t) \\ &\quad - P(X_n < k, Y_n \leq \ell | X_{n-1} = u, Y_{n-1} = t) \\ &\quad - P(X_n \leq k, Y_n < \ell | X_{n-1} = u, Y_{n-1} = t) \\ &\quad + P(X_n < k, Y_n < \ell | X_{n-1} = u, Y_{n-1} = t) \\ &= P(X_n \leq k, Y_n \leq \ell | X_{n-1} = u, Y_{n-1} = t) \\ &\quad - P(X_n \leq k - 1, Y_n \leq \ell | X_{n-1} = u, Y_{n-1} = t) \\ &\quad - P(X_n \leq k, Y_n \leq \ell - 1 | X_{n-1} = u, Y_{n-1} = t) \\ &\quad + P(X_n \leq k - 1, Y_n \leq \ell - 1 | X_{n-1} = u, Y_{n-1} = t) \end{aligned}$$

$$\begin{aligned}
&= F_{Z,W}(k,\ell)F_{\alpha o u,\beta o t}(k,\ell) \\
&\quad -F_{Z,W}(k-1,\ell)F_{\alpha o u,\beta o t}(k-1,\ell) \\
&\quad -F_{Z,W}(k,\ell-1)F_{\alpha o u,\beta o t}(k,\ell-1) \\
&\quad +F_{Z,W}(k-1,\ell-1)F_{\alpha o u,\beta o t}(k-1,\ell-1)\,.
\end{aligned}$$

So, since the process (3) is a Markov chain,

$$\begin{aligned}
&P(X_1 = x_1, Y_1 = y_1, X_2 = x_2, Y_2 = y_2, ..., X_n = x_n, Y_n = y_n) \\
&= P(X_1 = x_1, Y_1 = y_1)P(X_2 = x_2, Y_2 = y_2|X_1 = x_1, Y_1 = y_1) \times \\
&\quad \times P(X_3 = x_3, Y_3 = y_3|X_1 = x_1, Y_1 = y_1, X_2 = x_2, Y_2 = y_2) \times ... \times \\
&\quad \times P(X_n = x_n, Y_n = y_n|X_1 = x_1, Y_1 = y_1, ..., X_{n-1} = x_{n-1}, Y_{n-1} = y_{n-1}) \\
&= P(X_1 = x_1, Y_1 = y_1)\prod_{i=2}^{n} P(X_i = x_i, Y_i = y_i|X_{i-1} = x_{i-1}, Y_{i-1} = y_{i-1})
\end{aligned}$$

and the result follows. □

Now, applying the result of Lemma 1 to any finite sequence of random variables $(X_{1+k}, Y_{1+k}, X_{2+k}, Y_{2+k}, ..., X_{n+k}, Y_{n+k})$, $k \geq 1$, we conclude that the process is strictly stationary if it is i.d..

We emphasize the difficulty of characterizing analytically the class of stationary distributions $F_{X,Y}$ satisfying

$$F_{Z,W}(x,y) = \frac{F_{X,Y}(x,y)}{F_{\alpha o X,\beta o Y}(x,y)}\,. \tag{4}$$

Indeed, we are not able to discuss the limit behaviour of $\frac{1-F_{\alpha o X,\beta o Y}(x,y)}{1-F_{X,Y}(x,y)}$ from the general relationship (4). So, we choose the particular case of the bivariate geometric distribution defined in [2] by

$$1 - F_{X,Y}(x,y) = p_1^{[x]+1} + p_2^{[y]+1} - p_1^{[x]+1}p_2^{[y]+1}\left(\frac{p_3}{p_1p_2}\right)^{\min([x],[y])+1} \tag{5}$$

for all $(x, y) \in (\mathbb{R}_0^+)^2$ and with $p_3 < \min\{p_1, p_2\}$ and $p_3 > p_1 + p_2 - 1$.

Theorem 1 *Consider the d.f in (5) and the normalizations* $u_n = x - 1 - \frac{\ln n}{\ln p_1}$ *and* $v_n = y - 1 - \frac{\ln n}{\ln p_2}$. *Then we have*

$$\begin{cases}
\limsup\limits_{n\to\infty} F^n_{X,Y}(u_n, v_n) \leq \exp\{-p_1^x - p_2^y\} \\
\liminf\limits_{n\to\infty} F^n_{X,Y}(u_n, v_n) \geq \exp\{-p_1^{x-1} - p_2^{y-1}\}
\end{cases}$$

for all $(x, y) \in \mathbb{R}^2$.

Proof Indeed, since $\min([x],[y]) \le [x]$, we get

$$
\begin{aligned}
n\left(1 - F_{X,Y}\left(x - 1 - \tfrac{\ln n}{\ln p_1}, y - 1 - \tfrac{\ln n}{\ln p_2}\right)\right) &= np_1^{[x-1-\frac{\ln n}{\ln p_1}]+1} \\
+ np_2^{[y-1-\frac{\ln n}{\ln p_2}]+1} &- np_1^{[x-1-\frac{\ln n}{\ln p_1}]+1} p_2^{[y-1-\frac{\ln n}{\ln p_2}]+1} \left(\frac{p_3}{p_1p_2}\right)^{[x-1-\frac{\ln n}{\ln p_1}]+1} \\
:= \Sigma_n^{(1)} + \Sigma_n^{(2)} - \Sigma_n^{(3)} .
\end{aligned}
$$

We now prove that $\Sigma_n^{(3)} \longrightarrow 0$, as $n \to +\infty$. In fact, due to $p_i^{-\frac{\ln n}{\ln p_i}} = \frac{1}{n}$, it holds

$$
\begin{aligned}
\Sigma_n^{(3)} &\le np_1^{[x-\frac{\ln n}{\ln p_1}]} p_2^{[y-\frac{\ln n}{\ln p_2}]} \left(\frac{p_3}{p_1p_2}\right)^{[x-\frac{\ln n}{\ln p_1}]} \\
&\le np_1^{x-1-\frac{\ln n}{\ln p_1}} p_2^{y-1-\frac{\ln n}{\ln p_2}} \left(\max\{1, \tfrac{p_3}{p_1p_2}\}\right)^{x-\frac{\ln n}{\ln p_1}} \\
&= nO\left(1/n^{1+\gamma}\right) \longrightarrow 0,\ n \to +\infty ,
\end{aligned}
\tag{6}
$$

where

$$
\gamma = \begin{cases} 1 & \text{if } p_3 \le p_1p_2 \\ \frac{\ln(p_3/p_2)}{\ln p_1} > 0 & \text{if } p_3 > p_1p_2 \end{cases} .
$$

We also have $\Sigma_n^{(1)} \le np_1^{x-2-\frac{\ln n}{\ln p_1}+1} = p_1^{x-1}$ and $\Sigma_n^{(1)} \ge np_1^{x-1-\frac{\ln n}{\ln p_1}+1} = p_1^x$. The same for $\Sigma_n^{(2)}$. □

In the rest of this section, we characterize the distribution of the innovations $\{(Z_n, W_n)\}$.

The joint d.f of (X, Y) has the following relation with the joint d.f of (Z, W) and $(\alpha \circ X, \beta \circ Y)$:

$$
\begin{aligned}
1 - F_{X,Y}(x, y) &= 1 - F_{\alpha\circ X,\beta\circ Y}(x, y)F_{Z,W}(x, y) \\
&= 1 - F_{Z,W}(x, y) + F_{Z,W}(x, y)(1 - F_{\alpha\circ X,\beta\circ Y}(x, y)) .
\end{aligned}
\tag{7}
$$

Considering that $\alpha \circ X$ and $\beta \circ Y$ are independent given X and Y, in [15] the asymptotic behaviour of the tail $1 - F_{\alpha\circ X,\beta\circ Y}$ is established. To do so, that authors started by proving that the probability generating function

$$
P_{X,Y}(s_1, s_2) := \sum_{k=0}^{\infty}\sum_{\ell=0}^{\infty} P(X = k, Y = \ell)s_1^k s_2^\ell
$$

satisfies

$$
P_{\alpha\circ X,\beta\circ Y}(s_1, s_2) = P_{X,Y}(\alpha s_1 + 1 - \alpha, \beta s_2 + 1 - \beta)
$$

where the series converges. In addition, the same authors proved also that the tail probability generating function

$$Q_{X,Y}(s_1, s_2) = \sum_{k=0}^{\infty}\sum_{\ell=0}^{\infty} \left(1 - F_{(X,Y)}(k, \ell)\right) s_1^k s_2^\ell$$

satisfies

$$(1 - s_1)(1 - s_2)Q_{X,Y}(s_1, s_2) = 1 - P_{X,Y}(s_1, s_2)$$

as well as

$$Q_{\alpha\circ X,\beta\circ Y}(s_1, s_2) = \alpha\beta Q_{X,Y}(\alpha s_1 + 1 - \alpha, \beta s_2 + 1 - \beta)$$

under the convergence of the series. As a corollary, we can find also in [15] that

$$\begin{aligned}
&1 - F_{\alpha\circ X,\beta\circ Y}(x, y)\\
&= \sum_{k=x}^{+\infty}\sum_{\ell=y}^{+\infty} \binom{k}{x}\binom{\ell}{y}(1-\alpha)^{k-x}(1-\beta)^{\ell-y}\alpha^{x+1}\beta^{y+1}(1 - F_{X,Y}(k, \ell)) \quad (8)
\end{aligned}$$

for any non-negative integers x and y. Now, consider that (X, Y) has a bivariate geometric distribution given above. Taking into account (8) and

$$\sum_{k=0}^{+\infty}\binom{k+x}{k} z^k = \frac{1}{(1-z)^{x+1}}, \; |z| < 1 ,$$

it results in

$$\begin{aligned}
&1 - F_{\alpha\circ X,\beta\circ Y}(x, y) =\\
&= \sum_{k=[x]}^{+\infty}\sum_{\ell=[y]}^{+\infty} \binom{k}{[x]}\binom{\ell}{[y]}(1-\alpha)^{k-[x]}(1-\beta)^{\ell-[y]}\alpha^{[x]+1}\beta^{[y]+1}(p_1^{k+1} + p_2^{\ell+1})\\
&\quad - \sum_{k=[x]}^{+\infty}\sum_{\ell=[y]}^{+\infty} \binom{k}{[x]}\binom{\ell}{[y]}(1-\alpha)^{k-[x]}(1-\beta)^{\ell-[y]}\alpha^{[x]+1}\beta^{[y]+1} \times\\
&\quad \times p_1^{k+1} p_2^{\ell+1} \left(\tfrac{p_3}{p_1 p_2}\right)^{\min(k,\ell)+1} \quad (9)\\
&= \left(\tfrac{p_1\alpha}{1-(1-\alpha)p_1}\right)^{[x]+1} + \left(\tfrac{p_2\beta}{1-(1-\beta)p_2}\right)^{[y]+1} - P(\alpha\circ X > x, \beta\circ Y > y)
\end{aligned}$$

for any $(x, y) \in \mathbb{R}_+^2$.

Given the difficulty to obtain an explicit expression for $P(\alpha \circ X > x, \beta \circ Y > y)$ (second sum in (9)), we will obtain an appropriated upper bound. Note that

$$\left(\tfrac{p_3}{p_1 p_2}\right)^{\min([x],[y])} \leq \begin{cases} \left(\tfrac{p_3}{p_1 p_2}\right)^x & \text{if } p_3 > p_1 p_2 \\ 1 & \text{if } p_3 \leq p_1 p_2 \end{cases} .$$

Consequently, for any non-negative integers x and y, we deduce

$$P(\alpha \circ X > x, \beta \circ Y > y) \leq (\alpha p_3/p_2)^{x+1}(\beta p_2)^{y+1} \times$$

$$\times \sum_{k=0}^{+\infty}\sum_{\ell=0}^{+\infty} \binom{k+x}{x}\binom{\ell+y}{y}(1-\alpha)^k(1-\beta)^\ell p_1^k p_2^\ell \left(\frac{p_3}{p_1 p_2}\right)^k$$

$$= \left(\frac{\alpha p_3/p_2}{1-(1-\alpha)p_3/p_2}\right)^{x+1} \left(\frac{\beta p_2}{1-(1-\beta)p_2}\right)^{y+1}$$

when $p_3 > p_1 p_2$, and

$$P(\alpha \circ X > x, \beta \circ Y > y) \leq \left(\frac{\alpha p_1}{1-(1-\alpha)p_1}\right)^{x+1} \left(\frac{\beta p_2}{1-(1-\beta)p_2}\right)^{y+1}$$

when $p_3 \leq p_1 p_2$.

Write $A = \dfrac{\alpha p_1}{1-(1-\alpha)p_1}$, $B = \dfrac{\beta p_2}{1-(1-\beta)p_2}$ and $C = \dfrac{\alpha p_3/p_2}{1-(1-\alpha)p_3/p_2}$ when $p_3 > p_1 p_2$ and $C = A$ when $p_3 \leq p_1 p_2$. With some straightforward calculus, we conclude that

$$\frac{P(\alpha \circ X > x, \beta \circ Y > y)}{A^{[x]+1} + B^{[y]+1}} \leq \frac{1}{\left(\frac{A}{C}\right)^{[x]+1} + \frac{1}{C^{[x]+1}}} \longrightarrow 0, \ x, y \to +\infty$$

and

$$\frac{p_1^{[x]+1} p_2^{[y]+1} \left(\frac{p_3}{p_1 p_2}\right)^{\min([x],[y])+1}}{p_1^{[x]+1} + p_2^{[y]+1}} \longrightarrow 0, \ x, y \to +\infty\,.$$

As a consequence, it results in

$$\begin{aligned} \frac{1 - F_{\alpha\circ X, \beta\circ Y}(x, y)}{1 - F_{X,Y}(x, y)} &\sim \frac{A^{[x]+1} + B^{[y]+1}}{p_1^{[x]+1} + p_2^{[y]+1}} \\ &\leq \frac{A^{[x]+1}}{p_1^{[x]+1}} + \frac{B^{[y]+1}}{p_2^{[y]+1}} \longrightarrow 0, \ x, y \to +\infty\,. \end{aligned} \quad (10)$$

Then, combining (7) and (10), we can establish that $F_{Z,W}$ is asymptotically the d.f. of a bivariate geometric distribution. Namely,

$$1 - F_{Z,W}(x, y) \sim p_1^{[x]+1} + p_2^{[y]+1} - p_1^{[x]+1} p_2^{[y]+1} \left(\frac{p_3}{p_1 p_2}\right)^{\min([x],[y])+1}, \ x, y \to +\infty\,,$$

with $p_3 < \min\{p_1, p_2\}$ and $p_3 > p_1 + p_2 - 1$.

3 Limiting Distribution of the Bivariate Maximum

Let $M_n^{(1)} = \max\{X_1, ..., X_n\}$ and $M_n^{(2)} = \max\{Y_1, ..., Y_n\}$. In order to obtain the limiting distribution of the bivariate maxima $(M_n^{(1)}, M_n^{(2)})$, under linear normalization, we prove that the sequence $\{(X_n, Y_n)\}$ satisfies the condition $D(u_n, v_n)$ and some local dependence condition, in this case $D'(u_n, v_n)$. The conditions $D(u_n, v_n)$ and $D'(u_n, v_n)$ presented next were proposed in [3], and are extensions of Leadbetter's conditions $D(u_n)$ and $D'(u_n)$ in [16]. The long-range condition $D(u_n, v_n)$ states that exceedances occurring in block of random vectors ℓ_n separated are asymptotically independent.

Definition 1 The sequence of random vectors $\{(X_n, Y_n)\}$ satisfies condition $D(u_n, v_n)$ if for any integers $1 \le i_1 < ... < i_p < j_1 < ... < j_q \le n$, for which $j_1 - i_p > \ell_n$, we have

$$\left| P\left(\bigcap_{s=1}^{p}\{X_{i_s} \le u_n, Y_{i_s} \le v_n\}, \bigcap_{m=1}^{q}\{X_{j_m} \le u_n, Y_{j_m} \le v_n\}\right) - P\left(\bigcap_{s=1}^{p}\{X_{i_s} \le u_n, Y_{i_s} \le v_n\}\right) P\left(\bigcap_{m=1}^{q}\{X_{j_m} \le u_n, Y_{j_m} \le v_n\}\right)\right| \le \alpha_{n,\ell_n} ,$$

where $\lim_{n\to\infty} \alpha_{n,\ell_n} = 0$ for some sequence $\ell_n = o_n(n)$.

Condition $D'(u_n, v_n)$ prevents the existence of clusters of exceedances in blocks of size at most $[n/s_n]$ in both margins of $\{(X_n, Y_n)\}$ as well as together in the two components.

Definition 2 Let $\{s_n\}$ and $\{\ell_n\}$ be sequences of positive integers such that

$$\lim_{n\to\infty} \frac{1}{s_n} = \lim_{n\to\infty} \frac{s_n \ell_n}{n} = \lim_{n\to\infty} s_n \alpha_{n,\ell_n} = 0 .$$

The sequence of random vectors $\{(X_n, Y_n)\}$ satisfies condition $D'(u_n, v_n)$ if

$$\lim_{n\to\infty} n \sum_{j=2}^{[n/s_n]} \big[P(X_1 > u_n, X_j > u_n) + P(X_1 > u_n, Y_j > v_n) + P(Y_1 > v_n, X_j > u_n) + P(Y_1 > v_n, Y_j > v_n)\big] = 0 .$$

Since the conditions $D(u_n, v_n)$ and $D'(u_n, v_n)$ hold for the strictly stationary bivariate max-INAR(1) model, the limiting d.f. of the bivariate maximum of the associated sequence can be directly inferred from the limiting d.f. of the bivariate maximum of i.i.d. random vectors with the same marginals [3].

Theorem 2 *Let $\{(X_n, Y_n)\}$ be the bivariate max-INAR(1) sequence defined by*

$$(X_n, Y_n) = (\max\{\alpha \circ X_{n-1}, Z_n\}, \max\{\beta \circ Y_{n-1}, W_n\}) ,$$

where $\{(X_n, Y_n)\}$ *has the bivariate geometric distribution given by (5) and the innovations* $\{(Z_n, W_n)\}$ *are i.i.d. and independent of* (X_1, Y_1). *For all* $(x, y) \in \mathbb{R}^2$, *consider* $u_n = x - 1 - \frac{\ln n}{\ln p_1}$ *and* $v_n = y - 1 - \frac{\ln n}{\ln p_2}$. *Then* $\{(X_n, Y_n)\}$ *is a stationary sequence that satisfies* $D(u_n, v_n)$, $D'(u_n, v_n)$ *and, therefore*

$$\begin{cases} \limsup_{n\to\infty} P\left(M_n^{(1)} \le u_n, M_n^{(2)} \le v_n\right) \le \exp\left\{-p_1^x - p_2^y\right\} \\ \liminf_{n\to\infty} P\left(M_n^{(1)} \le u_n, M_n^{(2)} \le v_n\right) \ge \exp\left\{-p_1^{x-1} - p_2^{y-1}\right\} \end{cases} .$$

Proof To prove that the process $\{(X_n, Y_n)\}$ satisfies condition $D(u_n, v_n)$, with u_n and v_n as proposed in the theorem, consider the events

$$A_n = \bigcap_{k=1}^{p} \left\{X_{i_k} \le u_n, Y_{i_k} \le v_n\right\} \quad \text{and} \quad B_n = \bigcap_{k=1}^{q} \left\{X_{j_k} \le u_n, Y_{j_k} \le v_n\right\} ,$$

where $j_1 - i_p > \ell_n$, with $\ell_n = o(n)$. Consider also

$$C_n = \bigcap_{m=i_p+1}^{j_1} \{Z_m < \alpha \circ X_{m-1}\} \quad \text{and} \quad D_n = \bigcap_{m=i_p+1}^{j_1} \{W_m < \beta \circ Y_{m-1}\} .$$

Observe that for any events A, B and C, such that $P(C) \neq 0$, we have

$$\begin{aligned} &|P(A \cap B) - P(A)P(B)| \\ &\le |P((A \cap B \cap C) - P(A \cap C)P(B \cap C)| + 4P(\overline{C}) \\ &= P(C)\left|P(A \cap B|C) - P(A|C)P(B|C)P(C)\right| + 4P(\overline{C}) \\ &\le \left|P(A \cap B|C) - P(A|C)P(B|C)\right| + 5P(\overline{C}) . \end{aligned}$$

Then we get

$$\begin{aligned} &\left|P(A_n \cap B_n) - P(A_n)P(B_n)\right| \\ &\le \left|P(A_n \cap B_n|\overline{C}_n \cap \overline{D}_n) - P(A_n|\overline{C}_n \cap \overline{D}_n)P(B_n|\overline{C}_n \cap \overline{D}_n)\right| \\ &\quad +5P(C_n) + 5P(D_n) . \end{aligned} \tag{11}$$

Let us prove that

$$\left|P(A_n \cap B_n|\overline{C}_n \cap \overline{D}_n) - P(A_n|\overline{C}_n \cap \overline{D}_n)P(B_n|\overline{C}_n \cap \overline{D}_n)\right| \longrightarrow 0 , \tag{12}$$

as $n \to +\infty$.

Notice that $\alpha \circ \max(X, Y) \neq \max(\alpha \circ X, \alpha \circ Y)$.

In what concerns the event $\overline{C}_n$, we have $Z_m > \alpha \circ X_{m-1}$ at least for some $m \in \{i_p + 1, ..., j_1\}$. Then

$$\begin{cases} X_m = Z_m \\ X_{m+1} = \max(\alpha \circ X_m, Z_{m+1}) \\ \qquad = \max(\alpha \circ Z_m, Z_{m+1}) \\ \qquad = f_m^{(1)}(Z_m, Z_{m+1}) \\ X_{m+2} = \max(\alpha \circ X_{m+1}, Z_{m+2}) \\ \qquad = f_m^{(2)}(Z_m, Z_{m+1}, Z_{m+2}) \\ \quad \cdots \\ X_{j_1} = \max(\alpha \circ X_{j_1-1}, Z_{j_1}) \\ \qquad = f_m^{(j_1-m)}(Z_m, Z_{m+1}, ..., Z_{j_1}) \end{cases}$$

where $f_m^{(\ell)}$, $\ell \in \{1, 2, ..., j_1 - m\}$, are measurable functions of the subset of independent random variables $\{Z_m, Z_{m+1}, ..., Z_{m+\ell}\}$.

In the same way, we can prove that Y_{j_1} can be written as a measurable function of the independent random variables $\{W_{m'}, W_{m'+1}, ..., W_{j_1}\}$, for some $m' \in \{i_p + 1, i_p + 2, ..., j_1\}$.

Consequently, under the occurrence of $\overline{C}_n \cap \overline{D}_n$, $\{X_{j_1}, ..., X_{j_q}, Y_{j_1}, ..., X_{j_q}\}$ are measurable functions of $\{Z_{m^*}, ..., Z_{j_1}, ..., Z_{j_q}, W_{m^*}, ..., W_{j_1} ..., W_{j_q}\}$, with $m^* = \max\{m, m'\}$, which implies that A_n and B_n are independent given $\overline{C}_n \cap \overline{D}_n$. Then (12) is proved.

In the following, we prove that $P(C_n) \longrightarrow 0$, as $n \to +\infty$. For $\delta \in]0, 1[$, consider the event

$$E_n = \{Z_{i_p+[\ell_n^\delta]} = \ldots = Z_{j_1-1} = Z_{j_1} = 0\}$$

where

$$P(E_n) = P(Z = 0)^{j_1 - i_p - \ell_n^\delta + 1} \leq P(Z = 0)^{\ell_n - \ell_n^\delta + 1} \longrightarrow 0, \ n \to +\infty\,.$$

Moreover, with $\alpha^{(k)} \circ X_{i_p} = \underbrace{\alpha \circ \alpha \circ \ldots \circ \alpha \circ}_{k \text{ thinning operators}} X_{i_p}$,

$$\begin{aligned} P(C_n \cap \overline{E}_n) &= P\left(C_n \cap \left(\bigcup_{k=[\ell_n^\delta]}^{j_1-i_p} \{Z_{i_p+k} > 0\}\right)\right) \\ &\leq \sum_{k=[\ell_n^\delta]}^{j_1-i_p} P(X_{i_p+1} = \alpha \circ X_{i_p}, X_{i_p+2} = \alpha \circ X_{i_p+1}, \ldots, \\ &\qquad X_{j_1} = \alpha \circ X_{j_1-1}, 0 < Z_{i_p+k} < \alpha \circ X_{i_p+k-1}) \\ &\leq \sum_{k=[\ell_n^\delta]}^{j_1-i_p} P(X_{i_p+1} = \alpha \circ X_{i_p}, X_{i_p+2} = \alpha^{(2)} \circ X_{i_p}, \ldots, \end{aligned}$$

$$
\begin{aligned}
& X_{j_1} = \alpha^{(j_1-i_p)} \circ X_{i_p}, 0 < Z_{i_p+k} < \alpha \circ X_{i_p+k-1}) \\
\leq & \sum_{k=[\ell_n^\delta]}^{j_1-i_p} P(0 < Z_{i_p+k} < \alpha^{(k)} \circ X_{i_p}) \\
= & \sum_{k=[\ell_n^\delta]}^{j_1-i_p} \sum_{z=1}^{+\infty} P(\alpha^{(k)} \circ X_{i_p} > z) P(Z = z) \\
= & \sum_{k=[\ell_n^\delta]}^{j_1-i_p} \sum_{z=1}^{+\infty} P(\alpha^{k} \circ X_{i_p} > z) P(Z = z) \, ,
\end{aligned}
$$

because $\alpha^{(k)} \circ X_{i_p} =^d \alpha^k \circ X_{i_p}$. Using Markov's inequality and the fact that $E(\alpha^k \circ X_{i_p}) = \alpha^k E(X_{i_p})$, we achieve the following result:

$$
\begin{aligned}
P(C_n \cap \overline{E}_n) & \leq E(X_{i_p}) \sum_{k=[\ell_n^\delta]}^{j_1-i_p} \alpha^k \sum_{z=1}^{+\infty} z^{-1} P(Z = z) \\
& \leq E(X_{i_p}) \frac{\alpha^{\ell_n^\delta - 1}}{1-\alpha} C \longrightarrow 0, \; n \to +\infty \, ,
\end{aligned}
$$

where C bounds the convergent series $\sum_{z=1}^{+\infty} z^{-1} P(Z = z)$. Then, taking into account that

$$
P(C_n) \leq P(E_n) + P(C_n \cap \overline{E}_n) \, ,
$$

it results in $P(C_n) \longrightarrow 0$, as $n \to +\infty$.

Similarly, we prove that $P(D_n) \longrightarrow 0$, as $n \to +\infty$, considering the set

$$
F_n = \{W_{i_p+[\ell_n^\delta]} = \ldots = W_{j_1-1} = W_{j_1} = 0\} \, .
$$

Since all terms in (11) converge to zero, we conclude that

$$
|P(A_n \cap B_n) - P(A_n)P(B_n)| \longrightarrow 0, \; n \to +\infty \, .
$$

Condition $D(u_n, v_n)$ is satisfied. To show that condition $D'(u_n, v_n)$ holds, for the margins we have $P(X_1 > u_n, X_j > u_n) = O\left(1/n^2\right)$ and, similarly, $P(Y_1 > v_n, Y_j > v_n) = O\left(1/n^2\right)$, from the results in [1].

With respect to $P(X_1 > u_n, Y_j > v_n)$, we start by observing that due to (6) we have

$$
P(X_1 > u_n, Y_1 > v_n) = O\left(1/n^{1+\gamma}\right) \, ,
$$

where $\gamma = 1$ if $p_3 \leq p_1 p_2$ and $\gamma = \frac{\ln(p_3/p_2)}{\ln p_1} > 0$ if $p_3 > p_1 p_2$. Also, for $j \geq 2$, we get

$$
\begin{aligned}
P(X_1 > u_n, Y_j > v_n) &= P(X_1 > u_n) - P(X_1 > u_n, Y_j \le v_n) \\
&= \overline{F}_X(u_n) - P(X_1 > u_n, \beta \circ Y_{j-1} \le v_n, W_{j-1} \le v_n) \\
&= \overline{F}_X(u_n) - F_W(v_n) P(X_1 > u_n, \beta \circ Y_{j-1} \le v_n) \\
&= \overline{F}_X(u_n) - F_W(v_n)[P(X_1 > u_n) - P(X_1 > u_n, \beta \circ Y_{j-1} > v_n)] \\
&= \overline{F}_X(u_n) - F_W(v_n)\overline{F}_X(u_n) \\
&\quad + F_W(v_n) P(X_1 > u_n, \beta \circ Y_{j-1} > v_n, Y_{j-1} > v_n) \\
&\le \overline{F}_W(v_n)\overline{F}_X(u_n) + F_W(v_n) P(X_1 > u_n, Y_{j-1} > v_n) ,
\end{aligned}
$$

where $\overline{F} := 1 - F$. So, since $P(X_1 > u_n, Y_1 > v_n) = O(1/n^{1+\gamma})$, we prove that

$$
\begin{aligned}
P(X_1 > u_n, Y_2 > v_n) &\le \overline{F}_W(v_n)\overline{F}_X(u_n) + F_W(v_n) P(X_1 > u_n, Y_1 > v_n) \\
&= O\left(1/n^2\right) + O\left(1/n^{1+\gamma}\right) = O\left(1/n^{1+\gamma}\right) ,
\end{aligned}
$$

because $\gamma \in]0, 1]$. Recursively, for $j \ge 3$ it follows that $P(Y_1 > v_n, X_j > u_n) = O\left(1/n^{1+\gamma}\right)$.

In the same way, we deduce that $P(Y_1 > v_n, X_j > u_n) = O\left(1/n^{1+\gamma}\right)$.

Then

$$
\begin{aligned}
n \sum_{j=2}^{[n/s_n]} \big[& P(X_1 > u_n, X_j > u_n) + P(X_1 > u_n, Y_j > v_n) \\
& + P(Y_1 > v_n, X_j > u_n) + P(Y_1 > v_n, Y_j > v_n) \big] \\
\le\ & 4n[n/s_n] O(1/n^{1+\gamma}) \longrightarrow 0,\ n \to +\infty ,
\end{aligned}
$$

with $s_n = [n^{\psi}]$ for $\psi \in]0, 1[$ such that $\psi + \gamma > 1$.

Condition $D'(u_n, v_n)$ holds and the theorem is proved. □

The results of Theorems 1 and 2 deserve the following relevant remarks.

In the rich field of models based on bivariate sequences of real-valued random variables (with continuous d.f.), the dependence structure of the innovations margins (and process margins) is usually reflected in the limit results on bivariate maxima. However, in the bivariate integer context of our model (and [15] as well), even starting with dependent margins, X_n and Y_n, we arrive at the asymptotic independence of the marginal maxima $M_n^{(1)}$ and $M_n^{(2)}$, displayed in the upper and lower limiting bounds. Although surprising, this is due to the fact that

$$
nP(X > u_n, Y > v_n) \longrightarrow 0,\ n \to \infty .
$$

Indeed we established this limit in the proof of Theorem 1 by proving that $\Sigma^{(3)} \longrightarrow 0,\ n \to \infty$.

We also point out that instead of a well-defined limit of the double maxima, we only obtain limiting bounds because the geometric d.f. does not belong to any max-stable domain of attraction. That is, it is impossible to construct a normalization

$u_n(x)$ (linear or not) such that $n(1 - F_X(u_n(x)) \longrightarrow -\log G(x),\ n \to \infty$, for a non-degenerate d.f. G. As we can see, since the pioneering work of Anderson [9], we always have

$$p_1^x \leq n\left(1 - F_X\left(x + \frac{\log n}{\log p_1}\right)\right) \leq p_1^{x-1},$$

and the same for F_Y.

Acknowledgements The authors would like to thank the reviewer for his/her useful comments and suggestions.

The work of the first author was partially supported by Center for Computational and Stochastic Mathematics, Instituto Superior Técnico, University of Lisbon—UIDB/04621/2020, funded by the Portuguese Government through FCT/MCTES. The work of the second author was partially supported by the Centre for Mathematics of the University of Coimbra—UIDB/00324/2020, funded by the Portuguese Government through FCT/MCTES.

References

1. Scotto, M.G., Weiss, C.H., Möller, T.A., Gouveia, S.: The max-INAR(1) model for count processes. TEST **27**, 850–870 (2018). https://doi.org/10.1007/s11749-017-0573-z
2. Marshall, A.W., Olkin, I.: A family of bivariate distributions generated by the bivariate Bernoulli distribution. J. Amer. Stat. Assoc. **80**, 332–338 (1985). https://doi.org/10.2307/2287890
3. Hüsler, J.: Multivariate extreme values in stationary random sequences. Stoch. Proc. Appl. **35**, 99–108 (1990). https://doi.org/10.1016/0304-4149(90)90125-C
4. Steutel, F.W., van Harn, K.: Discrete analogues of self-decomposability and stability. Ann. Probab. **7**, 893–899 (1979)
5. McKenzie, E.: Some simple models for discrete variate time series. J. Amer. Water Resour. Assoc. **21**, 645–650 (1985). https://doi.org/10.1111/j.1752-1688.1985.tb05379.x
6. Al-Osh, M.A., Alzaid, A.A.: First-order integer-valued autoregressive (INAR(1)) process. J. Time Ser. Anal. **8**, 261–275 (1987). https://doi.org/10.1111/j.1467-9892.1987.tb00438.x
7. Pedeli, X., Karlis, D.: A bivariate INAR(1) process with application. Stat. Model. **11**(4), 325–349 (2011). https://doi.org/10.1177/1471082X1001100403
8. Silva, I., Silva, M.E., Torres, C.: Inference for bivariate integer-valued moving average models based on binomial thinning operation. J. Appl. Stat. **47**, 2546–2564 (2020). https://doi.org/10.1080/02664763.2020.1747411
9. Anderson, C.W.: Extreme value theory for a class of discrete distribution with applications to some stochastic processes. J. Appl. Probab. **7**, 99–113 (1970). https://doi.org/10.2307/3212152
10. Dias, S., Temido, M.G.: On the maxima of integer models based on a new thinning operator. In: Oliveira, T., Kitsos, C., Oliveira, A., Grilo, L. (eds.) Recent Studies on Risk Analysis and Statistical Modeling. Contributions to Statistics, pp. 213–226. Springer, Cham (2018). https://doi.org/10.1007/978-3-319-76605-8_15
11. Hall, A.: Extremes of integer-valued moving average models with exponential type tails. Extremes **6**, 361–379 (2003). https://doi.org/10.1007/s10687-004-4725-z
12. Hall, A., Scotto, M.G.: Extremes of periodic integer-valued sequences with exponential type tails. REVSTAT **4**(3), 249–273 (2006)
13. Hall, A., Temido, M.G.: On the maximum term of MA and Max-AR models with margins in Anderson's class. Theory Probab. Appl. **51**, 291–304 (2007). https://doi.org/10.1137/S0040585X97982347

14. Hall, A., Temido, M.G.: On the max-semistable limit of maxima of stationary sequences with missing values. J. Stat. Plan. Infer. **3**, 875–890 (2009). https://doi.org/10.1016/j.jspi.2008.05.038
15. Hüsler, J., Temido, M.G., Valente-Freitas, A.: On the maximum term of a bivariate infinite MA model with integer innovations. Methodol. Comput. Appl. Probab. (2022). https://doi.org/10.1007/s11009-021-09920-3
16. Leadbetter, M.R., Lindgren, G., Rootzén, H.: Extremes and Related Properties of Random Sequences and Processes. Springer, Berlin (1983)

The Performance of a Combined Distance Between Time Series

Margarida G. M. S. Cardoso and Ana Alexandra Martins

Abstract This paper presents the comparison of a proposed measure of dissimilarity between time series (COMB) with three baseline measures. COMB is a convex combination of Euclidean distance, a Pearson-correlation-based distance, a Periodogram-based measure and a distance between estimated autocorrelation structures. The comparison resorts to 1-Nearest Neighbour classifier (1NN) since the effectiveness of the dissimilarity measures is directly reflected on the performance of 1NN. Data considered is available in the University of California Riverside (UCR) Time-Series Archive which includes datasets from a wide variety of application domains and have been used in similar studies. The COMB measure shows promising results: a good trade-off performance-computation time when compared to the alternative distances considered.

Keywords Clustering · Distance measures · Time series

1 Introduction

The use of dissimilarity measures between time series is critical in several data analysis tasks which range from simple querying to classification, clustering and anomaly detection. The role of dissimilarity measures in these contexts has been acknowledged by several works, e.g. [1–3].

Recently, in [4], we proposed a new dissimilarity measure, COMB, a convex combination of four (normalized) distance measures which offer complementary perspectives on the differences between two time series: the Euclidean distance which

M. G. M. S. Cardoso (✉)
University Institute of Lisbon (ISCTE-IUL), Business Research Unit (BRU-IUL), Lisbon, Portugal
e-mail: margarida.cardoso@iscte-iul.pt

A. Alexandra Martins
CIMOSM, ISEL, Polytechnic of Lisbon, Lisbon, Portugal

R. Bispo et al. (eds.), *Recent Developments in Statistics and Data Science*,
Springer Proceedings in Mathematics & Statistics 398,
https://doi.org/10.1007/978-3-031-12766-3_6

captures differences in scale; a Pearson-correlation-based measure that takes into account linear increasing and decreasing trends over time; a Periodogram-based measure that expresses the dissimilarities between frequencies or cyclical components of the series and a distance between estimated autocorrelation structures, comparing the series in terms of their dependence on past observations.

COMB achieved quite good results when clustering electricity market prices time series in European regions and also when clustering electricity loads time series (Portuguese Transmission System Operator data)—[4, 5].

In this work, we conduct an experimental analysis to evaluate the comparative performance of the proposed combined distance measure.

The remainder is structured as follows: first we present the Methodology used to provide the comparison of COMB with alternative distance measures; then, the Data Analysis and Results section brings some insights regarding the comparative analysis and, finally, we end with Discussion and Future Research of the presented work.

2 Methodology

2.1 UCR Repository

We resort to the University of California Riverside (UCR) Time-Series Archive where we can find time series of diverse lengths and numbers of target classes, with corresponding test and train sets—[6]. The UCR time-series datasets are from a wide variety of application domains and have been used to study the comparative performance of time-series classifiers—e.g. [2]—and specifically used in comparative studies of dissimilarity measures between time series, e.g. [7].

We limit the datasets considered to 57 taking into account computational cost. This is a criterion that has been invoked in similar studies—e.g. [8]. In our study we found that, for example, the script routine, when referring to the analysis of the "GesturePebbleZ2" UCR dataset, took 18:45 h to run (using a PC with processor Intel(R) Core(TM) i7-10750H CPU @ 2.60 2.59 GHz with a RAM of 32 GB). Nevertheless, we tried to include dissimilar datasets, namely, in what regards the number of target classes: 28 datasets have 2 target classes while 29 have more than 2 target classes. The selected datasets are presented in the Appendix. As in previous studies—e.g. [7]—and although this can limit the analysis, z-standardization is adopted for fairness, since many of the UCR series are presented in their z-standardized form.

2.2 Using the 1NN Classifier

We follow a methodology suggested in previous studies that were conducted to compare several dissimilarity measures and their variants—e.g. [7]: we use one nearest neighbour (1NN) classifier on labelled data to evaluate the performance of the distance measures. In fact, since the distance measure used is critical to 1NN accuracy, this indicator directly reflects the effectiveness of the dissimilarity measure used. According to [7] p. 1890, *1NN classifiers are suitable methods for distance measure evaluation for several reasons:*

1. *resemble the problem solved in time-series similarity search;*
2. *are parameter-free and easy to implement;*
3. *are dependent on the choice of distance measure;*
4. *provide an easy-to-interpret (classification) accuracy measure which captures if the query and the nearest neighbour belong to the same class.*

2.3 Dissimilarity Measures

We compare COMB [4] with three alternative dissimilarity measures between time series. Comparisons are provided with three baseline measures: Euclidean distance, DTW (Dynamic Time-Warping with Sakoe-Chiba band [9] windowing considering 20% of the time-series length) and Complexity Invariance Distance (CID).

COMB Distance. Considering two time series x_t and y_t, $(t = 1, \ldots, T)$, the COMB distance is a convex combination of four distances: Euclidean (d_{Euclid}), a Pearson-correlation-based measure ($d_{Pearson}$), a Periodogram-based measure (d_{Period}) and an autocorrelation-based measure ($d_{Autocorr}$).

The Euclidean distance, d_{Eucl}, yields the sum of Euclidean distances corresponding to each pair (x_t, y_t) capturing the differences in scale:

$$d_{Eucl} = \left(\sum_{t=1}^{T} (x_t - y_t)^2 \right)^{\frac{1}{2}}. \tag{1}$$

The Pearson-correlation-based measure takes into account linear increasing and decreasing trends over time. The following measure was suggested by [10]:

$$d_{Pearson} = \sqrt{\frac{1 - r_{x_t, y_t}}{2}}, \tag{2}$$

where r_{x_t, y_t} represents the Pearson correlation.

The Periodogram-based measure [11] considers the Euclidean distances between the Periodograms expressing the contribution of the various frequencies or cyclical components to the variability of the series,

$$d_{Period} = \left(\sum_{j=1}^{\left[\frac{T}{2}\right]} \left(P_x\left(w_j\right) - P_y\left(w_j\right)\right)^2 \right)^{\frac{1}{2}}, \tag{3}$$

where $P_x\left(w_j\right)$ is the Periodogram of time series x_t at frequencies $w_j = 2\pi_j/n$, $j = 1, \ldots, [n/2]$ in the range 0 to π, being $[n/2]$ the largest integer less or equal to $n/2$,

$$P_x\left(w_j\right) = \left(\frac{1}{n}\right) \left| \sum_{t=1}^{T} x_t e^{-itw_j} \right|^2. \tag{4}$$

The autocorrelation-based distance [12] calculates Euclidean distances between autocorrelation structures, comparing the series in terms of their dependence on past observations

$$d_{Autocorr} = \left(\sum_{l=1}^{L} \left(r_l\left(x_t\right) - r_l\left(y_t\right)\right)^2 \right)^{\frac{1}{2}}, \tag{5}$$

where $r_l\left(x_t\right)$ and $r_l\left(y_t\right)$ represent the estimated autocorrelations of lag l of (x_t) and (y_t), respectively.

In this study, we specifically use an uniform convex combination, all four weights being equal.

Eucl—Euclidean Distance. The comparison with the performance of the Euclidean distance is unavoidable in all studies of this type. Even because, despite its simplicity, this distance can obtain surprisingly good results *especially if the size of the training set/database is relatively large*, [13], p. 281.

DTW—Dynamic Time-Warping. DTW is an elastic measure that computes the optimal alignment between two time series to minimize the sum of distances between aligned elements.

Considering two time series x_t and y_t, $(t = 1, \ldots, T)$, let M be the $T \times T$ matrix where each element is a dissimilarity $d_{i,j}$ (commonly the Euclidean distance is considered) between any pair of elements x_i and y_j $(i, j = 1, \ldots, T)$.
A warping path $P = ((i_1, j_1), (i_2, j_2))$ is a series of indexes of M defining a mapping from each element of one time series to one, or more than one, or even none, of the elements of the other time series. A valid path should satisfy several conditions, for example, $i_{k+1} \geq i_k$ ensures the path does not go back in time. For other step patterns constrains see, e.g. [14]. For each path P, through M, the total sum of the distances along it is

$$D(P) = \sum_{k=1}^{K} d_{i_k, j_k}. \tag{6}$$

For example, the Euclidean distance is the total distance along the diagonal of M. The goal of the DTW measure is to find a path P^* that minimizes the total distances $D(P)$:

$$P^* = \min_{P} D(P). \tag{7}$$

To improve the efficiency of the procedure, it is a common practice to limit the time distortion (e.g. considering 20% of the time-series length). For example, the Sakoe-Chiba band [9] limits the warping path to a band of size T_0 directly above and to the right of the diagonal of the matrix M, by enforcing the constraint $|i_k - j_k| < T_0$.

CID—Complexity Invariance Distance. CID measure was proposed by [15]. The time series' complexity is measured by stretching them and measuring the length of the resulting lines.

$$CID(x_t, y_t) = d_{Eucl}.CF(x_t, y_t), \tag{8}$$

where

$$CF(x_t, y_t) = \frac{max(CE(x_t), CE(y_t))}{min(CE(x_t), CE(y_t))} \tag{9}$$

is the Complexity Factor, and

$$CE(x_t) = \left(\sum_{t=1}^{T-1} (x_t - x_{t+1})^2 \right)^{\frac{1}{2}} \tag{10}$$

is the Complexity Estimate of time series x_t.

We resort to the R package "TSclust" [12] where the four distances that compose the COMB distance, the CID and the DTW (using the "dtw" package [14]) are implemented.

2.4 *Evaluating the Classification Results*

The evaluation of performance of the 1NN classifiers regards the test sets of the UCR time series considered. Balanced accuracy measure (average between sensitivity and specificity) when dealing with unbalanced sets is suggested by [6]. We propose using the Huberty index (HI)—e.g. [16], as a measure of classification performance:

$$HI = \sum_{k=1}^{K} \frac{p^c - p^{def}}{1 - p^{def}}, \tag{11}$$

where p^c and p^{def} are the proportion of observations correctly classified and the proportion of observations in the modal class, respectively. This measure is clearly useful for the evaluation of performance in unbalanced datasets. Furthermore, it provides a fair and interpretable view of the success of classification tasks which could be overestimated when high accuracy results are obtained in strongly unbalanced sets, e.g. a 90% accuracy result when a target class includes 95% of observations yields a negative Huberty index (one should do better by simply allocating all observations to the modal class). In addition, the computational time is also taken into account in the evaluation of the 1NN results referring to the four dissimilarity measures considered.

After the evaluation of aggregated results, comparisons referring to specific datasets are considered to get some dissimilarities' performance-related insights. On a "closer look to specific problems", [2] resorts to the selection of some time series from each target class, trying to capture the main differences between these classes on specific datasets. We propose using the medoids of each class as defined by each dissimilarity measure to obtain those insights. The medoid definition is the observations that minimize the sum of all distances to elements in the same class—[17].

3 Data Analysis and Results

3.1 General Comparisons

A brief exploratory data analysis leads to the conclusion that, in the datasets considered, DTW generally provides better classification results than the alternative distances, followed by COMB—Table 1. COMB comparative results are illustrated in Fig. 1. However, for time series with two target classes (K=2) only, COMB provides slightly better results—see Table 1. In what regards the computation time DTW clearly provides the worst results—see Table 2.

According to the Friedman test's results, there are no significant differences between the distributions of HI regarding the four dissimilarity measures (see Table 3). However, significant differences can be found when analysing data with more than two classes (K>2), which, after pairwise comparison of Dunn's test, can be referred to the significant difference between HI.Eucl and HI.DTW (see Table 4).

The differences between computation times regarding the four dissimilarity measures are all significant according to Friedman's test—see Table 5.

Table 1 All time-series results

	Hubert index				Computation time (seconds)			
	HI.Eucl	HI.DTW	HI.CID	HI.COMB	t.Eucl	t.DTW	t.CID	t.COMB
Mean	**0.581**	**0.631**	**0.599**	**0.603**	**0.01**	**7846.60**	**47.53**	**651.27**
Std. Dev.	0.279	0.268	0.273	0.261	0.01	15500.13	66.81	959.48
Coef. Var.	0.480	0.425	0.456	0.433	1	1.98	1.41	1.47
Perc. 25th	0.385	0.460	0.448	0.448	0.00	313.80	5.23	49.64
Perc. 50th	**0.633**	**0.679**	**0.609**	**0.636**	**0.00**	**1117.40**	**13.00**	**157.96**
Perc. 75th	0.799	0.842	0.830	0.791	0.02	7241.48	88.95	1047.15
IQR	0.414	0.382	0.382	0.343	0.02	6927.68	83.72	997.51

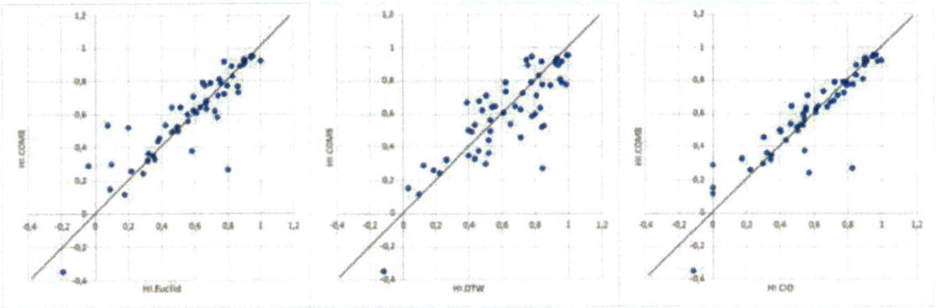

Fig. 1 Plot of Huberty index results: COMB versus Euclidean, DTW and CID

Table 2 Huberty index results: time series with two target classes versus more than two target classes

	Two target classes				More than two target classes			
	HI.Eucl	HI.DTW	HI.CID	HI.COMB	HI.Eucl	HI.DTW	HI.CID	HI.COMB
Mean	**0.516**	**0.547**	**0.544**	**0.562**	**0.642**	**0.712**	**0.651**	**0.643**
Std. Dev.	0.346	0.298	0.321	0.314	0.179	0.212	0.210	0.194
Coef. Var.	0.669	0.544	0.591	0.559	0.278	0.297	0.323	0.302
Perc. 25th	0.211	0.394	0.337	0.323	0.511	0.528	0.533	0.496
Perc. 50th	**0.546**	**0.579**	**0.551**	**0.612**	**0.662**	**0.722**	**0.622**	**0.636**
Perc. 75th	0.827	0.799	0.842	0.809	0.778	0.925	0.803	0.790
IQR	0.616	0.405	0.505	0.486	0.267	0.397	0.270	0.294

Table 3 Friedman test's results regarding Huberty index

	Test statistic (p-value)
All sample	7.062 (0.07)
K = 2	4.375 (0.228)
k > 2	12.761 (0.005)

Table 4 Dunn's pairwise comparison tests regarding Huberty index for data with more than two classes ("Adj. Sig" are p-values adjusted by Bonferroni correction)

	Test statistic	Sig.	Adj. Sig.
HI.Eucl-HI.CID	−0.328	0.334	1.000
HI.Eucl-HI.COMB	−0.414	0.222	1.000
HI.Eucl-HI.DTW	−1.121	0.001	0.006
HI.CID-HI.COMB	−0.086	0.799	1.000
HI.CID-HI.DTW	0.793	0.019	0.116
HI.COMB-HI.DTW	0.707	0.037	0.222

Table 5 Friedman test's results regarding computation time

	Test statistic (p-value)
All sample	171.0 (0.000)
K = 2	84.0 (0.000)
K > 2	87.0 (0.000)

3.2 COMB "Wins" and "Looses" Examples

In an attempt to understand the data conditions that could (un)favour COMB, we looked for some insights regarding a "COMB wins example" and a "COMB looses example": ToeSegmentation2 and Herring time series, respectively. ToeSegmentation2 was originated in the CMU Graphics Lab Motion Capture Data, referring to right toe movements, with target classes "Walk Normally" and "Walk Abnormally". Herring data refers to calcium carbonate structures from two classes of Herring: North sea or Thames. In Table 6, we present the details of data referring to these two datasets.

On the assumption that exploring the target classes in the test set could bring some insights into the performance of 1NN classifier, we obtained the medoids of target classes according to each of the four dissimilarity measures. The ToeSegmentation2 test set classes' medoids are depicted in Fig. 2. The COMB measure reveals not only scale differences between the medoids (as Euclidean distance does, with the poorest results) but it is also apparent (for example) how the medoids' tendencies diverge from each other, which, conjugated with the additional differences captured by COMB, results in its best performance, according to the HI.

Table 6 COMB "wins" and "looses" datasets

Name	Train	Test	Class	Length	HI.Eucl	HI.DTW	HI.CID	HI.COMB
ToeSegmentation2	36	130	2	343	−0.0416	0.1252	0.0001	0.2915
Herring	64	64	2	512	−0.192	−0.115	−0.115	−0.346

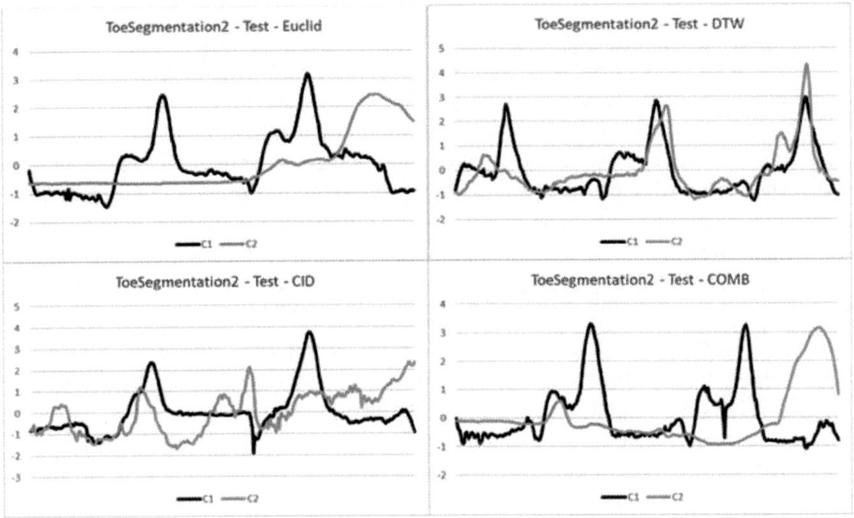

Fig. 2 Medoids of ToeSegmentation2 test set classes, according to dissimilarity measures Eucl, DTW, CID and COMB

The Herring test set classes' medoids coincide for all dissimilarity measures except DTW which presents slightly different medoids. Nevertheless, a negative HI was obtained for all measures (revisit Table 6).

In an attempt to explore the potential of COMB measure, in a worst-case scenario, we performed a brief sensitivity analysis manipulating the COMB's weights. After some trials, when considering the COMB weights regarding d_{Period} and $d_{Autocorr}$ as nine times the weights regarding d_{Euclid} and $d_{Pearson}$, we managed to cross the "waterline", obtaining a HI slightly positive which the alternative measures could not. Note, however, that a customized parametrization of DTW could eventually obtain better results also, but we believe that it would also bring a relevant increase in computation time.

4 Discussion and Future Research

We conducted experiments on 57 time-series datasets from diverse application domains to compare the proposed dissimilarity measure, COMB, with three baseline alternative measures: Euclidean, Dynamic Time-Warping and Complexity Invariance Distance. We resorted to the 1-Nearest Neighbour classifier, using the four dissimilarities, to compare their effectiveness. Huberty index was used as a classification metric providing more informative analysis results than the simple Accuracy measure, adopted in previous studies to evaluate performance (ignoring prevalence). Experimental results obtained indicate that there are no significant differences between the classification performance (Huberty index measures) of the four dissimilarity measures. Nevertheless, it appears COMB can produce better results regarding time series with two target classes. Furthermore, there is also the potential to improve the results obtained with COMB by changing the weights in the convex combination: an example was provided for the Herring dataset where the COMB with uniform weights provided the worst classification results, while COMB with tuned weights was able to provide the best results. In what regards the computation time, Dynamic Time-Warping, which appears to be the most direct COMB competitor regarding classification performance, presented the (significantly) worst results. Considering the classification performance-runtime results we conclude that the proposed combined measure can be seen as competitive in several settings.

In future research, we aim to extend the present analysis to all (128) UCR datasets which will require to explore hardware-aware implementations and/or algorithmic solutions to turn the measures' implementation the most efficient. We also think the Complexity Invariance Distance, which revealed to be a competitive measure, should definitely play a role in future similar studies (along with the unavoidable Euclidean and Dynamic Time-Warping dissimilarities and other eventual baseline measures). An investigation of the process to determine COMB weights should also be considered. Finally, the experimental design should include additional characteristics of the time-series data, besides the number of target classes, namely, we think that the inclusion of a measure of separation between classes should be considered.

Acknowledgements This work was supported by Fundação para a Ciência e a Tecnologia, grant UIDB/00315/2020.

5 Appendix: The Datasets

The characteristics of the 57 datasets used in this work are presented in Tables 7 and 8. Several time series have missing values which were treated with linear interpolation. In order to make all time series of the same dataset with equal length, low-amplitude random noise was imputed to the end of time series with smallest length. For more details, see web page https://www.cs.ucr.edu/~eamonn/time_series_data_2018/.

Table 7 The datasets' dimensions

Name	Train	Test	No. Classes	Length
ArrowHead	36	175	3	251
Beef	30	30	5	470
BeetleFly	20	20	2	512
BirdChicken	20	20	2	512
BME	30	150	3	128
Car	60	60	4	577
CBF	30	900	3	128
Chinatown	20	343	2	24
Coffee	28	28	2	286
DiatomSizeReduction	16	306	4	345
DodgerLoopDay	78	80	7	288
DodgerLoopGame	20	138	2	288
DodgerLoopWeekend	20	138	2	288
ECG200	100	100	2	96
ECGFiveDays	23	861	2	136
FaceFour	24	88	4	350
Fish	175	175	7	463
FreezerSmallTrain	28	2850	2	301
Fungi	18	186	18	201
GestureMidAirD1	208	130	26	360
GestureMidAirD2	208	130	26	360
GestureMidAirD3	208	130	26	360
GesturePebbleZ1	132	172	6	455
GesturePebbleZ2	146	158	6	455
GunPoint	50	150	2	150
GunPointAgeSpan	135	316	2	150
GunPointMaleVersusFemale	135	316	2	150
GunPointOldVersusYoung	136	315	2	150
Ham	109	105	2	431
Herring	64	64	2	512
HouseTwenty	40	119	2	2000
InsectEPGRegularTrain	62	249	3	601

Table 8 The datasets' dimensions (continuation)

Name	Train	Test	No. Classes	Length
InsectEPGSmallTrain	17	249	3	601
ItalyPowerDemand	67	1029	2	24
Lightning2	60	61	2	637
Lightning7	70	73	7	319
Meat	60	60	3	448
MoteStrain	20	1252	2	84
OliveOil	30	30	4	570
OSULeaf	200	242	6	427
PickupGestureWiimoteZ	50	50	10	361
Plane	105	105	7	144
PowerCons	180	180	2	144
Rock	20	50	4	2844
ShakeGestureWiimoteZ	50	50	10	385
ShapeletSim	20	180	2	500
SmoothSubspace	150	150	3	15
SonyAIBORobotSurface1	20	601	2	70
SonyAIBORobotSurface2	27	953	2	65
Symbols	25	995	6	398
ToeSegmentation1	40	228	2	277
ToeSegmentation2	36	130	2	343
Trace	100	100	4	275
TwoLeadECG	23	1139	2	82
UMD	36	144	3	150
Wine	57	54	2	234
WormsTwoClass	181	77	2	900

References

1. Ding, H., Trajcevski, G., Scheuermann, P., Wang, X., Keogh, E.: Querying and mining of time series data: experimental comparison of representations and distance measures. In: Proceedings of the VLDB Endowment, vol. 1, pp. 1542–1552 (2008)
2. Bagnall, A., Lines, J., Bostrom, A., Large, J., Keogh, E.: The great time series classification bake off: a review and experimental evaluation of recent algorithmic advances. Data Min. Knowl. Disc. **31**(3), 606–660 (2017)
3. Javed, A., Lee, B.S., Rizzo, D.M.: A benchmark study on time series clustering. In: Machine Learning with Applications, vol. 1, p. 100001 (2020)
4. Cardoso, M., Martins, A., Lagarto, J.: Combining various dissimilarity measures for clustering electricity market prices. In: Milheiro, P., Pacheco, A., de Sousa, B., Alves, I.F., Pereira, I., Polidoro, M.J., Ramos, S. (eds.) Estatística: Desafios Transversais ás Ciências dos Dados—Atas do XXIV Congresso da Sociedade Portuguesa de Estatística (), Edições SPE, pp. 197–212 (2021)

5. Martins, A., Lagarto, J., Canacsinh, H., Reis, F., Cardoso, M.: Short-term load forecasting using time series clustering. In: Proceedings of 16th Conference on Sustainable Development of Energy, Water and Environment Systems (2021). ISSN: 1847-7178
6. Dau, H.A., Bagnall, A., Kamgar, K., Yeh, C.-C.M., Zhu, Y., et al.: The UCR time series archive. IEEE/CAA J. Autom. Sin. **6**(6), 1293–1305 (2019)
7. Paparrizos, J., Liu, C., Elmore, A.J., Franklin, M.J.: Debunking four long-standing misconceptions of time-series distance measures. In: Proceedings of the 2020 ACM SIGMOD International Conference on Management of Data. ACM (2020)
8. Hills, J., Lines, J., Baranauskas, E., Mapp, J., Bagnall, A.: Classification of time series by shapelet transformation. Data Min. Knowl. Disc. **28**(4), 851–881 (2013)
9. Sakoe, H., Chiba, S.: Dynamic programming algorithm optimization for spoken word recognition. IEEE Trans. Acoust. Speech Signal Process. **26**(1), 43–49 (1978)
10. Rodrigues, P., Gama, J., Pedroso, J.: Hierarchical clustering of time-series data streams. IEEE Trans. Knowl. Data Eng. **20**(5), 615–627 (2008)
11. Caiado, J., Crato, N., Peña, D.: A periodogram-based metric for time series classification. Comput. Stat. Data Anal. **50**(10), 2668–2684 (2006)
12. Montero, P., Vilar, J.A.: TSclust: an R package for time series clustering. J. Stat. Softw. **62**(1) (2014)
13. Wang, X., Mueen, A., Ding, H., Trajcevski, G., Scheuermann, P., et al.: Experimental comparison of representation methods and distance measures for time series data. Data Min. Knowl. Disc. **26**(2), 275–309 (2012)
14. Giorgino, T.: Computing and visualizing dynamic time warping alignments in R: the `dtw` package. J. Stat. Softw. **31**(7) (2009)
15. Batista, G., Wang, X., Keogh, E.: A complexity-invariant distance measure for time series. In: Proceedings of the 2011 SIAM International Conference on Data Mining, pp. 699–710 (2011)
16. Sharma, S.: Applied Multivariate Techniques. Wiley, New York (1996)
17. Kaufman, L., Rousseeuw, P.J.: Finding Groups in Data: An Introduction to Cluster Analysis. Wiley, New York (2009)

Zero-Distorted Generalized Geometric Distribution with Application to Time Series of Counts

Esmeralda Gonçalves and Diogo Sousa

Abstract We consider a recently introduced discrete distribution [1] that generalizes the geometric law and that, through an additional parameter, allows changing the probability attributed to observation zero. After referring to some characteristics of this distribution, we establish the asymptotic behaviour, according to different types of convergence, of the estimators of the parameters obtained using three methods, and their performance is compared by means of numerical studies in medium- and large-sized samples. The study proceeds with the introduction of a model for time series of integer values in which the law conditional to the past belongs to this family of laws. The first-order stationarity of this model is established. Modelling the number of new Hantavirus infection cases per week reported in a German state between 2005 and 2018 concludes this study.

Keywords Asymptotic behaviour of estimators · Generalized geometric distribution · INGARCH time series · Zero-distorted law

1 Introduction

We have witnessed a growing interest in the study of time series of integer values, also called counting time series. As examples of such series, we can mention the number of infections by a virus and deaths recorded daily, the number of daily transactions on a stock market, the strikes in a social sector or the sales of a certain product in a store per day, coming from areas as diverse as Medicine or Economics or even Actuarial or Biology. It is therefore important to introduce probabilistic models to describe the dynamics of these time series and their future evolution.

E. Gonçalves (✉)
Department of Mathematics, CMUC, University of Coimbra, Coimbra, Portugal
e-mail: esmerald@mat.uc.pt

D. Sousa
Department of Mathematics, University of Coimbra, Coimbra, Portugal

R. Bispo et al. (eds.), *Recent Developments in Statistics and Data Science*, Springer Proceedings in Mathematics & Statistics 398,
https://doi.org/10.1007/978-3-031-12766-3_7

The integer-valued models presented in the literature have underlying distributions which allow the count time series in the study to be zero, which means that zero is a possible value of the model.

It may happen, however, that the expected number of zeros according to the underlying distribution is not compatible with those actually occurring. We have in this case an inflation or deflation situation of zero value and, in order to correct this situation, we have to provide for the possibility to mix the underlying distribution with a point probability. This is for example the case of integer-valued zero-inflated models, studied in particular by Zhu [2], and Gonçalves, Mendes Lopes and Silva [3], involving Poisson, generalized Poisson, negative binomial and compound Poisson distributions.

Motivated by this problem, we consider a generalized geometric distribution recently proposed [1] which permits inflation or deflation of the zero count probability, analyse some of its statistical properties and use it to introduce a new model for integer-valued time series.

In Sect. 2, we recall the definition of the zero-distorted generalized geometric distribution [1], denoted as ZDGGD, Sect. 3 includes the estimation of the parameters of the ZDGGD by the proportions of zeros and ones, the moments method and by maximum likelihood, stating the asymptotic behaviour of the corresponding estimators. A simulation study illustrates the behaviour of these estimators in moderate and large samples. In Sect. 4, we introduce the INARCH model with conditional ZDGG distribution for time series, state its first-order stationarity and illustrate its interest in the modelling of the number of new cases of Hantavirus infection per week recorded in a German state between 2005 and 2018.

2 The Zero-Distorted Generalized Geometric Distribution

We begin this section with the definition of the zero-distorted generalized geometric distribution, proposed by [1].

Definition 1 A discrete random variable X with support $S_X = \mathbf{N}_0 = \{0, 1, ...\}$ follows a zero-distorted generalized geometric distribution with parameters $q \in]0, 1[$ and $\alpha \in [-1, +\infty[$, briefly $X \sim ZDGGD\,(q, \alpha)$, if

$$P\,(X = k) = \begin{cases} 1 - q^{\alpha+1}, & k = 0 \\ (1 - q)\, q^{k+\alpha}, & k \in \mathbf{N}. \end{cases} \tag{1}$$

If $\alpha = 0$ then $P\,(X = k) = (1 - q)\, q^k$, $k \in \mathbf{N}_0$, that is, X follows a Geometric distribution with parameter q, denoted as $X \sim G\,(q)$.

The effect of parameter α is enhanced in Table 1, becoming clear that the new distribution is able to take into account characteristics that are not covered by the geometric one. For example, for some values of q and α the new distribution presents

Table 1 The effect of parameter α

	$G(q)$	$ZDGGD(q,\alpha)$
$P(X=0) > P(X=1)$	$\forall q$	$\exists(q,\alpha)$
$P(X=0) < P(X=1)$	–	$\exists(q,\alpha)$
Positive asymmetry	$\forall q$	$\exists(q,\alpha)$
Negative asymmetry	–	$\exists(q,\alpha)$
Dispersion index > 1	$\forall q$	$\exists(q,\alpha)$
Dispersion index < 1	–	$\exists(q,\alpha)$

negative asymmetry and the dispersion index, defined as the quotient $V(X)/E(X)$, is no longer only greater than 1.

Sastry et al. [1] propose this generalized geometric distribution which permits inflation or deflation of the zero count probability and derive certain distributional results such as its distribution function, generating functions, moments, relations with other distributions and also the explicit form of the estimators of parameters q and α by three methods. In particular, all moments exist and we have $E(X) = \frac{q^{\alpha+1}}{1-q}$, $E(X^2) = \frac{q^{\alpha+1}(q+1)}{(1-q)^2}$.

We naturally compare this new distribution with that of the random variable Y such that

$$P(Y=k) = w\partial_{o,k} + (1-w)(1-q)q^k,\ k \in \mathbf{N}_0,$$

known as Geometric distribution inflated in zero with parameters $q \in]0,1[$ and $w \in]0,1[$, briefly $Y \sim ZIG(q,w)$, where $\partial_{o,k} = 1$ if $k=0$ and $\partial_{o,k} = 0$ if $k \neq 0$. We have

$$E(Y) = (1-w)\frac{q}{1-q},\ V(Y) = (1-w)\frac{q(1+wq)}{(1-q)^2}.$$

We note that if $X \sim ZDGGD(q,\alpha)$ and we take $w = 1-q^{\alpha}$, then $X \sim ZIG(q,w)$. Nevertheless, the two families of laws do not coincide because if $Y \sim ZIG(q,w)$ its dispersion index is

$$\frac{V(Y)}{E(Y)} = 1 + q\frac{1+w}{1-q} > 1, \forall q, w \in]0,1[.$$

3 Estimators of ZDGG Distribution Parameters

Sastry et al. [1] presents the estimators of parameters q and α of ZDGG distribution using the proportions of zeros and ones as well as those based on the moments and maximum likelihood methods. In this section, after remembering their expressions we state the corresponding asymptotic behaviour and present numerical studies on its behaviour in moderate and large samples.

Consider the statistical model associated with a n-sample $(X_1, ..., X_n)$ of $X \sim ZDGGD(q, \alpha)$

$$\left(R^n, \mathcal{B}_n, ZDGGD(q, \alpha)^{(n)}\right)_{(q,\alpha) \in]0,1[\times[-1,+\infty[}$$

where $ZDGGD(q, \alpha)^{(n)}$ is a discrete law with probability function

$$g_{q,\alpha}(x_1, x_2, .., x_n) = \left[\prod_{i=1}^{n}\left[(1-q^{\alpha+1})\right]^{\mathbf{I}_{x_i=0}} \prod_{i=1}^{n}\left[(1-q)q^{x_i+\alpha}\right]^{\mathbf{I}_{x_i>0}}\right] \mathbf{I}_{\mathbf{N}_0}(x_1, \ldots, x_n),$$

with $(x_1, x_2, .., x_n) \in \mathbf{R}^n$.

The estimator of (q, α) of the ZDGG distribution obtained using the proportions of zeros and ones is given by

$$\left(\dot{Q}_n, \dot{A}_n\right) = \left(\frac{P_{1,n}}{1-P_{0,n}}, \frac{2\log(1-P_{0,n}) - \log(1-P_{0,n}-P_{1,n})}{\log(1-P_{0,n}-P_{1,n}) - \log(1-P_{0,n})}\right) \tag{2}$$

where $P_{0,n} = \frac{1}{n}\sum_{i=1}^{n} \mathbf{1}_{X_i=0}$ and $P_{1,n} = \frac{1}{n}\sum_{i=1}^{n} \mathbf{1}_{X_i=1}$.

Considering the empirical moments of orders 1 and 2, $M_1 = \frac{1}{n}\sum_{i=1}^{n} \mathbf{X}_i$ and $M_2 = \frac{1}{n}\sum_{i=1}^{n} \mathbf{X}_i^2$, the estimator of (q, α) obtained by the method of moments is

$$\left(\widetilde{Q}_n, \widetilde{A}_n\right) = \left(\frac{M_2 - M_1}{M_2 + M_1}, \frac{\log\left(2M_1^2\right) - \log\left(M_2 - M_1\right)}{\log\left(M_2 - M_1\right) - \log\left(M_2 + M_1\right)}\right). \tag{3}$$

The maximum likelihood estimator of (q, α) is given by

$$\left(\hat{Q}_n, \hat{A}_n\right) = \left(1 - \frac{n - \sum_{i=1}^{n} \mathbf{I}_{X_i=0}}{\sum_{i=1}^{n} X_i \mathbf{I}_{X_i>0}}, \frac{\log\left(1 - \frac{1}{n}\sum_{i=1}^{n} \mathbf{I}_{X_i=0}\right)}{\log\left(1 - \frac{n - \sum_{i=1}^{n} \mathbf{I}_{X_i=0}}{\sum_{i=1}^{n} \mathbf{I}_{X_i>0} X_i}\right)} - 1\right). \tag{4}$$

3.1 Asymptotic Behaviour of the Estimators of (q, α)

3.1.1 Proportions of Zeros and Ones Method

Theorem 1 *The estimators $\dot{Q}_n$ and $\dot{A}_n$ given in (2) verify $\dot{Q}_n \longrightarrow q$, in probability, $\dot{A}_n \longrightarrow \alpha$ in probability, and*

$$\sqrt{n}\left(\begin{bmatrix}\dot{Q}_n\\ \dot{A}_n\end{bmatrix}-\begin{bmatrix}q\\ \alpha\end{bmatrix}\right)\longrightarrow Z,\ in\, law,\ Z\sim N\left(0, B\left(q,\alpha\right)\Sigma\left(q,\alpha\right)B\left(q,\alpha\right)^T\right)$$

where $B(q,\alpha)=\left[b_{i,j}\right]_{1\le i,j\le 2}$, $\Sigma(q,\alpha)=\left[\sigma_{i,j}\right]_{1\le i,j\le 2}$ are given by

$$b_{1,1}=-\frac{p_1}{(1-p_0)^2},\ b_{1,2}=-\frac{1}{1-p_0},$$

$$b_{2,1}=\frac{(1-p_0-p_1)\log(1-p_0-p_1)+(1-p_0)\log(1-p_0)}{(p_0-1)(p_0+p_1-1)\left[\log(1-p_0-p_1)-\log(1-p_0)\right]^2}$$

$$b_{2,2}=\frac{\log(1-p_0)}{(1-p_0-p_1)\left[\log(1-p_0-p_1)-\log(1-p_0)\right]^2}$$

$$\sigma_{1,1}=p_0\left(1-p_0\right),\ \sigma_{1,2}=\sigma_{2,1}=-p_0p_1,\ \sigma_{2,2}=p_1\left(1-p_1\right),$$

with $p_0=1-q^{\alpha+1}$ and $p_1=(1-q)\,q^{\alpha+1}$.

Proof Let us prove the convergence in probability as $n\rightarrow+\infty$. The random variables $\left(\mathbf{1}_{X_n=0}\right)_{n\in\mathbf{N}}$ are independent and identically distributed according to a Bernoulli distribution with parameter p_0, with $E\left(\mathbf{1}_{X_n=0}\right)=p_0$ and, analogously, $\left(\mathbf{1}_{X_n=1}\right)_{n\in\mathbf{N}}$ are independent and identically distributed with a Bernoulli distribution with parameter p_1, with $E\left(\mathbf{1}_{X_n=1}\right)=p_1$. So, by Kolmogorov theorem, $P_{0,n}\longrightarrow p_0$ almost surely (a.s.), and $P_{1,n}\longrightarrow p_1$ a.s., and we have $P_{0,n}\longrightarrow p_0$ and $P_{1,n}\longrightarrow p_1$, in probability. Using the properties of convergence in probability, we deduce that $\dot{Q}_n=1-\frac{P_{1,n}}{1-P_{0,n}}\longrightarrow 1-\frac{(1-q)q^{\alpha+1}}{1-1+q^{\alpha+1}}=q$, in probability. Otherwise, $1-P_{0,n}\longrightarrow q^{\alpha+1}$ and $1-P_{0,n}-P_{1,n}\longrightarrow q^{\alpha+2}$, in probability. Since $\log(x)$ is a continuous function in $]0,+\infty[$, then $\log\left(1-P_{0,n}\right)\longrightarrow\log\left(q^{\alpha+1}\right)$ and $\log\left(1-P_{0,n}-P_{1,n}\right)\longrightarrow\log q^{\alpha+2}$, in probability. Again by the properties of convergence in probability, we conclude that $\dot{A}_n\longrightarrow\frac{2(\alpha+1)\log q-(\alpha+2)\log q}{(\alpha+2)\log q-(\alpha+1)\log q}=\alpha$, in probability.

Since $Y_n=\left(\mathbf{1}_{X_n=0},\mathbf{1}_{X_n=1}\right), n\in N$, are independent and identically distributed random variables with mean $E\left(Y_n\right)=\left(p_0,p_1\right)$ and matrices of variances-covariances given by

$$\Sigma=\begin{bmatrix}V\left(\mathbf{1}_{X_n=0}\right) & Cov\left(\mathbf{1}_{X_n=0},\mathbf{1}_{X_n=1}\right)\\ Cov\left(\mathbf{1}_{X_n=0},\mathbf{1}_{X_n=1}\right) & V\left(\mathbf{1}_{X_n=1}\right)\end{bmatrix}=\begin{bmatrix}p_0\left(1-p_0\right) & -p_0p_1\\ -p_0p_1 & p_1\left(1-p_1\right)\end{bmatrix}$$

then, by [4, p. 61],

$$\sqrt{n}\left(\begin{bmatrix} P_{0,n} \\ P_{1,n} \end{bmatrix} - \begin{bmatrix} p_0 \\ p_1 \end{bmatrix}\right) \longrightarrow Z,\ in\, law,\ Z \sim N\left(0, \Sigma\right).$$

Considering now the functions

$$h_1\left(p_0, p_1\right) = 1 - \frac{p_1}{1-p_0}, \qquad h_2\left(p_0, p_1\right) = \frac{2\log\left(1-p_0\right) - \log\left(1-p_0-p_1\right)}{\log\left(1-p_0-p_1\right) - \log\left(1-p_0\right)},$$

we obtain

$$\sqrt{n}\left(\begin{bmatrix} h_1\left(P_{0,n}, P_{1,n}\right) \\ h_2\left(P_{0,n}, P_{1,n}\right) \end{bmatrix} - \begin{bmatrix} h_1\left(p_0, p_1\right) \\ h_2\left(p_0, p_1\right) \end{bmatrix}\right) \longrightarrow Z,\ in\, law,\ Z \sim N\left(0, B\Sigma B^T\right)$$

where $B = \left[\frac{\partial h_i}{\partial p_{j-1}}\right]_{1\le i,j\le 2}$, that is,

$$\frac{\partial h_1}{\partial p_0} = -\frac{p_1}{(1-p_0)^2}, \frac{\partial h_1}{\partial p_1} = -\frac{1}{1-p_0},$$

$$\frac{\partial h_2}{\partial p_0} = \frac{\left(1-p_0-p_1\right)\log\left(1-p_0-p_1\right) + \left(1-p_0\right)\log\left(1-p_0\right)}{\left(p_0-1\right)\left(p_0+p_1-1\right)\left[\log\left(1-p_0-p_1\right) - \log\left(1-p_0\right)\right]^2},$$

$$\frac{\partial h_2}{\partial p_1} = \frac{\log\left(1-p_0\right)}{\left(1-p_0-p_1\right)\left[\log\left(1-p_0-p_1\right) - \log\left(1-p_0\right)\right]^2}. \qquad \square$$

3.1.2 Moments Method

The estimators obtained by the method of moments $\widetilde{Q}_n$ and $\widetilde{A}_n$ are almost surely (a.s.) convergent. In fact, we state the following result.

Theorem 2 *The estimators $\widetilde{Q}_n$ and $\widetilde{A}_n$ given in (3) verify $\left(\widetilde{Q}_n, \widetilde{A}_n\right) \longrightarrow (q, \alpha)$ a.s. and*

$$\sqrt{n}\left(\begin{bmatrix} \widetilde{Q}_n \\ \widetilde{A}_n \end{bmatrix} - \begin{bmatrix} q \\ \alpha \end{bmatrix}\right) \longrightarrow Z,\ in\, law,\ Z \sim N\left(0, D\left(q,\alpha\right) A\left(q,\alpha\right) D\left(q,\alpha\right)^T\right)$$

where $A\left(q,\alpha\right) = \left[a_{i,j}\right]_{1\le i,j\le 2}$, $D\left(q,\alpha\right) = \left[d_{i,j}\right]_{1\le i,j\le 2}$ are such that

$$a_{1,1} = \frac{q^{\alpha+1}\left(1+q-q^{\alpha+1}\right)}{(1-q)^2},$$

$$a_{1,2} = a_{2,1} = \frac{q^{\alpha+1}\left(1+4q+q^2\right)}{(1-q)^3} - \frac{q^{\alpha+1}\left(1+q\right)}{\left(1-q^2\right)}\frac{q^{\alpha+1}}{1-q},$$

$$a_{2,2} = \frac{q^{\alpha+1}\left(1+11q+11q^2+q^3\right) - q^{2\alpha+2}\left(1+q\right)^2}{\left(1-q\right)^4},$$

$$d_{1,1} = -\frac{2m_2}{\left(m_1+m_2\right)^2},\ d_{1,2} = \frac{2m_1}{\left(m_1+m_2\right)^2},$$

$$d_{2,1} = \frac{\frac{1}{m_2-m_1}\log\left(\frac{2m_1^2}{m_2+m_1}\right) + \frac{2}{m_1}\log\left(\frac{m_2-m_1}{m_2+m_1}\right) + \frac{1}{m_2+m_1}\log\left(\frac{2m_1^2}{m_2-m_1}\right)}{\left[\log\left(m_2-m_1\right) - \log\left(m_2+m_1\right)\right]^2},$$

$$d_{2,2} = \frac{-\frac{1}{m_2-m_1}\left[\log\left(2m_1^2\right) - \log\left(m_1+m_2\right)\right] + \frac{1}{m_2+m_1}\log\left(\frac{2m_1^2}{m_2-m_1}\right)}{\left[\log\left(m_2-m_1\right) - \log\left(m_2+m_1\right)\right]^2}$$

and $m_1 = \frac{q^{\alpha+1}}{1-q}$, $m_2 = \frac{q^{\alpha+1}(1+q)}{(1-q)^2}$.

Proof We have the asymptotic normality since X has fourth-order moments, and this estimator verifies $\left(\widetilde{Q}_n, \widetilde{A}_n\right) = \left(f_1\left(M_1, M_2\right), f_2\left(M_1, M_2\right)\right)$ with $f_1\left(m_1, m_2\right) = \frac{m_2-m_1}{m_2+m_1}$ and $f_2\left(m_1, m_2\right) = \frac{\log\left(2m_1^2\right) - \log\left(m_2-m_1\right)}{\log\left(m_2-m_1\right) - \log\left(m_2-m_1\right)}$. The normal distribution is centred with matrice of variances-covariances given by $D\left(q,\alpha\right) A\left(q,\alpha\right) D\left(q,\alpha\right)^T$ where $A\left(q,\alpha\right) = \left[Cov\left(X^j, X^l\right)\right]_{1\le j,l\le 2}$, that is,

$$Cov\left(X,X\right) = V\left(X\right) = \frac{q^{\alpha+1}\left(1+q-q^{\alpha+1}\right)}{\left(1-q\right)^2}$$

$$Cov\left(X,X^2\right) = Cov\left(X^2,X\right) = E\left(X^3\right) - E\left(X^2\right)E\left(X\right)$$

$$= \frac{q^{\alpha+1}\left(1+4q+q^2\right)}{\left(1-q\right)^3} - \frac{q^{\alpha+1}\left(1+q\right)}{\left(1-q^2\right)}\frac{q^{\alpha+1}}{1-q}$$

$$Cov\left(X^2,X^2\right) = E\left(X^4\right) - E\left(X^2\right)E\left(X^2\right)$$

$$= \frac{q^{\alpha+1}\left(1+11q+11q^2+q^3\right) - q^{2\alpha+2}\left(1+q\right)^2}{\left(1-q\right)^4}$$

and $D = \left[\frac{\partial f_i}{\partial m_j}\right]_{1\le i,j\le 2}$, that is,

$$\frac{\partial f_1}{\partial m_1} = -\frac{2m_2}{\left(m_1+m_2\right)^2},\ \frac{\partial f_1}{\partial m_2} = \frac{2m_1}{\left(m_1+m_2\right)^2}$$

$$\frac{\partial f_2}{\partial m_1} = \frac{\frac{1}{m_2-m_1}\log\left(\frac{2m_1^2}{m_2+m_1}\right) + \frac{2}{m_1}\log\left(\frac{m_2-m_1}{m_2+m_1}\right) + \frac{1}{m_2+m_1}\log\left(\frac{2m_1^2}{m_2-m_1}\right)}{\left[\log\left(m_2-m_1\right) - \log\left(m_2+m_1\right)\right]^2},$$

$$\frac{\partial f_2}{\partial m_2} = \frac{-\frac{1}{m_2-m_1}\left[\log\left(2m_1^2\right) - \log\left(m_1+m_2\right)\right] + \frac{1}{m_2+m_1}\log\left(\frac{2m_1^2}{m_2-m_1}\right)}{\left[\log\left(m_2-m_1\right) - \log\left(m_2+m_1\right)\right]^2}.$$

□

3.1.3 Maximum Likelihood Method

Theorem 3 *The estimators* $\widehat{Q}_n$ *and* $\widehat{A}_n$ *given in (4) verify* $\widehat{Q}_n \longrightarrow q$, $\widehat{A}_n \longrightarrow \alpha$ *in probability and*

$$\sqrt{n}\left(\begin{bmatrix}\widehat{Q}_n\\ \widehat{A}_n\end{bmatrix} - \begin{bmatrix} q \\ \alpha \end{bmatrix}\right) \longrightarrow Z,\ in\, law,\ Z \sim N\left(0, \left(I\left(q,\alpha\right)\right)^{-1}\right)$$

where $I\left(q,\alpha\right) = \left[I_{i,j}\right]_{1\leq i,j\leq 2}$ *is such that*

$$I_{1,1} = q^{\alpha-1} \frac{\left(1-q^2\right)\left(\alpha+1\right)^2 + \left(1-q^{\alpha+1}\right)\left[1-\left(1-q\right)^2\right]}{\left(1-q^{\alpha+1}\right)\left(1-q\right)^2},$$

$$I_{1,2} = I_{2,1} = q^{\alpha}\frac{\left(\alpha+1\right)\log q}{1-q^{\alpha+1}},\ I_{2,2} = \frac{q^{\alpha+1}\left(\log q\right)^2}{1-q^{\alpha+1}}.$$

Proof The proof of this result follows from ([4], pp. 461–465). The verification of conditions is quite technical and a detailed proof may be found in [5]. □

3.2 Numerical Studies: Behaviour of Estimators in Moderate and Large Sample Sizes

In this section, we illustrate by several forms the finite sample performance of the estimation methods previously referred. We evaluate the average values produced and the corresponding variability, and the evolution of these summaries with the sample size. In this sense, we generated a sample of a ZDGG (q, α) distribution of dimension $n \in \{100, 500\}$ and calculated parameter estimates by the three estimation methods. We repeated this procedure 1000 times with $q \in \{0.4, 0.8\}$ and $\alpha \in \{-0.7, -0.3, 0.5\}$.

Tables 2, 3 and 4 include the empirical means and standard deviations, respectively $E_{est}(.)$ and $SD_{est}(.)$, of the estimates of parameters. We note that, as expected, the estimates of the parameters seem to converge to the corresponding true parameter

Table 2 Estimators based on zeros and ones proportions

Parameters		$n = 100$				$n = 500$			
α	q	$E_{est}(\dot{\alpha}_n)$	$SD_{est}(\dot{\alpha}_n)$	$E_{est}(\dot{q}_n)$	$SD_{est}(\dot{q}_n)$	$E_{est}(\dot{\alpha}_n)$	$SD_{est}(\dot{\alpha}_n)$	$E_{est}(\dot{q}_n)$	$SD_{est}(\dot{q}_n)$
−0.7	0.4	−0.6950	0.0818	0.3990	0.0571	−0.6987	0.0347	0.4005	0.0252
	0.8	−0.6830	0.1568	0.7998	0.0425	−0.6931	0.0636	0.8007	0.0184
−0.3	0.4	−0.2822	0.1835	0.3992	0.0675	−0.2966	0.0737	0.4004	0.0298
	0.8	−0.2631	0.2896	0.7976	0.0446	−0.2915	0.1169	0.7999	0.0189
0.5	0.4	0.5874	0.5073	0.4015	0.0986	0.5213	0.2035	0.4010	0.0432
	0.8	0.6300	0.6560	0.7997	0.0488	0.5265	0.2284	0.8003	0.0220

Table 3 Estimators based on the moments method

Parameters		$n = 100$				$n = 500$			
α	q	$E_{est}(\widetilde{\alpha}_n)$	$SD_{est}(\widetilde{\alpha}_n)$	$E_{est}(\widetilde{q}_n)$	$SD_{est}(\widetilde{q}_n)$	$E_{est}(\widetilde{\alpha}_n)$	$SD_{est}(\widetilde{\alpha}_n)$	$E_{est}(\widetilde{q}_n)$	$SD_{est}(\widetilde{q}_n)$
−0.7	0.4	−0.7014	0.1080	0.3935	0.0506	−0.7014	0.0461	0.3985	0.0230
	0.8	−0.7098	0.4345	0.7957	0.0246	−0.7049	0.1875	0.7992	0.0110
−0.3	0.4	−0.3049	0.1950	0.3908	0.0598	−0.3025	0.0855	0.3981	0.0274
	0.8	−0.3067	0.5167	0.7955	0.0256	−0.3056	0.2224	0.7991	0.0115
0.5	0.4	0.4771	0.4469	0.3830	0.0841	0.4928	0.2024	0.3955	0.0380
	0.8	0.4826	0.6348	0.7955	0.0274	0.4938	0.3009	0.7988	0.0122

Table 4 Estimators of maximum likelihood

Parameters		$n = 100$				$n = 500$			
α	q	$E_{est}(\widehat{\alpha}_n)$	$SD_{est}(\widehat{\alpha}_n)$	$E_{est}(\widehat{q}_n)$	$SD_{est}(\widehat{q}_n)$	$E_{est}(\widehat{\alpha}_n)$	$SD_{est}(\widehat{\alpha}_n)$	$E_{est}(\widehat{q}_n)$	$SD_{est}(\widehat{q}_n)$
−0.7	0.4	−0.6984	0.0738	0.3969	0.0434	−0.6998	0.0321	0.3996	0.0195
	0.8	−0.7004	0.1216	0.7982	0.0188	−0.6969	0.0556	0.7999	0.0082
−0.3	0.4	−0.2953	0.1513	0.3958	0.0519	−0.2994	0.0637	0.3995	0.0230
	0.8	−0.2969	0.1986	0.7980	0.0197	−0.2980	0.0901	0.7998	0.0086
0.5	0.4	0.5252	0.3772	0.3938	0.0776	0.5062	0.1609	0.3986	0.0327
	0.8	0.5181	0.3514	0.7986	0.0219	0.5032	0.1452	0.7996	0.0094

Table 5 Empirical and theoretical variances and covariances of the ZDGG distribution with $(q, \alpha) = (0.4, -0.7)$, for the proportions method [5]

	$n = 100$	$n = 500$	Theoretical values
$nV_{est}(\dot{q}_n)$	0.3264	0.3179	0.3159
$nV_{est}(\dot{\alpha}_n)$	0.6690	0.6022	0.5885
$nCov_{est}(\dot{q}_n, \dot{\alpha}_n)$	0.2806	0.2655	0.2586

values as the sample size increases. Further, the standard deviations of the estimates decrease when the sample size increases.

We also constructed confidence regions for the parameters, based on the limit laws of the estimators, and compared the degree of confidence set with the so-called coverage probability, that is, with the proportion of generated samples whose estimated confidence region contains the true values of the parameters. The numerical results support the theoretical findings regarding the consistency of the estimators.

Next, we considered the parameter $(q, \alpha) = (0.4, -0.7)$ and compared the theoretical values $nV(\dot{q}_n)$, $nV(\dot{\alpha}_n)$ and $nCov(\dot{q}_n, \dot{\alpha}_n)$, related to the method of proportions of zeros and ones, with the empirical ones, respectively $nV_{est}(\dot{q}_n)$, $nV_{est}(\dot{\alpha}_n)$ and $nCov_{est}(\dot{q}_n, \dot{\alpha}_n)$.

In Table 5 (in [5]), we observe that for $n = 100$ the estimates of the elements of the variance-covariance matrices of the asymptotic law are close to the theoretical values, unless those related to the variance of the α estimator. For $n = 500$, the estimates behave better than in the case $n = 100$ with all of them very close to the

Table 6 Empirical and theoretical variances and covariances of the ZDGG distribution with $(q, \alpha) = (0.4, -0.7)$, for the moments method

	$n = 100$	$n = 500$	Theoretical values
$nV_{est}(\widetilde{q}_n)$	0.2556	0.2641	0.2654
$nV_{est}(\widetilde{\alpha}_n)$	1.1673	1.0648	1.0313
$nCov_{est}(\widetilde{q}_n, \widetilde{\alpha}_n)$	0.3667	0.3619	0.3551

Table 7 Empirical and theoretical variances and covariances of the ZDGG distribution with $(q, \alpha) = (0.4, -0.7)$, for the maximum likelihood method

	$n = 100$	$n = 500$	Theoretical values
$nV_{est}(\widehat{q}_n)$	0.1883	0.1899	0.1896
$nV_{est}(\widehat{\alpha}_n)$	0.5450	0.5150	0.5038
$nCov_{est}(\widehat{q}_n, \widehat{\alpha}_n)$	0.1624	0.1617	0.1552

theoretical values. We have repeated the process using the estimators of moments and maximum likelihood methods, and we note that similar conclusions were observed, as illustrated in Tables 6 and 7.

4 The INARCH Model with Conditional ZDGG Distribution

In this section, we introduce a model for time series with integer values such that its conditional law given the past belongs to the ZDGG distribution and states its first-order stationarity.

4.1 *Definition and First-order Stationarity*

Definition 2 A stochastic process $X = (X_t, t \in Z)$ follows a zero-distorted generalized geometric integer-valued ARCH model with order $p \in \mathbf{N}$ and parameters $q_t \in]0, 1[$ and $\alpha_t \in [-1, +\infty[$, briefly ZDGGD-INARCH(p), if for all $t \in \mathbf{Z}$,

$$\begin{cases} X_t | \underline{X}_{t-1} \sim ZDGGD\,(q_t, \alpha_t) \\ E\left(X_t | \underline{X}_{t-1}\right) = \lambda_t = \dfrac{q_t^{\alpha_t+1}}{1-q_t} = a_0 + \displaystyle\sum_{i=1}^{p} a_i X_{t-i} \end{cases}$$

where $a_0 > 0$ and $a_i \geq 0$ for $i = 1, ..., p$. For all $t \in \mathbf{Z}$, $\underline{X}_{t-1}$ denotes the σ-field generated by $\{X_{t-k}, k \in \mathbf{N}\}$.

Theorem 4 *A stochastic process* $X = (X_t, t \in \mathbf{Z})$ *following a ZDGGD-INARCH(p) model is first-order stationary if and only if* $\sum_{i=1}^{p} a_i < 1$.

Proof We have to verify that $E(X_t)$ exists and is independent of t, for any $t \in \mathbf{Z}$. As X_t is a positive measurable function, we can write formally

$$\mu_t = E(X_t) = E\left(E\left(X_t|\underline{X}_{t-1}\right)\right) = E(\lambda_t) = E\left(a_0 + \sum_{i=1}^{p} a_i X_{t-i}\right)$$
$$\Leftrightarrow \mu_t = a_0 + \sum_{i=1}^{p} a_i \mu_{t-i},$$

taking into account that the involved sums exist although they may be non-finite. This non-homogenous difference equation has a stable solution, which is independent of t and finite, if and only if all roots of the equation $1 - \sum_{i=1}^{p} a_i z^i$ lie outside the unit circle, that is, if and only if $\sum_{i=1}^{p} a_i < 1$.

□

In these conditions, we have $E(X_t) = \mu = \dfrac{a_0}{1 - \sum_{i=1}^{p} a_i}$, $t \in \mathbf{Z}$.

In the general case, the second-order stationarity of a ZDGGD-INARCH(p) model is an open question. There are studies [2, 3] in some sub-families like in the geometric INARCH model, which is obtained when we consider $\alpha_t = 0$ in the general one. This G-INARCH model is also a member of the ZIG-INARCH family, defined as a stochastic process $X = (X_t, t \in \mathbf{Z})$ satisfying

$$\begin{cases} X_t|\underline{X}_{t-1} \sim ZIG(1 - p_t, w) \\ E\left(X_t|\underline{X}_{t-1}\right) = (1 - w)\dfrac{1 - p_t}{p_t} = (1 - w)\lambda_t \\ \lambda_t = a_0 + \sum_{i=1}^{p} a_i X_{t-i} \end{cases}$$

with $w \in [0, 1[$, $a_0 > 0$ and $a_i \geq 0$ for $i = 1, ..., p$. If $w = 0$ we get the G-INARCH(p) model.

4.2 *Real-Data Application: Number of New Hantavirus Infections Per Week in a German State*

We study now the modelling of a dataset related to the number of new cases of Hantavirus infection per week in the federal state Eslésvico-Holsácia of Germany between 2005 and 2018, totaling 742 observations (obtained from the database of Robert-Koch Institute, https://survstat.rki.de). We intend to identify, among some of the models here discussed, which are the most compatible with the evolution of this series. In this study, we will use the log-likelihood (-Log L), Akaike (AIC) and Bayesian (BIC) criteria as well as the comparison between theoretical summaries of the models and the corresponding summaries of the observed series and a residual analysis.

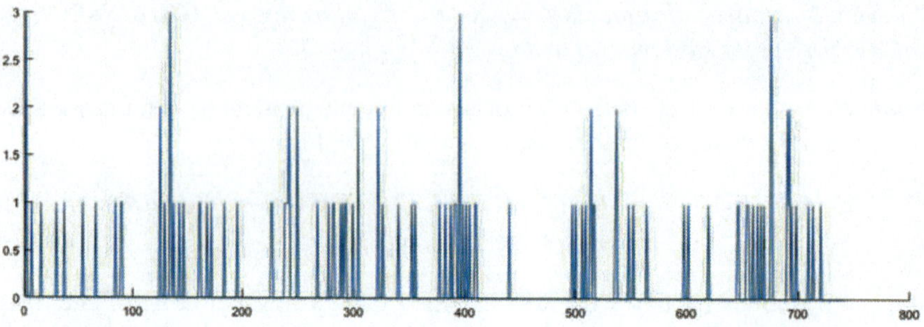

Fig. 1 Hantavirus infections per week: trajectory

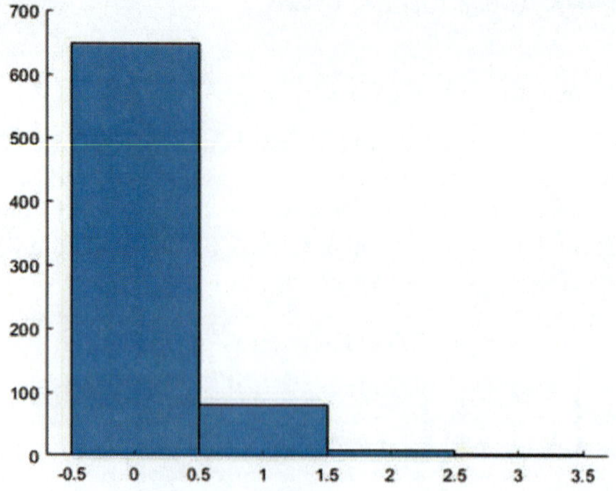

Fig. 2 Hantavirus infections per week: histogram

Figure 1 presents the trajectory of the series and in Fig. 2, we have its histogram. Autocorrelation and partial autocorrelation empirical values are in Fig. 3. The maximum observed is 3 and the empirical mean and variance are 0.1509 and 0.1877, respectively. The proportion of zero observations is 0.8733 and the autocorrelations of order two or greater are not significant.

Since the partial autocorrelations are not significant for lag 2 or greater, we choose G-INARCH(1) and Poisson-INARCH(1) models. Taking into account the large number of zeros present in the observed series, we decided to consider also the zero-inflated Geometric and Poisson INARCH(1) models (ZIG-INARCH and ZIP-INARCH, respectively).

Taking into account the smaller values of the criteria, as visible in Table 8 (in [5]), we note that the G-INARCH and ZIG-INARCH models perform better than the others. Also, from Table 9 (in [5]) we conclude that the ZIG-INARCH(1) presents, in general, the best results and so we decide to analyse the residual series produced.

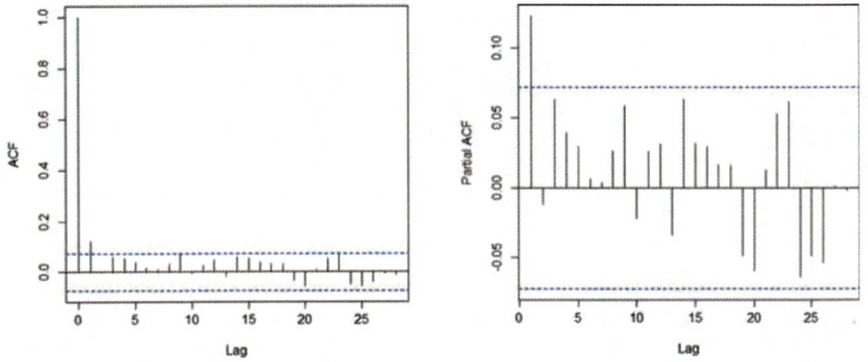

Fig. 3 Hantavirus infections per week: autocorrelation (left) and partial autocorrelation (right) values

Table 8 Estimates of models parameters and values of -Log L, AIC and BIC criteria [5]

Model	Estimates			Criteria		
	α_0	α_1	w	- log L	AIC	BIC
G-INARCH(1)	0.1320	0.1269		327.1165	658.2330	667.4517
INARCH(1)	0.1321	0.1259		332.2810	668.5619	677.7806
ZIG-INARCH(1)	0.1508	0.1441	0.1238	326.9672	659.9343	673.7624
ZIP-INARCH(1)	0.2800	0.2480	0.5259	327.6763	661.3525	675.1806

Table 9 Theoretical values of mean, variance and autocorrelation of order 1 for estimated models and for the Hantavirus infections data. Mean (Mr) and variance (Vr) of Pearson residuals for each model [5]

Model	G-INARCH(1)	INARCH(1)	ZIG-INARCH(1)	ZIP-INARCH(1)	Hantavirus series
Mean	0.1512	0.1511	0.1512	0.1505	0.1509
Variance	0.1799	0.1536	0.1873	0.1808	0.1877
ACF(1)	0.1269	0.1259	0.1262	0.1176	0.1227
Mr	0.0000	0.001	0.0001	0.0006	0
Vr	1.0858	1.2450	1.0482	1.0699	1

Figure 4 shows the correlogram and partial correlogram of the Pearson residuals. The compatibility with white noise is clear.

Finally, a model for the X series of the new cases of Hantavirus infection per week in the federal state Eslésvico-Holsácia of Germany is then

$$\begin{cases} X_t|\underline{X}_{t-1} \sim ZIG\,(1-p_t, 0.1238) \\ E\left(X_t|\underline{X}_{t-1}\right) = (1-0.1238)\lambda_t \\ \lambda_t = \frac{1-p_t}{p_t} = 0.1508 + 0.1441X_{t-1}. \end{cases}$$

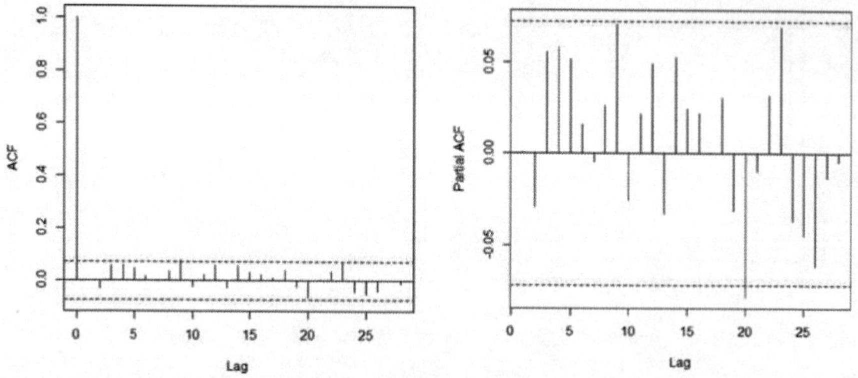

Fig. 4 Pearson residuals related to the ZIG-INARCH(1) model: autocorrelation (left) and partial autocorrelation (right) values

5 Conclusion

After recalling the definition of the ZDGG distribution, we stated the asymptotic behaviour of the estimators of its parameters deduced using three approaches (proportions of zeros and ones, moments and maximum likelihood). We illustrated by numerical studies the corresponding behaviour in moderate and large samples, concluding the coherency with the theoretical results. Finally, we have introduced the INARCH model with a ZDGG conditional distribution for the study of counting time series, stated its first-order stationarity and evaluated the performance of some members of this family in the modelling of the number of new cases of Hantavirus infection recorded in a German state. Further studies in the general ZDGGD-INARCH model are in progress, in particular on the second-order stationarity.

Acknowledgements This work was partially supported by the Centre for Mathematics of the University of Coimbra—UIDB/00324/2020 funded by the Portuguese Government through FCT/MEC.

References

1. Sastry, D.V.S., Bhati, D., Rattihalli, R.N., Gómez-Déniz, E.: On zero-distorted generalized geometric distribution. Commun. Stat.-Theory Methods **45**(18), 5427–5442 (2015)
2. Zhu, F.: Zero-inflated poisson and negative binomial integer-valued GARCH models. J. Stat. Plan. Inference **142**(4), 826–839 (2012)
3. Gonçalves, E., Mendes-Lopes, N., Silva, F.: Zero-inflated compound Poisson distributions in integer-valued GARCH models. Statistics **50**, 558–578 (2015). Dec
4. Lehmann, E.L., Casella, G.: Theory Theory of Point Estimation, 2nd edn. Springer, New York (1998)
5. Sousa, D.: Modelos para séries temporais de contagem com perturbação em zero. M.Sc. Thesis, Universidade de Coimbra (2021)

Uncovering Abnormal Water Consumption Patterns for Sustainability's Sake: A Statistical Approach

Ana Borges, Clara Cordeiro, and M. Rosário Ramos

Abstract Monitoring domestic water usage may help the water utilities uncover abnormal water consumption. In this context, it is necessary to improve and develop tools based on data analysis of households' meter readings. This study contributes to this goal by using a statistical methodology that detects abnormal water consumption patterns, namely, significant increases or decreases. This approach relies on a combination of methods that analyse billed water consumption time series. The first step is to decompose the time series using Seasonal-Trend decomposition based on Loess. Next, breakpoint analysis is performed on the seasonally adjusted time series to look for changes in the pattern over time. Afterwards, the Mann–Kendall test and Sen's slope estimator are applied to assess whether there are significant increases or decreases in water consumption. The strategy is applied to water consumption data from the Algarve, Portugal, successfully detecting breakpoints associated with significant increasing or decreasing trends.

Keywords Breakpoints · Time series decomposition · Trend analysis · Water consumption

A. Borges (✉)
CIICESI, ESTG, Politécnico do Porto, Porto, Portugal
e-mail: aib@estg.ipp.pt

Department of Natural and Exact Sciences, ESTG, Politécnico do Porto, Porto, Portugal

C. Cordeiro
Department of Mathematics, Faculty of Science and Technology, Universidade do Algarve, Faro, Portugal

M. Rosário Ramos
Department of Science and Technology, Universidade Aberta, Lisbon, Portugal

C. Cordeiro · M. Rosário Ramos
CEAUL, Faculty of Science, Universidade de Lisboa, Lisbon, Portugal

M. Rosário Ramos
CEG, Universidade Aberta, Lisbon, Portugal

R. Bispo et al. (eds.), *Recent Developments in Statistics and Data Science*, Springer Proceedings in Mathematics & Statistics 398,
https://doi.org/10.1007/978-3-031-12766-3_8

1 Introduction

In the last decades, water has been recognised as an essential resource for guaranteeing economic development and maintaining living standards. Water stress makes it indispensable to acknowledge water as a scarce resource and to enhance focus on managing demand [1]. In the context of water scarcity, [2] alert to the importance of assessing losses in water distribution systems since the compensation of water losses increases water demand. Enhancing water use efficiency and conservation are priorities to ensure, for example, universal access to drinking water and reduce the population suffering from its scarcity.

Water companies' awareness for the responsible use of water has gained importance, with climate changes emphasising this need. The analysis of urban water consumption patterns and the estimation of the corresponding water demand are expected to be among the top priorities for water companies in the near future [3]. In this sense, controlling domestic water usage can help reduce both water consumption and protect the environment [4]. Therefore, investigating water consumption patterns will provide a better understanding at a household level. This will promote water use efficiency and help to reduce non-revenue water (NRW). Detecting an anomalous increase will allow companies to take measures, such as alerting their consumers to have sustainable behaviours.

The Portuguese region of Algarve is known for registering the highest values of water consumption [5]. This region faces an enormous challenge in optimising water management and usage standards due to long periods of drought. Consequently, water utilities feel the need to develop mechanisms for water planning based on data analysis. Overall, they concentrate their efforts on addressing the consequences of climate change. Therefore, managing Portuguese water resources is likely to become challenging due to the potential decrease of water availability and the increase of the seasonal hydrological asymmetries [6].

This paper presents an application of a procedure capable of detecting significant changes in a time series anchored on statistical methods. The aim is the assessment of abnormal increasing and decreasing trends in water consumption. The methodology is an extension of the work developed by [7] that detects significant decreasing trends in water consumption time series. This approach can be synthesised in four steps: the first step consists of time series decomposition using Seasonal-Trend decomposition based on Loess [8]; on the second step, a breakpoint analysis is performed on the seasonally adjusted time series; the third step consists of the search for decreasing or increasing changes in the periods between breakpoints through the Mann–Kendall [9] test, and Sen's [10] slope estimator. In the end, an indicator for the magnitude of change is presented. Monthly time series of billed water consumption from Loulé Municipality, located in Algarve—the southern region of Portugal, is used.

The paper is organised as follows: the Methodology section describes the statistical methods that underlie the procedure and how they are connected; the following section presents the data set used to exemplify the procedure; the results are detailed in the next section and it ends with the Conclusion and Future Work section.

2 Methodology

A time series is a set of consecutive observations indexed in time t, $t = 1, \cdots n$, during regular intervals. Often time series exhibit seasonal behaviour, and adequate "control" for a seasonal component is essential before using any statistical model. Also, the time series may exhibit patterns such as an upward or downward movement (trend). The irregular component is the remaining time series behaviour that is not attributed to trend or seasonality. Both trend and seasonality components are potential confounding features in analysis, so identification and removal are important.

The methodology is organised into four steps described below.

In the first step, the Seasonal-Trend decomposition procedure based on Loess (STL) [8] is applied to decompose each time series into a trend (T_t), seasonal (S_t) and irregular or residual (I_t) components using nonparametric regression. Assuming the additive model, the time series is decomposed into

$$Y_t = T_t + S_t + I_t, \tag{1}$$

where $t = 1, \cdots n$, is the time period and n its length. This method was chosen over other decomposition methods in the literature because it has attractive modelling features, such as the seasonal component being allowed to change over time and being robust in the presence of outliers. This procedure is available in the R software through function `stl()` [11]. However, this procedure requires a subjective selection of two smoothing parameters: the seasonal (*s.window*) and trend (*t.window*) window widths. Therefore, the algorithm used was proposed by [12], named as `stl.fit()` [13], which overcomes this drawback. The latter selects the best STL model with the smallest error measure achieved with a specific combination of the smoothing parameters. In this study, the Mean Absolute Error (MAE) is used. For more details, see [12].

The second step consists of the detection of breakpoints in the seasonally adjusted time series of water consumption given by

$$Y_t^* = Y_t - S_t \tag{2}$$

$t = 1, \cdots, n$. The R package *strucchange* [14] is used to obtain the breakpoints. This package features methods from the generalised fluctuation and F-test (Chow test) frameworks. That includes methods to fit, plot and test fluctuation processes (e.g. CUSUM, MOSUM, recursive/moving estimates and F-statistics, respectively). This procedure tests for structural changes in linear regression models, estimating the number of segments (m) and the set of the breakpoints $bp = \{t_1^*, t_2^*, \cdots, t_{m-1}^*\}$, minimising the Bayesian information criterion and the residual sum of squares [15]. The present study uses the two expressions proposed in [7] for obtaining the minimum length between consecutive breaks (*min.h*) and the maximum number of breaks (*max.breaks*).

In a third step, the change identified in the previous procedure is submitted to a nonparametric analysis through Mann–Kendall (MK) test [9], and Theil–Sen's (TS) Slope [10]. The choice of these methods is linked to the fact that they can handle situations where the segments correspond to short periods of asymmetric distributions and allow assess of the underlying increase or decrease through robust methods [16]. If the result is significant, positive or negative, then the breakpoint adjacent to the segment is considered relevant. To obtain these statistics, the function `sen.slope()`, available in the R package *trend* [17] is used.

In the last step, the magnitude of the change in water consumption before and after the significant break is obtained by the Relative Magnitude of the Change (RMC) proposed by [7]. This indicator is a ratio that compares the water consumption pattern before and after a breakpoint as follows:

$$RMC = \frac{slp_{after} - slp_{before}}{|slp_{before}|}, \tag{3}$$

where slp_{after} and slp_{before} are the nonparametric Sen's slopes in the neighbourhood of a specific breakpoint $t_k^* \in bp^*$. Higher negative values of RMC represent a higher decreasing change in water consumption after the considered breakpoint. While high positive values of RMC represent a higher increase in water consumption after the considered breakpoint.

For more details about each step, see [7].

3 Data

The empirical analysis uses billed water consumption data from residential households (**RH**) from a municipality located in the Portuguese region of Algarve. The municipality occupies about 200 km^2 and has an estimated population of around 5,000 inhabitants. It is characterised by an elderly population and an agricultural-based economy.

Two case studies will be presented to exemplify the procedure. Both cases refer to household's monthly water consumption (m^3) from February 2011 until December 2017, registered by two water meters: **RH1** and **RH2**.

On meter **RH1**, the higher values of water consumption (see Fig. 1a) were registered in the summer months of July and August. This is consistent with a strong seasonal behaviour, with the higher temperatures justifying the need for higher water consumption, related to Algarve's tourism period. Moreover, a decrease in the trend until 2016 was followed by an increase more pronounced during 2017, as seen in Fig. 1. The latter might be explained by its replacement on 8 November 2016. The consumption registered by this meter showed a noticeable abrupt increase in 2018, reaching a value higher than 30 m^3.

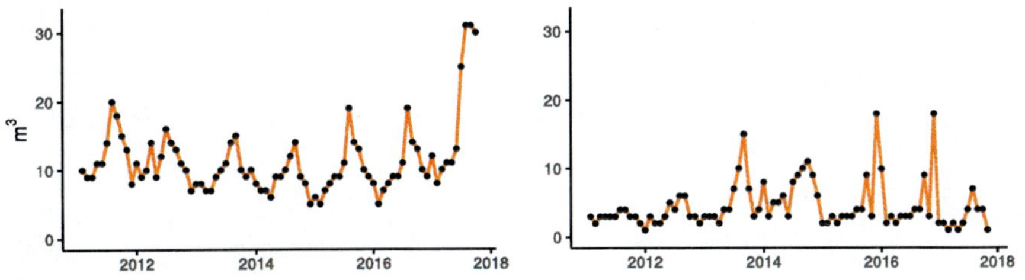

(a) RH1 (b) RH2

Fig. 1 Time series of water consumption

In contrast, meter **RH2** did not present a seasonal pattern as regular as in the previous case. In addition, it showed the highest values of water consumption in months such as October 2014, December 2016 and December 2017, as shown in Fig. 1b.

4 Results

The proposed strategy was applied to two case studies showing different water consumption patterns.

The first step was the decomposition of the water consumption time series into its components: trend, seasonal and remainder. STL [8] has already been successfully applied in studies of water consumption such as [18] and more recently [7]. Since STL is robust against outliers, the detection of these observations was done according to [8]. From Fig. 2, the robust approach of the STL was applied to **RH1** and **RH2**.

The `stl.fit()` proposed by [12] was applied, and the decomposition plots are shown in Fig. 3a and b. Note that this function searches for the best combination of the parameters (s.window and s.trend) minimising an error measure, which in this case

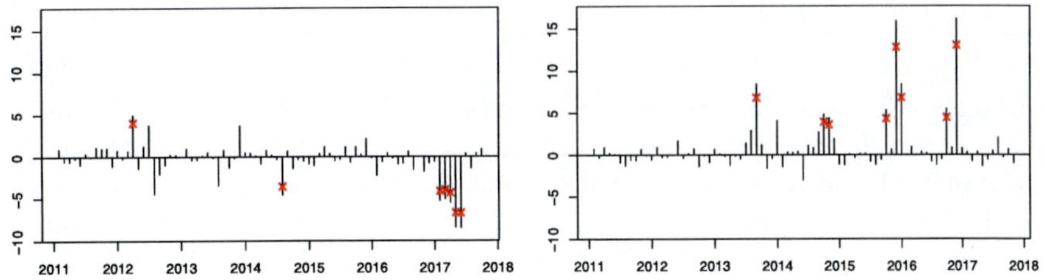

(a) RH1 (b) RH2

Fig. 2 Detecting outliers according to [8]

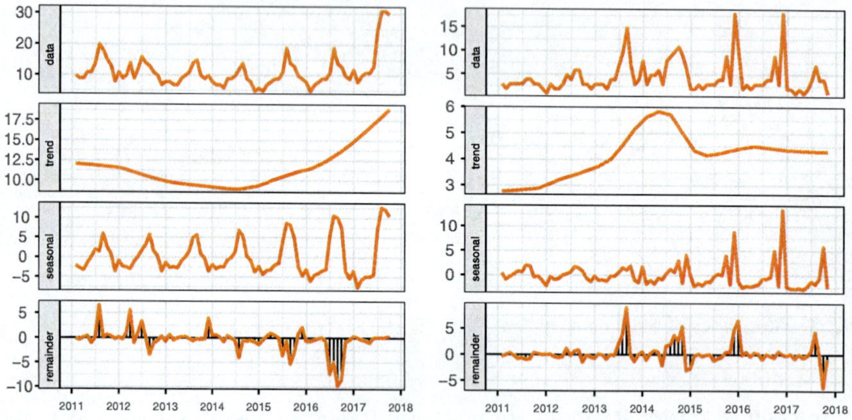

(a) RH1 (b) RH2

Fig. 3 Water consumption decomposition plots

Table 1 MAE results

RH	stl	stl.fit
1	1.33	1.25
2	1.57	1.09

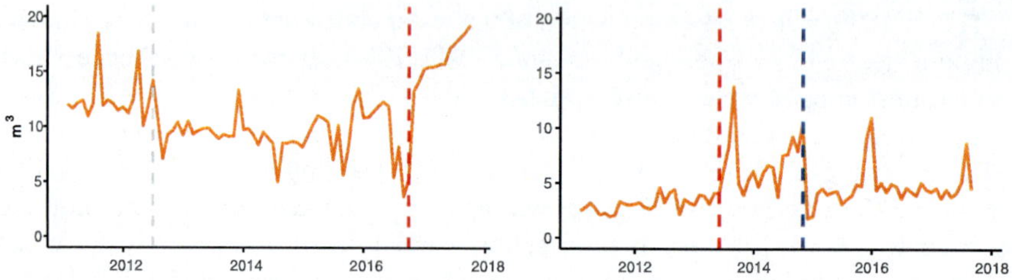

(a) RH1 (b) RH2

Fig. 4 Breakpoints analysis

was the MAE. Table 2 presents the results of the `stl()`, with s.window="periodic" (fixed seasonality), and the `stl.fit()` that search for the "best" combination, in terms of MAE. Therefore, based on these results, the latter was chosen (Table 1).

The breakpoint algorithm was applied to the seasonally adjusted water consumption, considering *min.h* = 0.15 (12.2 months) and *max.breaks* = 4. The relevance of each breakpoint was detected through MK and TS methods that infer the significance of the adjacent trends before and after the breakpoint.

For **RH1**, the procedure detected two breakpoints in water consumption in July 2012 and in October 2016 (Fig. 4a and Table 2). However, the estimated Theil–Sen's

Table 2 Breakpoints & Trend analysis

RH	Breakpoints	Theil–Sen's slopes			RMC
		Segment 1	Segment 2	Segment 3	
1	2012 (Jul), 2016 (Oct)	0.009 (0.880)	−0.016 (0.533)	**0.536 (<0.001)**	34.5
2	2013 (Jun), 2014 (Nov)	**0.052 (0.002)**	**0.236 (0.005)**	0.004 (0.744)	3.538, −0.983

Note 1 Statistically significant trend **slope (p-value)** in boldface
Note 2 All values are rounded with three decimal places

slopes of the segments, before and after the breakpoint in 2012, were not significant (p-values of 0.880 and 0.533, respectively). This means that the breakpoint was not considered as a relevant one by the procedure. Hence, the water utility should not be concerned with the pattern of water consumption of this household at that moment. Nonetheless, regarding the second breakpoint in October 2016, the segment slope estimated after it was positive (0.536) and statistically significant (p-value < 0.001). This represented an increased pattern in water consumption after that moment, with a magnitude RMC = 34.5.

Regarding **RH2**, the strategy implemented was able to detect two relevant breakpoints in June 2013 and November 2014 (Fig. 4b and Table 1). The estimated Theil–Sen's slope of the segment before the first breakpoint was positive with the low value of 0.052 (p-value = 0.0017), and the slope of the segment after the breakpoint was higher with the value of 0.236 (p-value = 0.0489). This represents an increase in water consumption pattern, with a magnitude of RMC = 3.538 (lower than the change in consumption of water meter **RH1**). In a deeper inspection, we can deduce that this result may be associated with a change in the mean value between the two periods (before and after the break). For the second breakpoint detected in November 2014, a decrease in water consumption was detected since the estimated segment slope before it was 0.236 and the estimated slope after the breakpoint was 0.004 and non-significant. Thus, the indicator RMC = –0.983, i.e. negative, as expected.

5 Conclusion

Trend and breakpoint analysis of water consumption—at an individual level—are important for decision-making in a broad sense, including in environmental, health and sustainability concerns.

This study presents an integrated statistical approach to analyse water consumption time series within the framework of water sustainability. The goal is to detect the moment (or moments) when a significant increase or decrease in consumption occurs.

Several studies have adopted time series decomposition and breakpoint detection methodologies, such as [7, 18–21]. The classical methods of decomposition of time series allow identifying the trend, the seasonality and the irregular components. However, these methodologies do not allow for a flexible specification of the seasonal component, and the trend component is generally represented by a deterministic time function, which is easily affected by the existence of outliers. The nonparametric Seasonal-Trend decomposition by Loess can identify a seasonal component that changes over time, a non-linear trend, and it can be robust in the presence of outliers. Similar to all nonparametric regression methods, STL requires the subjective selection of smoothing parameters. The two main parameters are the seasonal (*s.window*) and trend (*t.window*) window widths. Therefore, to overcome this limitation, the `stl.fit()` procedure [12] was used since it allows an "objective" choice of STL smoothing parameters. This procedure has been developed to obtain "automatically" the seasonal and trend smoothing parameters by minimising an error measure.

After estimating the components using STL, the seasonality was removed. Afterwards, a combination of methods was applied on the seasonally adjusted time series to detect breakpoints, using the algorithm implemented in the R package *strucchange* [14]. Subsequently, statistically significant decreasing and increasing segments of water consumption were analysed using robust nonparametric methods such as MK and TS.

Additionally, a water consumption change indicator, the RMC, was calculated. The RMC is unitless, allowing to compare different types of consumption. It allows the water utility to understand and compare consumption patterns between households (or other buildings) and between different periods. The water company can also choose threshold values for RMC, at which the consumption is considered problematic. Overall, the idea is to quantify the change of the decrease or increase in water consumption for each consumer and identify which ones the water company should investigate.

This strategy was applied to real data of billed water consumption from households located in the municipality of Loulé, characterised as an agriculturally based economy region with tourism activity. The methodology successfully detected breakpoints linked to a significant increase or decrease in water consumption. Moreover, the difference in household water consumption patterns justifies the importance of implementing a procedure at an individual level able to capture consumption specificities.

The detection of an abnormal increase will allow the water utility to alert its consumers of less environmentally sustainable behaviour. This is important since the impacts of climate change on water demand may be particularly relevant in the case of agricultural water use. In fact, the water needs for crop production increase as a consequence [6].

In conclusion, this integrated strategy may also contribute to the assessment of losses in water distribution systems as well as apparent losses and NRW. Furthermore, the application of the methodology is not limited to the time series of water consumption. The flexibility of the procedure allows, in each step, to regulate parameters such as the seasonal and trend windows in STL decomposition, the minimum length (*min.h*) of the segment and the maximum number of breaks (*max.breaks*).

In the future, an alternative approach could be a prior application of time series clustering on households' water consumption to group the consumers by pattern similarity. Afterwards, the proposed strategy would be implemented only to the most problematic consumer profiles.

Acknowledgements The authors are grateful to Loulé Municipality (http://www.cm-loule.pt), for providing the water consumption data and inside technical guidance. Ana Borges work has been supported by national funds through FCT—Fundação para a Ciência e Tecnologia through projects UIDB/04728/2020. Clara Cordeiro and M. Rosário Ramos are partially financed by national funds through FCT under the project UIDB/00006/2020.

References

1. Cámara, Á., Llop, M.: Defining sustainability in an input-output model: an application to spanish water use. Water **13**(1), 1 (2021)
2. Oviedo-Ocaña, E., Dominguez, I., Celis, J., Blanco, L., Cotes, I., et al.: Water-loss management under data scarcity: case study in a small municipality in a developing country. J. Water Resour. Plan. Man. **146**(3), 05020001 (2020)
3. Ioannou, A.E., Creaco, E.F., Laspidou, C.S.: Exploring the effectiveness of clustering algorithms for capturing water consumption behavior at household level. Sustainability **13**(5), 2603 (2021)
4. Abid, I., Khattak, H.A., Khan, R.W.A.: Water conservation and environmental sustainability approach. In: Collaboration and Integration in Construction, Engineering, Management and Technology, pp. 485–490. Springer, Berlin (2021)
5. Reynaud, A.: Modelling household water demand in Europe. Insights From a Cross-country Econometric Analysis of EU, vol. 28 (2015)
6. Ferreira, J.P.L., Vieira, J.M., et al.: Water in Celtic Countries: Quantity, Quality and Climate Variability. IAHS Press, Wallingford (2007)
7. Cordeiro, C., Borges, A., Ramos, M.R.: A strategy to assess water meter performance. J. Water Resour. Plan. Manag. **148**(2), 05021027 (2022)
8. Cleveland, R.B., Cleveland, W.S., McRae, J.E., Terpenning, I.: STL: a seasonal-trend decomposition. J. Off. Stat. **6**(1), 3–73 (1990)
9. Kendall, M.: Rank Correlation Methods. Griffin, London (1975)
10. Sen, P.K.: Estimates of the regression coefficient based on Kendall's tau. J. Amer. Stat. Assoc. **63**(324), 1379–1389 (1968)
11. R Core Team: R: A Language and Environment for Statistical Computing. R Foundation for Statistical Computing, Vienna, Austria (2021)
12. Cristina, S., Cordeiro, C., Lavender, S., Costa Goela, P., Icely, J., et al.: Meris phytoplankton time series products from the SW Iberian Peninsula (Sagres) using seasonal-trend decomposition based on loess. Remote Sens. **8**(6), 449 (2016)
13. Cordeiro, C.: `stl.fit()`: Function developed in Cristina et al. (2016)
14. Zeileis, A., Leisch, F., Hornik, K., Kleiber, C.: `strucchange`: an R package for testing for structural change in linear regression models. J. Stat. Softw. **7**(2), 1–38 (2002)
15. Zeileis, A., Kleiber, C., Krämer, W., Hornik, K.: Testing and dating of structural changes in practice. Comput. Stat. & Data Anal. **44**, 109–123 (2003)
16. Helsel, D.R., Hirsch, R.M.: Statistical Methods in Water Resources, vol. 323. US Geological Survey Reston, VA (2002)
17. Pohlert, T.: trend: Non-Parametric Trend Tests and Change-Point Detection (2020). R package version 1.1.4

18. Hester, C.M., Larson, K.L.: Time-series analysis of water demands in three North Carolina cities. J. Water Resour. Plan. Manag. **142**(8), 05016005 (2016)
19. Gelažanskas, L., Gamage, K.A.: Forecasting hot water consumption in residential houses. Energies **8**(11), 12702–12717 (2015)
20. Quesnel, K.J., Ajami, N.K.: Changes in water consumption linked to heavy news media coverage of extreme climatic events. Sci. Adv. **3**(10), e1700784 (2017)
21. Ohana-Levi, N., Munitz, S., Ben-Gal, A., Schwartz, A., Peeters, A., et al.: Multiseasonal grapevine water consumption-drivers and forecasting. Agric. For. Meteorol. **280**, 107796 (2020)

Modeling and Forecasting Wind Energy Production by Stochastic Differential Equations

Paulo Cabral and Paula Milheiro–Oliveira

Abstract Renewable energies are on the rise and their impact on the sustainability of our planet is consensual. Adequate tools for modeling and forecasting production from different sources are needed, so that management of energy resources is automatic and efficient. This work addresses this issue by a first modeling attempt of the wind power production in Continental Portugal using Stochastic Differential Equations (SDEs), based on available hourly observations. We resort to parametric SDE models proposed in the literature on wind energy research (the Ornstein–Uhlenbeck model and a transformed Ornstein–Uhlenbeck model), we estimate the model parameters, we perform the residual analysis and the short-term forecasting. We found that SDEs have produced useful results for the management of wind energy production. However, there would be an interest in evolving toward SDEs models that better explain the data in short periods of time, in order to obtain more reliable forecasts.

Keywords Ornstein–Uhlenbeck process · Parameter estimation · Predictive modeling · Renewable energy · Stochastic differential equations · Wind power

1 Introduction

Renewable energies have increased their relevance in the composition of the world's energy matrix. In particular, in Portugal, wind energy corresponds to 27.5% of total energy production, being the second largest energy source in the country [1]. The diversification of the energy matrix requires adequate tools for forecasting production from different sources, so that the management of energy resources is automatic and

P. Cabral (✉)
Faculty of Sciences and Center for Mathematics, University of Porto, Porto, Portugal
e-mail: paulo.cabral.anjos@gmail.com

P. Milheiro–Oliveira
Faculty of Engineering and Center for Mathematics, University of Porto, Porto, Portugal
e-mail: poliv@fe.up.pt

R. Bispo et al. (eds.), *Recent Developments in Statistics and Data Science*,
Springer Proceedings in Mathematics & Statistics 398,
https://doi.org/10.1007/978-3-031-12766-3_9

efficient. Wind energy presents a particular challenge in this context, as it is a highly complex phenomenon with possibly non-linear behavior and with high variability [2].

Advanced computational and statistical methods should be able to provide a complete description of predictive densities of energy production with forecast horizons from seconds to days [3]. Forecasts should desirably be obtained in such a way that they can be used in smart grids and therefore need to be computed in real time. Forecasting wind energy production remains a challenge even after 25 years of research, from a statistical point of view. This is mainly due to the non-linear and doubly limited nature of the stochastic process that describes the variation over time in the amount of wind energy produced [4]. We are referring to a phenomenon that suffers influences as varied as those resulting from the speed of the wind that passes through the turbine up to the amount of debris stuck to the propellers during its operation.

The literature contains a diversity of approaches to the problem of modeling and forecasting wind energy production [5, 6]. Among this previous research, [3, 7–9] approach the problem using Stochastic Differential Equations (SDEs). The advantage of the approach via SDEs lies in that, once the model is judged adequate, it is possible to fully describe the phenomenon, including the characterization of its variability, independently of the time scale or the frequency of the collected observations, meeting state-of-the-art requirements.

This work discusses a first attempt at modeling the energy production of the wind turbines placed in continental Portugal using SDEs, based on available hourly observations. With this goal, we resort to parametric models of SDEs proposed in the literature of wind energy research, namely, the Ornstein–Uhlenbeck (O-U) model and a transformed Ornstein–Uhlenbeck model [9], we perform the estimation of the model parameters, the residual analysis, and the short-term forecasting. By short term we mean either the 24 or the 48 h ahead forecast. We find that tested SDEs produce useful results for the management of continental Portugal wind energy production. However, additional research addressing other alternative SDE models that would better explain data over short time periods would be recommended in order to try achieve more reliable forecasts.

The paper is organized as follows: in Sect. 2 we introduce the problem under study; in Sect. 3 we explore different SDE models that could fit the available data; in Sect. 4 we compare solutions to the problem under study by computing the 1 h, the 24 h, and the 48 h ahead forecasts of the hourly wind energy production in Continental Portugal. This is our main contribution to the subject. Finally, in Sect. 5 we present some final comments and main directions for future research.

2 The Problem Under Study

The amount of wind energy produced in Continental Portugal exhibits variability along time (see Fig. 1) and models representing its behavior, which can subsequently be used to derive good quality predictions of future values of wind energy production,

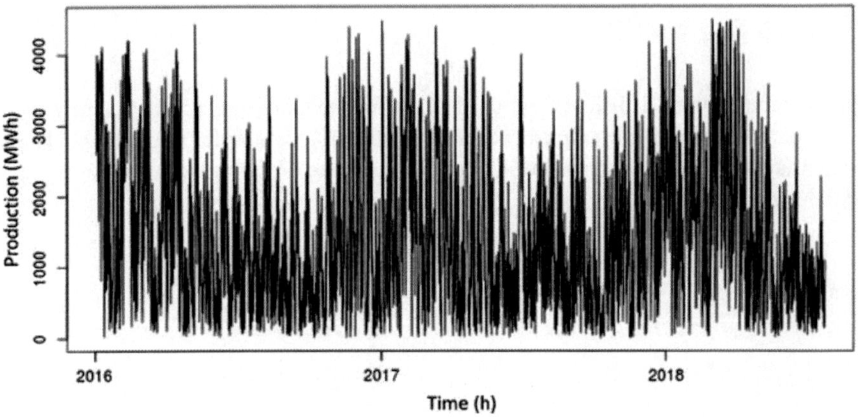

Fig. 1 Wind energy produced in Continental Portugal from January 3, 2016 until July 25, 2018

are needed. It is our intention to consider particular classes of SDEs to represent the dynamics of the wind energy production along time.

The problem under study can be formulated as follows. Let $\{\Omega, \mathcal{F}, \mathbf{P}\}$ be a probability space and $\{X_t\}_t$, with $t \geq 0$, a stochastic process representing the wind energy production along time. We assume that $\{X_t\}_t$ is the solution of a SDE

$$dX_t = b(t, X_t, \theta)dt + \sigma(t, X_t, \theta)dW_t, \tag{1}$$

where $\{W_t\}_t$ is a standard Wiener process and $X_0 = x_0$ represents the initial condition, in our case assumed known for simplification. Assume that $\{X_t\}_t$ is observed at discrete time instants $t_0, t_1, t_2, \ldots, t_n$ until time T. Denote by $\mathcal{F}_{t'}$ the σ-algebra of the observations until time $t' \in [0, T]$. Our goal is twofold:

- fit a parametric model of type (1) in which the families of functions $b(\cdot)$ and $\sigma(\cdot)$ are assumed to be known except for the dependency on a vector θ of unknown parameters, with $\theta \in \Theta$. We will use different models, that is, different forms of $b(\cdot)$ and $\sigma(\cdot)$, and we will estimate the parameters based on the available observations $\{X_{t_i}\}_{i=0}^n$;
- forecast the amount of energy produced by the set of wind turbines, that is, for the stochastic process $\{X_t\}_t$ with $t \geq T$, based on the values available up to time T.

In our case, we consider the data collected on the wind energy produced from January 3, 2016 until July 25, 2018. We separate the collected data in a training set consisting on the observations from January 3, 2016 until January 16, 2018, and a test set consisting on the observations from there on until July 25, 2018. The training set will be used to fit the SDE and the remaining data will be used to assess forecasting capability. Data has been hourly collected and our goal is to compute short horizon forecasts that could go from 1 to 48 h horizons.

3 Modeling via SDEs

The literature suggests different types of SDEs for the modeling of wind energy production: the Ornstein–Uhlenbeck process [10]; the Black–Scholes equation [11] and some transformation of a Ornstein–Uhlenbeck process [9]. We give a brief overview of the main points that are needed in the sequel.

Ornstein–Uhlenbeck process:

$$dX_t = \omega X_t dt + \nu dW_t \tag{2}$$

with $\omega \in \mathbb{R}$ and $\nu \in \mathbb{R}_+$.

We remind that the solution of (2) is a Gaussian process and one can easily write closed formulas for the conditional moments:

$$\mathbb{E}[X_t|\mathcal{F}_{t'}] = X_{t'} e^{\omega(t-t')} \tag{3a}$$

and

$$\mathbb{V}[X_t|\mathcal{F}_{t'}] = \frac{\nu^2}{2\omega}(e^{2\omega(t-t')} - 1)\,. \tag{3b}$$

An extension $dX_t = \omega(X_t - \lambda)dt + \nu dW_t$, with λ being an extra parameter, can also be considered.

Black–Scholes model:

$$dX_t = \theta_1 X_t dt + \theta_2 X_t dW_t \tag{4}$$

with $\theta_1 \in \mathbb{R}$, $\theta_2 \in \mathbb{R}_+$ and $X_0 = x_0 > 0$.

Closed formulas for the conditional moments of $Z_t = \ln\left(\frac{X_t}{x_0}\right)$ exist as well:

$$\mathbb{E}[Z_t|\mathcal{F}_{t'}] = Z_{t'} + \left(\theta_1 - \frac{\theta_2^2}{2}\right)(t - t') \tag{5a}$$

and

$$\mathbb{V}[Z_t|\mathcal{F}_{t'}] = \theta_2^2(t - t')\,. \tag{5b}$$

Also

$$X_t|\mathcal{F}_{t'} \sim Log\mathcal{N}\left(x_{t'} e^{\theta_1(t-t')},\quad x_{t'}^2 e^{2\theta_1(t-t')}(e^{\theta_2^2(t-t')} - 1)\right), \tag{5c}$$

where we have indicated, in parenthesis, the conditional mean and variance of this lognormal distribution.

Transformed Ornstein–Uhlenbeck process [9]:

$$dX_t = \left(\omega \ln(X_t) - \omega h + \frac{\nu^2}{2}\right) X_t dt + \nu X_t dW_t \,. \tag{6}$$

This means that

$$X_t = e^{U_t + h}, \tag{7}$$

where h is a parameter of the model which should guarantee that the paths remain close to the average of the observations, and $\{U_t\}_t$ is a Ornstein–Uhlenbeck process with parameters ω and ν.

Again closed formulas for the conditional moments can be derived by using the well-known expression for the expected value of an exponential of a Gaussian distribution:

$$\mathbb{E}[X_t|\mathcal{F}_{t'}] = \exp\left\{h + \mathbb{E}[U_t|\mathcal{F}_{t'}] + \frac{\mathbb{V}[U_t|\mathcal{F}_{t'}]}{2}\right\} \tag{8a}$$

and

$$\mathbb{V}[X_t|\mathcal{F}_{t'}] = \exp\{2h + 2\mathbb{E}[U_t|\mathcal{F}_{t'}] + \mathbb{V}[U_t|\mathcal{F}_{t'}]\} \left(\exp\{\mathbb{V}[U_t|\mathcal{F}_{t'}]\} - 1\right) \,. \tag{8b}$$

For a detailed reading on SDE modeling in general we refer to, e.g., [12–15].

3.1 Parameter Estimation

In this study, the available data consists on hourly observations of wind energy production. Therefore, the time unit will be from now on equal to 1 hour and the convention that zero will be the initial time (with known $X_0 = x_0$) is adopted, so that $t_i = i$. The wind energy production X will be expressed in MWh. Parameter estimates and other results reported in the present paper use these units of time and energy production.

The ML estimators of the previous models' parameters are consistent and normally distributed as $n \to \infty$ (e.g., [12, 15–17]). For model (2) one has

$$\hat{\omega}_n = \ln\left(\frac{\sum_{i=1}^{n} X_{i-1} X_i}{\sum_{i=1}^{n} X_{i-1}^2}\right) \tag{9a}$$

$$\hat{\nu}_n^2 = \frac{2\hat{\omega}_n}{n(e^{2\hat{\omega}_n} - 1)} \sum_{i=1}^{n} \left(X_i - X_{i-1} e^{\hat{\omega}_n}\right)^2 \,. \tag{9b}$$

Table 1 ML estimates of the model parameters

Model	Parameter estimates	Confidence interval (95%)
Model (2)	$\hat{\omega} = -0,0041$	(−0.0054; −0.0028)
	$\hat{\nu} = 154.48$	(152.89; 156.10)
Model (4)	$\hat{\theta}_1 = 0.0170$	(0.0143; 0.0197)
	$\hat{\theta}_2 = 0.1847$	(0.1828; 0.1866)
Model (6)	$\hat{\omega} = -0.0195$	(−0.0224; −0.0166)
	$\hat{\nu} = 0.1856$	(0.1837; 0.1876)

For model (4), denoting $\theta^* = \theta_1 - \frac{\theta_2^2}{2}$, one has

$$\hat{\theta}_n^* = \frac{1}{n}\sum_{i=1}^{n} \ln\left(\frac{X_i}{X_{i-1}}\right) \tag{10a}$$

$$\hat{\theta}_{2,n} = \frac{1}{n}\sum_{i=1}^{n}\left(\ln\left(\frac{X_i}{X_{i-1}}\right) - \hat{\theta}_n^*\right)^2 . \tag{10b}$$

For model (6), the transformation (7) is combined with (9a)–(9b), meaning that, since the process $\{X_t\}_t$ is transformed into process $\{U_t\}_t$ and $\{U_t\}_t$ is a Ornstein–Uhlenbeck process, the tools used with model (2) are also used on the transformed data. The value 6.908 has been used for h in (7). This corresponds to taking

$$\hat{h} = \frac{1}{n}\sum_{i=1}^{n} \ln X_i ,$$

given that $h = E[\ln X_t - U_t] = E[\ln X_t]$ (see [9]). Computation of the ML estimates and confidence intervals can be performed resorting to functions *mle* and *confint* available in the *R software*.

Table 1 shows the estimates of the model parameters for the models mentioned above. The extra parameter λ of the extended O-U process was dropped as it was not significant.

3.2 *Analysis of the Residuals*

Denoting by $\mathbb{E}[\cdot]$ and $\mathbb{V}[\cdot]$ as usual the expected value and variance, respectively, we analyze the standardized residuals [18]:

$$R_{t_i}(\theta) = \frac{x_{t_i} - \mathbb{E}[X_{t_i}|X_{t_{i-1}};\theta]}{\sqrt{\mathbb{V}[X_{t_i}|X_{t_{i-1}};\theta]}} . \tag{11}$$

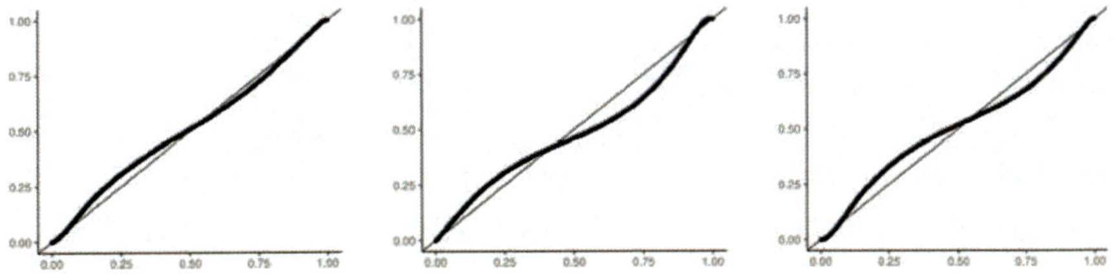

(a) model (2) (b) model (4) (c) model (6)

Fig. 2 *QQ-plot* of the standardized residuals

Since we do not know the true parameter values we estimate the residuals R_{t_i} by replacing the parameters by their ML estimates. In the case of models (4) and (6), we analyze the residuals of the Z_{t_i} and U_{t_i} predictions, respectively, instead of the X_{t_i} predictions. If the model fits the data, residuals should behave as Gaussian white noise.

The residuals have been analyzed for their concentration on the band $[-2, 2]$, their auto-correlation as well as their normality. Although statistical testing (Ljung-Box and significance of ACF and PACF) leads to the rejection of the assumptions underlying Gaussian white noise for the behavior of the residuals, we should remark that the data set contains more than 10,000 observations, thus the emphasis of analyzing the conformity of the residuals should not be placed on the strict violation of white noise model assumptions but rather on the degree of violation that can disrupt the good functioning, for the purpose of forecasting, of a statistical model that requires standard Gaussian white noise. The QQ-plots of the residuals are depicted in Fig. 2. We consider that model (4) does not fit the data well. Therefore this model will not be used for prediction.

4 Forecasting

Generally speaking, once model (1) has been fitted, the optimal predictor in terms of the root mean square error RMSE is given by

$$\hat{X}_{t|T} = \mathbb{E}[X_t|\mathcal{F}_T] \text{ for } t \geq T\,. \tag{12}$$

In the Gaussian case, one can also determine the approximate prediction interval for a 95% confidence level:

$$\hat{X}_{t|T} \pm 1.96\sqrt{\mathbb{V}[X_t|\mathcal{F}_T](1+\tau/T)} \tag{13}$$

with $\tau = t - T$. Since $\mathbb{V}[X_t|\mathcal{F}_T]$ is not known but the number of observations used to estimate the model is very large, in our problem the conditional variance has been

Table 2 1, 24, and 48 h ahead predictors

Model	Predictor ($\hat{\mu}_{t_i} = \hat{\mathbb{E}}[X_{t_i} \| \mathcal{F}_{t_{i-1}}]$)		
	1 h	24 h	48 h
Model (2)	$\hat{\mu}_{t_i} = x_{t_{i-1}} e^{-0.0041}$	$\hat{\mu}_{t_i} = x_{t_{i-1}} e^{-0.0981}$	$\hat{\mu}_{t_i} = x_{t_{i-1}} e^{-0.1962}$
Nodel (6)	$\hat{\mu}_{t_i} = 1017.8\, e^{0.9807\, u_{t_{i-1}}}$	$\hat{\mu}_{t_i} = 1308.8\, e^{0.6260\, u_{t_{i-1}}}$	$\hat{\mu}_{t_i} = 1454.0\, e^{0.3919\, u_{t_{i-1}}}$

replaced by its estimate. In the case of model (6), this expression (13) is used for the process U_t instead. Based on this model it is reasonable to compute an approximation of the prediction interval for X_t by applying transformation (7) to the bounds of the prediction interval for U_t.

Table 2 shows the expressions of the predictors of the selected models (2) and (6), for three different forecast horizons of interest. They stem from (3a) and (8a), which allow us to anticipate the expected behavior of predictors according to their analytic expression.

Figures 3, 4, 5 show the forecasts that were obtained for the first 480 h (20 d) of the test set.

Because $\hat{\omega} = -0.0041$ is small, we have that $e^{\hat{\omega}} \approx 1$ and the O-U process approaches a *martingale*. As a result, the obtained 1 h ahead forecasts closely follow the observed series (slight horizontal translation; see Fig. 3).

As an example, Table 3 presents the 95% confidence intervals for the 1 h ahead forecasts relative to January 17, 2018 at 12:00 a.m.

The forecast produced by model (2) appears to be closer to the test set trajectory. However, forecasts are still not able to follow the data when rapid ascents occur. This holds for the 24 h as well as for the 48 h ahead forecasts (Figs. 4 and 5). The results obtained with model (4) are also shown in Fig. 5 as a curiosity.

The following measures have been used to assess the error when producing forecasts:

$$MPE = \left(\frac{1}{m} \sum_{i=1}^{m} \frac{x_i - \hat{x}_i}{x_i} \right), \tag{14a}$$

$$MAPE = \left(\frac{1}{m} \sum_{i=1}^{m} \frac{|x_i - \hat{x}_i|}{|x_i|} \right), \tag{14b}$$

$$RMSE = \sqrt{\frac{1}{m} \sum_{i=1}^{m} (x_i - \hat{x}_i)^2}, \tag{14c}$$

where x_i denotes the ith observation after time T, m the forecasting horizon, and $\hat{x}_i$ the ith forecast. Table 4 presents the forecast errors obtained on the test set.

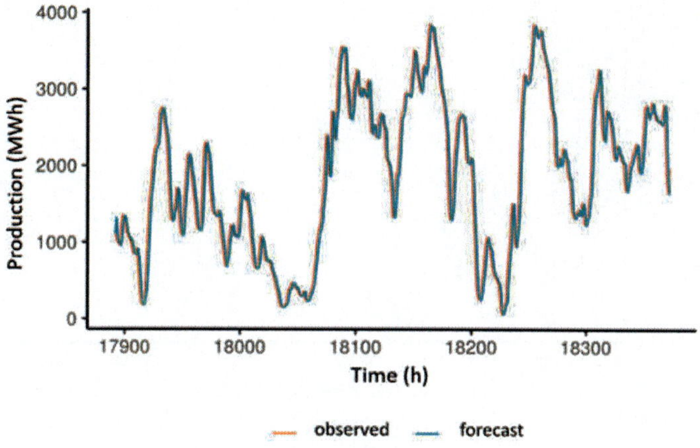

(a) model (2)

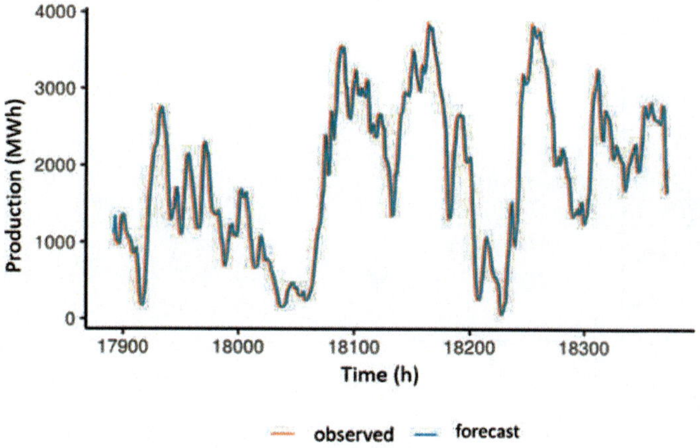

(b) model (6)

Fig. 3 1 h ahead forecasts for the first 480 h of the test set

Table 3 95% confidence intervals for the 1 h ahead forecasts relative to January 17, 2018 at 12:00 a.m.

Model	Forecast (MWh)	Prediction interval (MWh)
Model (2)	1313.69	(1011.52 ; 1615.87)
Model (6)	1334.41	(0.00 ; 2769.19)

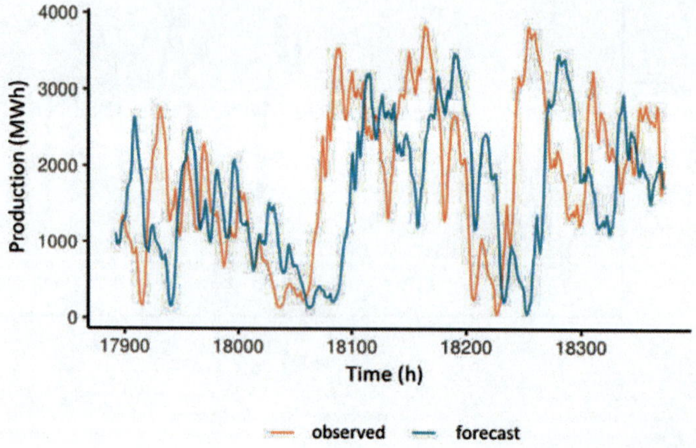

(a) model (2)

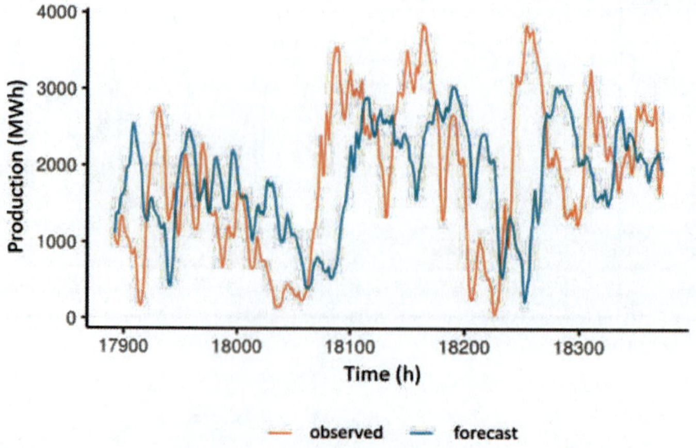

(b) model (6)

Fig. 4 24 h ahead forecasts for the first 480 h of the test set

From a statistical point of view, model (2), despite fitting the training set quite well, does not have a high predictive capability for 48 h horizons, as shown in our test set. Model (6) gives even worst results. However, from the engineering point of view, these results are still useful. It is also interesting to note that the forecast errors are in line with the quality of the residuals when we talk about the comparison between models fit.

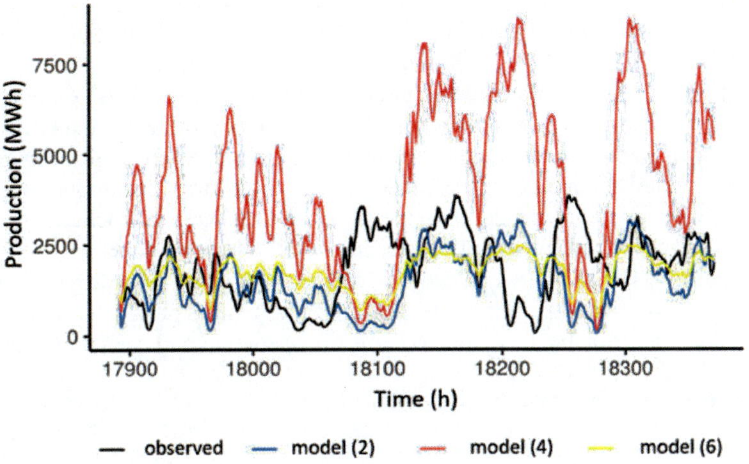

Fig. 5 48 h ahead forecasts for the first 480 h of the test set

Table 4 Forecast errors computed on the test set

Model	Prediction horizon (h)	*MAPE* (%)	*MPE* (%)	*RMSE*
Model (2)	1 h	23.7	−5.1	297.9
	24	91.0	−43.8	1023.0
	48	102.7	−45.7	1147.1
Model (6)	1 h	24.2	−7.1	297.2
	24	115.9	−89.2	947.9
	48	145.3	−120.1	1011.9

5 Final Comments

From the family of models that were examined, model (2) was the one that best fitted the data. In addition, according to most commonly used forecast error metrics, model (2) was also the model which gave the closest forecasts to the test set.

Assessing the predictive capacity of the models for the most relevant forecast horizons, 24 h ahead and specially 48 h ahead, all models showed large forecast errors, which reflects the high complexity of the task of predicting the phenomenon. Although the obtained forecasts have low precision they are still of use for engineering and management purposes. The results suggest that we should evolve toward more complex models which would be more likely to describe the inherent complexity. The fact that we are trying to model and predict the total production of Continental Portugal, encompassing individual productions subject to different climate and operational conditions, deserves further attention. If data could be made available on each wind tower or at least on each of the existing wind farms, the modeling and prediction of each of those and its contribution to predicting the total production would give a better solution to the problem at hand.

There are a couple of immediate directions for future work. The first is to seek better forecasts for hourly wind energy production based on non-parametric EDE models which can better adapt to the behavior of the observed data, allowing greater adherence to sudden ascents or descents (see, e.g., [14] for an introduction). The second is to incorporate wind data into the model as an exogenous stochastic process. Also it would be interesting to apply the techniques developed in this work to different time scales (and horizons). All approaches can be enriched by comparing these with other forecasting methods, such as classic time series models or other computational tools of *machine learning* as, for instance, *neural networks* and *random forests*.

Acknowledgements This research was partially supported by CMUP (UID/MAT/00144/2019) funded by FCT (Pt) with National and European structural funds through FEDER, under partnership agreement PT2020, and by project STRIDE (NORTE-01-0145-FEDER-000033) supported by NORTE2020. The authors are very grateful to Professor Dr. Eng. Cláudio Monteiro (University of Porto, FEUP) for his suggestions, for giving the authors access to the data and details of the problem under study. The authors are very grateful to reviewer 1 for his/her anonymous contribution to improve the paper.

References

1. APREN (2020). https://www.apren.pt/pt/energias-renovaveis/producao. Accessed 26 Oct 2020
2. Giebel, G., Brownsword, R., Kariniotakis, G., Denhard, M., Draxl, C.: The state-of-the-art in short-term prediction of wind power: a literature overview. Technical Report NEI-DK-5521 (2011)
3. Iversen, E.B., Morales, J.M., Møller, J.K., Madsen, H.: Short-term probabilistic forecasting of wind speed using stochastic differential equations. Int. J. Forecast. **32**(3), 981–990 (2016)
4. Pinson, P.: Very-short-term probabilistic forecasting of wind power with generalized logit-normal distributions. J. R. Stat. Soc. Ser. C **61**(4), 555–576 (2012)
5. Pinson, P., Madsen, H., Nielsen, H.A., Papaefthymiou, G., Klöckl, B.: From probabilistic forecasts to statistical scenarios of short-term wind power production. Wind. Energy: Int. J. Prog. Appl. Wind. Power Convers. Technol. **12**(1), 51–62 (2009)
6. Talari, S., Shafie-Khah, M., Osório, G.J., Aghaei, J., Catalão, J.P.: Stochastic modelling of renewable energy sources from operators' point-of-view: a survey. Renew. Sustain. Energy Rev. **81**, 1953–1965 (2018)
7. Møller, J.K., Zugno, M., Madsen, H.: Probabilistic forecasts of wind power generation by stochastic differential equation models. J. Forecast. **35**(3), 189–205 (2016)
8. Verdejo, H., Awerkin, A., Saavedra, E., Kliemann, W., Vargas, L.: Stochastic modeling to represent wind power generation and demand in electric power system based on real data. Appl. Energy **173**, 283–295 (2016)
9. Verdejo, H., Awerkin, A., Kliemann, W., Becker, C.: Modelling uncertainties in electrical power systems with stochastic differential equations. Int. J. Electr. Power Energy Syst. **113**, 322–332 (2019)
10. Ornstein, L.S., Uhlenbeck, G.E.: On the theory of the Brownian motion. Phys. Rev. **36**, 823–841 (1930). Sep
11. Black, F., Scholes, M.: The pricing of options and corporate liabilities. J. Polit. Econ. **81**(3), 637–54 (1973)

12. Iacus, S.M.: Simulation and Inference for Stochastic Differential Equations: With R Examples. Springer, New York (2009)
13. Kutoyants, Y.A.: Statistical Inference for Ergodic Diffusion Processes. Springer, New York (2013)
14. Kessler, M., Lindner, A., Sorensen, M.: Statistical Methods for Stochastic Differential Equations. Chapman and Hall/CRC, Boca Raton, FL (2019)
15. Braumann, C.A.: Introduction to Stochastic Differential Equations with Applications to Modelling in Biology and Finance. Wiley, New York (2019)
16. Pedersen, A.R.: A new approach to maximum likelihood estimation for stochastic differential equations based on discrete observations. Scand. J. Stat. **22**(1), 55–71 (1995)
17. Sorensen, H.: Parametric inference for diffusion processes observed at discrete points in time: a survey. Int. Stat. Rev. **72**(3), 337–354 (2004)
18. Pedersen, A.R.: Uniform residuals for discretely observed diffusion processes. Technical Report, vol. 292. Department of Theoretical Statistics, University of Aarhus (1994)

Intensity-Dependent Point Processes

Andreia Monteiro, Maria Lucília Carvalho, Ivone Figueiredo, Paula Simões, and Isabel Natário

Abstract A practical and theoretically interesting problem in the context of point processes are marked point patterns where the statistical properties of marks depend locally on point intensity. Such dependence can be observed, for example, in fishery data, where catches (marks) are certainly associated with the locations where the fisheries take place (points), in order to optimize capture effort. In intensity-marked point processes, the marks are allowed to be marginally correlated and the mark size depends locally on the point density. In this work, we analyse the relationship between these models and the geostatistical model under preferential sampling. Detecting dependence between marks and locations of marked point processes is an important issue because predictions of the process can be severely biased when standard statistical methodologies are applied to data where the distribution of a mark varies along the point density. The aforementioned relationship was explored in real data.

Keywords Log-Gaussian Cox process · Marked point process · Preferential sampling

A. Monteiro (✉) · P. Simões · I. Natário
NOVA MATH – Center for Mathematics and Applications (CMA), NOVA University of Lisbon, Lisbon, Portugal
e-mail: andreiaforte50@gmail.com

M. L. Carvalho · I. Figueiredo
Centre of Statistics and its Applications (CEAUL), Faculty of Sciences of the University of Lisbon, Lisbon, Portugal

I. Figueiredo
Portuguese Institute for Sea and Atmosphere (IPMA), Lisbon, Portugal

P. Simões
Military Academy Research Center - Military University Institute (CINAMIL), Lisbon, Portugal

I. Natário
Department of Mathematics, NOVA School of Science and Technology, Caparica, Portugal

R. Bispo et al. (eds.), *Recent Developments in Statistics and Data Science*, Springer Proceedings in Mathematics & Statistics 398,
https://doi.org/10.1007/978-3-031-12766-3_10

1 Introduction

Traditional geostatistical methods assume that sampling locations are either fixed or stochastically independent of the spatially continuous phenomenon under study. However, in practice, choice of sampling positions in a spatial network is often guided by budget and other practical requirements. For example, it is well known that in air pollution studies the monitors are, typically, placed near the most likely pollution sources and in areas of higher population density. In fisheries, where data are observed when and where the resource is available, this means sampling in locations that were deliberately chosen guided by a belief regarding the abundance of the species of interest. Thus, the aforementioned assumption fails since the process under study determines data locations. This problem, coined preferential sampling in the context of spatial statistics, has been discussed in a model-based approach by [1]. Diggle and co-authors demonstrate that ignoring the preferential nature of the sampling can lead to biased estimates and misleading inferences.

Watson [2] claims that predictions of the process can be severely biased when standard statistical methodologies are applied to preferentially sampled data without adjustment. Preferential sampling of sites chosen to observe a spatial process has been identified as a major problem in several fields. In species richness studies, preferential sampling may occur due to data being comprised of opportunistic sightings. Observers frequently focus their efforts in areas where they expect to find the species, [2]. Conn and colleagues [3] use geostatistical methods to model ecological data obtained by preferential sampling, referring to a special case of opportunistic sampling in which there is stochastic dependence between the sampling design and the reported species counts. Pennino and colleagues [4] present an approach for modelling the distribution of species using opportunistic data and show that predictive maps significantly improve the prediction of the target species when the model accounts for preferential sampling.

Geostatistical model [5], can be regarded from the perspective of a marked point process [6], modelling the marks the observed quantities and the points the sampling locations. In this context, Illian and colleagues [7] consider three types of models: Independent marks, which may be regarded as a null model, where the marks are drawn independently from a probability distribution; random field model, where the marks are correlated, meaning that marks of points close together are typically similar; however, there is no correlation between marks and points density. This is termed geostatistical marking. The third type is marked Cox process, the case where the marks depend linearly on local point density. Therefore, a practically and theoretically interesting problem are marked point patterns where the statistical properties of marks depend locally on point intensity. Myllymäki [8] considered a log-intensity marked Cox process to deal with intensity-dependent marks. Myllymäki [9] extend the family of intensity-dependent marked processes considering conditionally heteroscedastic intensity-dependent markings, meaning that not only the mean but also the variance of a mark depends on the local intensity.

In this work, we analyse and compare the model proposed by [1] to deal with preferential sampling in the context of Geostatistics and the model proposed by [8] to deal with intensity-dependent marks in the context of marked point processes.

For modelling preferential sampling directly, it is common to take a model-based approach, within a joint model framework for the observation process and sampling process. Due to the computational challenges of fitting joint models, detecting preferential sampling or dependence between marks and points is, therefore, an important issue. When there are covariates available, it is possible that when they are explicitly included in the model they are sufficient to account for this relationship between points and marks. The discovery of these covariates may justify the continued use of standard methodologies [10]. As such, it is also important to find this set of informative covariates.

In this study, we present a test proposed by [11] to detect preferential sampling and identify informative covariates that correct preferential sampling and compare it with another test proposed by [12] to analyse the independence of marks and points.

The paper is organized as follows. In Sect. 2, we analyse and compare the model for preferential sampling in Geostatistics and the model for intensity-dependent marks in marked point processes. Section 3 is dedicated to the presentation of two tests to detect the existence of preferential sampling. In Sect. 4, we show the application of the previously described tests to a real dataset provided by the Instituto Português do Mar e da Atmosfera (IPMA) which corresponds to the black scabbardfish catches in the fishing grounds of the south zone of Portugal, from 2009 to 2013. Section 5 is devoted to draw some conclusions and directions for future work.

2 Intensity-Dependent Processes

In this section, we present the models proposed by [1, 8] to deal with the situation where there is stochastic dependence between the spatial process under study and the sampling locations where it is observed. In addition, we analyse the relationship that exists between these two models.

2.1 Geostatistical Model for Preferential Sampling

Diggle and colleagues [1] developed a model for geostatistical data collected in a preferential way, where sampling locations and observations are jointly modelled depending on a common unobserved random field. The sampling points and the observations can also be considered as a marked point pattern [9].

The model for point locations is a log-Gaussian Cox process with intensity

$$\Lambda(x_i) = \exp\{\alpha + \beta S(x_i)\} \tag{1}$$

where S is a stationary Gaussian Process with mean μ_s and variance σ_s^2 and β controls the degree of preferentiality, the case $\beta = 0$ corresponds to a homogeneous Poisson process with intensity $\exp(\alpha)$.

A model for the data takes the following form:

$$Y(x_i) = S(x_i) + W_i \tag{2}$$

where $Y(x_i)$ denotes the measured value at the location x_i and W_i is a Gaussian random error with mean 0, variance τ^2 and $i = 1 \cdots n$, where n is the number of locations.

Diggle and colleagues [1] suggest a modelling approach that accounts for preferential sampling using likelihood-based inference with Monte Carlo methods but Bayesian inference based on an SPDE-INLA approach has more recently been used [13].

2.2 Log-Intensity Marked Cox Processes

In the context of marked point processes, [8] considered a log-intensity marked Cox process, in which point density and mark sizes are closely coupled.

The simple point pattern is a log-Gaussian Cox process with intensity

$$\Lambda(x_i) = \exp\{S(x_i)\}$$

Conditional on $\Lambda(x_i)$, the marks are provided by

$$Y(x_i) = a + bS(x_i) + W_i \tag{3}$$

where a and b are model parameters.

If $b < 0$, then the marks are small in regions of high point density, while positive b yields large marks in regions with high intensity.

2.3 Geostatistical Model for Preferential Sampling Versus Log-Intensity Marked Cox Processes

The geostatistical model presented in Sect. 2.1 equals the marks of the log-intensity marked Cox process up to parametrization with respect to the intensity of the point process. Indeed, the marks (2) can be rewritten as

$$Y(x_i) = -\frac{\alpha}{\beta} + \frac{1}{\beta}\log(\Lambda(x_i)) + W_i \tag{4}$$

with $\beta = \frac{1}{b}$, $\alpha = -\frac{a}{b}$ and $\Lambda(x_i)$ is given by (1).

The parameterization is a matter of interpretation of the model. In the geostatistical model, the interest is in the random field $S(x)$, while in the log-intensity marked Cox process model, the interest is in the mark. Parameter β controls the degree of preferentiality; if $\beta > 0$, this means that more sampling locations are collected in areas, where $S(x)$ is expected to get higher values. In analysing marked point patterns, $\beta > 0$ means that marks are larger in areas with high point density. Thus, in the geostatistical model, β can be interpreted similarly as b in the log-intensity marked Cox process. The importance of this relationship for this work is that it allows the use of methodologies developed in the context of point processes for the analysis of preferential sampling.

3 Test to Detect Preferential Sampling or Intensity-Dependent Marks

Not taking preferential sampling into account whenever it is present leads to biased results. As such, the application of a test that allows to identify its existence becomes of primordial importance in the analysis to be carried out.

3.1 Nearest Neighbour Test

Watson [11] developed a general test for the presence of preferential sampling. He uses the nearest neighbour distances (or averaged K-nearest neighbour distances for some chosen integer K) between points as a way to measure the local degree of clustering. In case of preferential sampling, a significant correlation should exist between the nearest neighbour distances and the observed response values at each of sampled locations. He computes Spearman's rank correlation coefficient between estimates of $S(x)$ at observed locations and the mean nearest neighbour distances. The method primarily requires that one is able to predict the values of $S(x)$, [2]. Preferential sampling often appears as a spatial clustering of locations chosen to observe and this test directly targets this excess clustering. A point process is fitted to the observed locations to capture the true sampling process under the null hypothesis of no preferential sampling. Then, Monte Carlo realizations of the point process under the null hypothesis are generated and an empirical p-value associated with any desired test statistic can be computed. If a stronger correlation is observed in the real data compared with the Monte Carlo samples, then evidence for preferential sampling has been found. The ranked nearest neighbour distances between the sampling locations provide a way to measure the local magnitude of clustering, [2].

A set of covariates can condition the choice of sampling locations, and these covariates can also be associated with the underlying process being modelled. When this occurs, the inclusion of the necessary covariates in the model can partially remove the effects of the preferential sampling [10]. The test can also be adjusted for covariates, allowing researchers to discover whether a given covariate is sufficient to control preferential sampling.

The nearest neighbour test can be used when the responses (marks) are non-Gaussian and even non-continuous and is available on the R package PStestR. For the algorithm and more details about the test, see [10].

3.2 Schlather Test

The independence of marks and points can be tested as suggested by [12]. They developed two Monte Carlo tests and their null hypothesis assumes that the data locations are a realization of a point process, the marks of the points are the values of a realization of a random field and they are independent processes.

To detect deviations from the null hypothesis, the authors define two characteristics of marked point processes, denoted $E(r)$ and $V(r)$. These represent respectively the conditional expectation and conditional variance of a mark, given that there exists another point of the process at a distance r. Under the null hypothesis, E and V should be constant. This approach requires the assumption of Gaussian observations and does not generalize to non-continuous marks. To assess deviations of E and V from constant function in this paper, we will use Envelope Tests. A brief description of envelope tests and global envelope tests is presented in the next subsection.

3.3 Envelope Tests

Envelope tests, proposed by [14], are Monte Carlo significance tests [15], based on some summary function $F(r)$, where r denotes distance. It is a common situation that distribution of $F(r)$ is unknown, and the use of Monte Carlo simulations is the only way to test a hypothesis [16].

The simulation envelope method works as follows. First, simulate s marked point patterns independently according to the null hypothesis of independence. Then, calculate $\hat{F}(r)$ for each simulated marked point pattern. Among the summary functions $\hat{F}_2(r), \cdots, \hat{F}_{s+1}(r)$ obtained, the kth largest and smallest $\hat{F}_i(r)$ for each r in some range of scales $[r_{min}, r_{max}]$ are taken to form the upper $F_{up}(r)$ and lower $F_{low}(r)$ envelopes. If the summary function $\hat{F}_1(r)$ obtained for the data is not completely between the envelopes, there is evidence against the null hypothesis.

However, the type I error probability is high, and this is related to the so-called multiple testing problem [17], because, in the envelope test, the null hypothesis is tested simultaneously for many distances r. Increasing the number of simulations from which the envelopes are calculated is a way to obtain a reasonable type I error. Grabarnik and colleagues [16] suggest carrying out 999 simulations.

The results for envelope tests are displayed in a graphical manner, but it is desirable to use them as a proper statistical test. In this way, we use a global envelope test, introduced by [18], a statistical test that rejects the null hypothesis if the observed function $\hat{F}_1(r)$ is not completely inside the envelope. This test provides p-values and a graphical representation. The $100(1-\alpha)\%$ global envelope complements the test result given by the p-values.

Global envelope tests are available in the R library GET, with detailed descriptions in [19].

4 Data Example

We illustrate the previously described tests on a real data provided by the Instituto Português do Mar e da Atmosfera (IPMA) on black scabbardfish catches in the fishing grounds of the south zone of Portugal, from 2009 to 2013.

4.1 Data

A subset of the original data described in [20] was taken for this data analysis: the fishing area with latitude minor than 39.3°, captures that occurred from September to February for the years between 2009 and 2013, resulting in a total set of 732 observations. The data not only include the Black Scabbardfish (BSF) catches (in kg) by a fishing haul of the longline fishing fleet but also include the location of each fishing haul (Fig. 1), the corresponding vessel identification and the depth of the locations where the fish was captured. A total of 12 vessels were grouped into two levels according to their tonnage (low and medium) that relates to the cargo capacity.

4.2 Application of Nearest Neighbour Test to BSF catches

The nearest neighbour test was applied to BSF catches. Initially, the presence of preferential sampling is tested without any covariate. A Box–Cox transformation of the catches was used

$$BSF^* = 2\sqrt{BSF} - 2$$

The R-INLA package with the SPDE approach is used to fit a standard geostatistical model. Following [2], PC priors were placed on the approximate Matern field parameters. A prior probability that the spatial range is below 30 km was set to 0.2, and the prior probability that the standard deviation of the field is above 10 was set to 0.01. Empirical p-values were computed using 1000 Monte Carlo samples. The empirical pointwise p-values of this test, for different values of K, where K is the

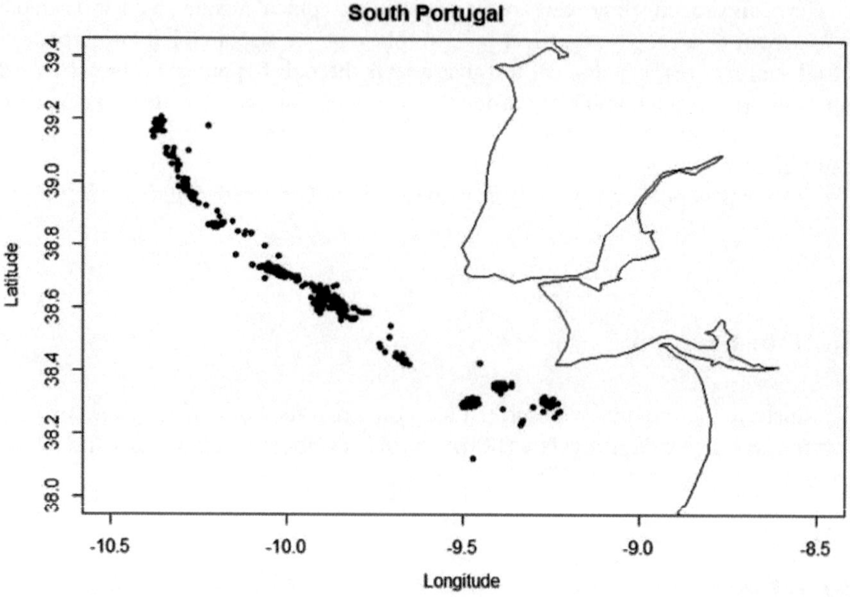

Fig. 1 Locations of the BSF catches

Table 1 Table of empirical p-values

K	1	2	3	4	...	11	12	13	14	15
p-value	0.001	0.001	0.001	0.001	...	0.002	0.002	0.002	0.002	0.003

number of neighbours considered, are shown in Table 1. Strong evidence of preferential sampling is found. A researcher would now have to decide whether to pursue a sufficient set of covariates or fit a joint model, [2].

Tonnage group (medium or low) was taken as an informative covariate and it was then investigated if preferential sampling remains unaccounted. Based on Fig. 2, to obtain the covariate in a fine grid, we considered that data points with latitude greater than or equal to 4280 were classified as corresponding to vessels of medium tonnage, with latitude less than or equal to 4250 are classified as low tonnage and points with latitude between 4250 and 4280 are random assignment of medium tonnage and low tonnage, respectively, according to the proportion of boats observed in that area.

The empirical pointwise p-values of this test are shown in Table 2. Preferential sampling is no longer detected after this adjustment. Tonnage group covariate has explained preferential sampling, so standard methods can be used.

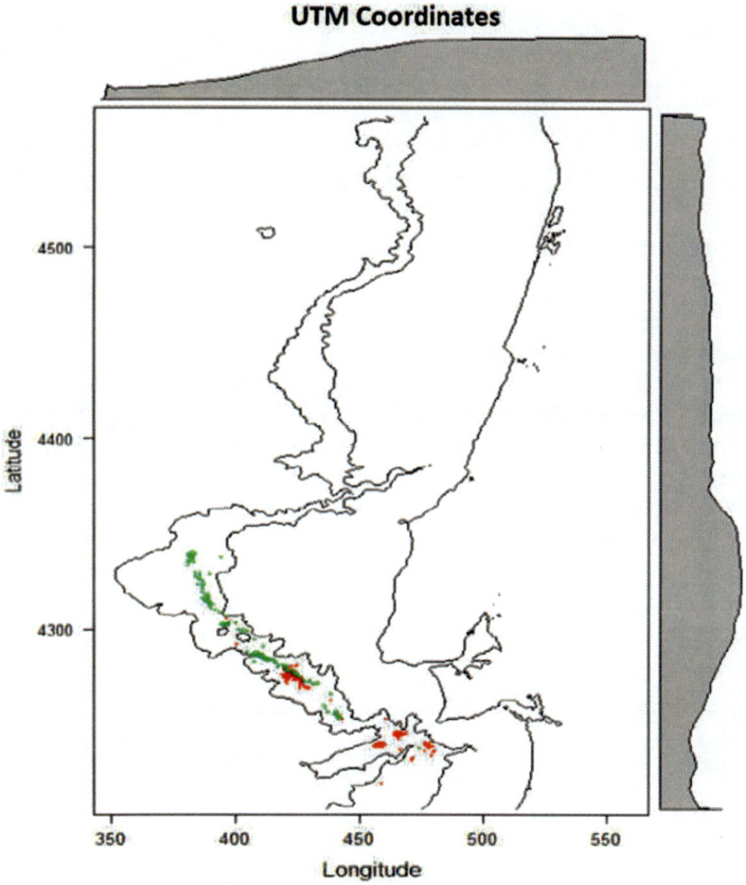

Fig. 2 Tonnage group, red—low; green—medium

Table 2 Table of empirical p-values

K	1	2	3	4	5	6	7	8	9
p-value	0.702	0.724	0.839	0.872	0.897	0.920	0.930	0.942	0.947

We also analysed depth as an informative covariate and whether its inclusion in the model was able to explain preferential sampling. The empirical pointwise p-values of this test are shown in Table 3. Depth fails to explain the observed preferential sampling seen in the data.

Table 3 Table of empirical p-values

K	1	2	3	4	...	9	...	29	...	40
p-value	0.001	0.001	0.001	0.001	...	0.003	...	0.002	...	0.002

4.3 Application of Schlater Test to BSF catches

Schlater Test was applied to BSF catches. $E(r)$ and $V(r)$ functions were built using *Emark* and *Vmark* functions in R-library spatstat. Options "isotropic", "Ripley" or "translate" specify the edge corrections to be applied. Ripley's isotropic correction is implemented only for rectangular and polygonal windows. In Fig. 3, we present $E(r)$ and $V(r)$ functions for BSF catches. $E(r)^{iso}$ and $V(r)^{iso}$ represent, respectively, the estimates of functions $E(r)$ or $V(r)$ obtained by the edge correction isotropic. $E(r)^{trans}$ and $V(r)^{trans}$ represent, respectively, the estimates of functions $E(r)$ or $V(r)$ obtained by the edge correction translate. $E^{iid}(r)$ and $V^{iid}(r)$ represent, respectively, constant value of $E(r)$ or $V(r)$ when the marks attached to different points are independent. If the marks and points are independent then we expect both $E(r)$ and $V(r)$ to be constant as the horizontal line $E^{iid}(r)$ and $V^{iid}(r)$, respectively.

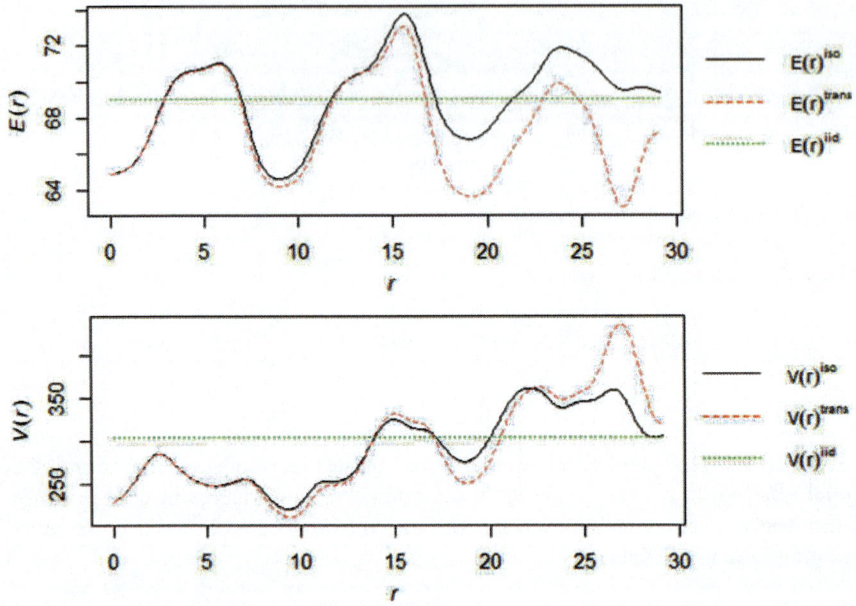

Fig. 3 $E(r)$ and $V(r)$ functions for BSF catches

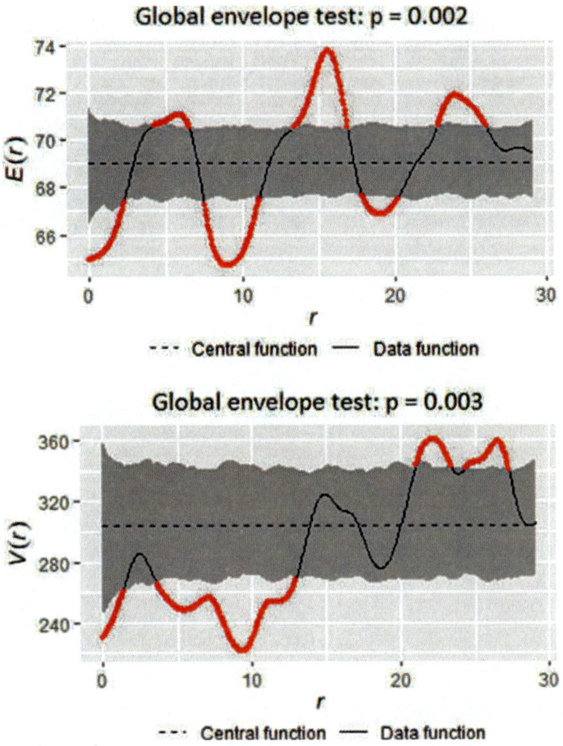

Fig. 4 Global envelope tests for $E(r)$ and $V(r)$ functions

To assess deviations of E and V from constant function, we use global envelope tests. The results are presented in Fig. 4. Envelope tests were based on 999 simulations, the grey areas show the 95% global envelopes, the solid black line is the data function, $\hat{F}_1(r)$, and the dashed line represents the (estimated) expectation. For $E(r)$, we obtained p-value = 0.002, and for $V(r)$, we obtained p-value = 0.003; thus, the null hypothesis was rejected at the significance level 0.05 by this test. Graphically, we can see that data function has not completely covered the envelopes in none of the situations. In this way, we reject the independence of marks and points.

To analyse the Tonnage group covariate effect, we construct $E(r)$ and $V(r)$ functions and the respective global envelope tests to data with only medium tonnage vessels, Fig. 5, and with only low tonnage vessels, Fig. 6. For data with only medium tonnage vessels, the null hypothesis was rejected at the significance level of 0.05 but was not rejected at the significance level of 0.01. Only for $E(r)$, data function was in a small part outside the envelopes. In this way, we accept the independence of marks and points for data with only medium tonnage vessels. In the case of data only with low tonnage vessels, the null hypothesis was rejected, for both $E(r)$ and $V(r)$ and, in this case, it seems to exist dependence between marks and points. We think that these results are possible due to a poor categorization of the Tonnage group covariate.

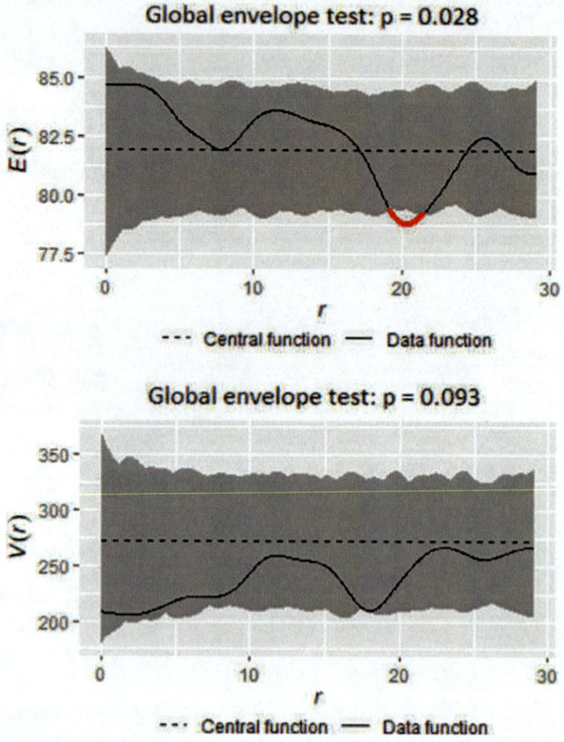

Fig. 5 Global envelope tests for $E(r)$ and $V(r)$ functions, for medium tonnage vessels

5 Final Remarks and Future Work

The main objectives of this work were centred on the analysis of how the geostatistical model can be understood from the point of view of marked point processes, namely considering log-intensity marked Cox processes, and the presentation of tests capable of identifying the existence of dependence between marks and the point process. Furthermore, we show that the preferential sampling model proposed by [1] in the geostatistics context equals the log-intensity marked Cox processes in the context of point processes, up to parametrization.

The two tests presented in Sect. 3 were applied to a set of real data related to BSF catches in the south zone of Portugal. Both tests revealed the existence of dependence between the marks and the point process. The existence of this dependency implies the use of more complex models, such as the joint model proposed by [1]. In an attempt to avoid the use of this type of technique, we looked for a set of informative covariates capable to explain the dependence between marks and points. The nearest neighbour test revealed that the covariate Tonnage group is sufficient for controlling the preferential sampling. On the other hand, depth fails to explain the observed preferential sampling seen in the data. Schlater test corroborated the conclusion

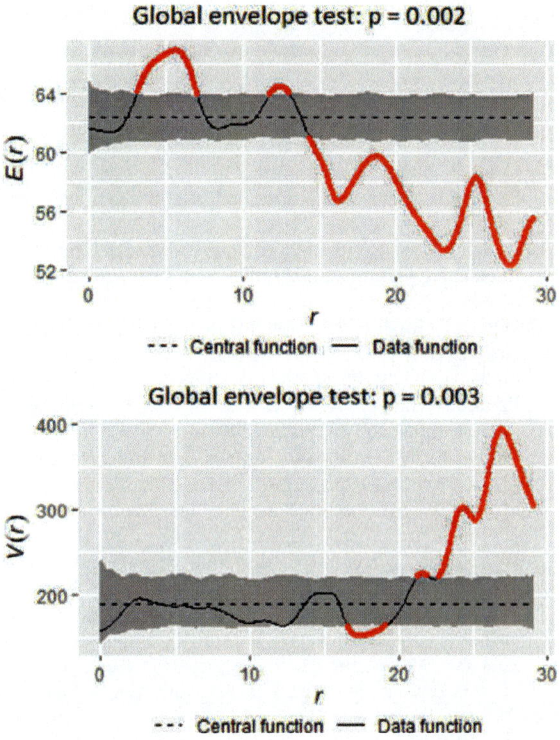

Fig. 6 Global envelope tests for $E(r)$ and $V(r)$ functions, for low tonnage vessels

obtained in the nearest neighbour test that the analysed fishery data present dependence between marks and points. However, the covariate Tonnage group, namely in the case of low tonnage vessels, fails to explain the observed preferential sampling. Other categorizations of this covariate can be analysed to see if the results change.

As a goal for future research, we plan to investigate the use of constructed covariates that are able to explain preferential sampling. Constructed covariates are summary characteristics defined for any location in the observation window reflecting spatial behaviour such as local interaction or competition. We intend to consider a construct covariate based on the distance to the kth nearest point. The objective is that the inclusion of this covariate is able to explain the dependence existing between the marks and the points. If this dependence is no longer detected after this adjustment, then we can use standard statistical techniques.

Acknowledgements This work is funded by the national funds through the FCT—Fundação para a Ciência e Tecnologia, I.P., under the scope of the projects PREFERENTIAL, PTDC/MAT-STA/28243/2017; UIDB/00297/2020 and UIDP/00297/2020 (Center for Mathematics and Applications); and UIDB/00006/2020 and UIDP/00006/2020 (CEAUL).

References

1. Diggle, P., Menezes, R., Su, T.: Geostatistical inference under preferential sampling. J. R. Stat. Soc. Ser. C (Appl. Stat.) **59**(2), 191–232 (2010)
2. Watson, J.: A fast monte carlo test for preferential sampling (2020). arXiv:2003.01319
3. Conn, P., Thorson, J., Johnson, D.: Confronting preferential sampling when analysing population distributions: diagnosis and model-based triage. Methods Ecol. Evol. **8**(11), 1535–1546 (2017)
4. Pennino, M.G., Paradinas, I., Illian, J., Muñoz, F., Bellido, J.M., López-Quílez, A., Conesa, D.: Accounting for preferential sampling in species distribution models. Ecol. Evol. **9**(1), 653–663 (2019)
5. Diggle, P., Ribeiro, P.J.: Model-Based Geostatistics. Springer (2007)
6. Ho, L.P., Stoyan, D.: Modelling marked point patterns by intensity-marked cox processes. Stat. Probab. Lett. **78**(10), 1194–1199 (2008)
7. Illian, J., Penttinen, A., Stoyan, H., Stoyan, D.: Statistical Analysis and Modelling of Spatial Point Patterns, vol. 70. Wiley (2008)
8. Myllymäki, M.: On intensity-dependent marking of log gaussian cox processes. Master's thesis, M. Sc. thesis in Mathematics. University of Jyväskylä, Finland (2006)
9. Myllymäki, M.: Statistical models and inference for spatial point patterns with intensity-dependent marks. Ph.D. thesis, University of Jyväskylä (2009)
10. Watson, J.: A perceptron for detecting the preferential sampling of locations and times chosen to monitor a spatio-temporal process. Spat. Stat. **43**, 100500 (2021)
11. Watson, J.: Accounting for preferential sampling in the statistical analysis of spatio-temporal data. Ph.D. thesis, University of British Columbia (2020)
12. Schlather, M., Ribeiro, P., Jr., Diggle, P.: Detecting dependence between marks and locations of marked point processes. J. R. Stat. Soc. Ser. B (Stat. Methodol.) **66**(1), 79–93 (2004)
13. Dinsdale, D., Salibian-Barrera, M.: Modelling ocean temperatures from bio-probes under preferential sampling. Ann. Appl. Stat. **13**(2), 713–745 (2019)
14. Ripley, B.: Modelling spatial patterns. J. R. Stat. Soc. Ser. B (Methodol.) **39**(2), 172–192 (1977)
15. Besag, J., Diggle, P.: Simple monte carlo tests for spatial pattern. J. R. Stat. Soc. Ser. C (Appl. Stat.) **26**(3), 327–333 (1977)
16. Grabarnik, P., Myllymäki, M., Stoyan, D.: Correct testing of mark independence for marked point patterns. Ecol. Model. **222**(23–24), 3888–3894 (2011)
17. Westfall, P., Young, S.: Resampling-Based Multiple Testing: Examples and Methods for p-Value Adjustment, vol. 279. Wiley (1993)
18. Myllymäki, M., Mrkvička, T., Grabarnik, P., Seijo, H., Hahn, U.: Global envelope tests for spatial processes. J. R. Stat. Soc. Ser. B (Stat. Methodol.) **79**(2), 381–404 (2017)
19. Myllymäki, M., Mrkvička, T.: Get: Global envelopes in R (2020)
20. André, L. M., Figueiredo, I., Carvalho, M. L., Simões, P., Natário, I.: Spatial modelling of black scabbardfish fishery off the portuguese coast. In: *International Conference on Computational Science and Its Applications*, pp. 332–344. Springer (2020)

Geostatistical Sampling Designs Under Preferential Sampling for Black Scabbardfish

Paula Simões, Maria Lucília Carvalho, Ivone Figueiredo, Andreia Monteiro, and Isabel Natário

Abstract In Portugal, the spatial distribution and abundance of the black scabbardfish (BSF) is mostly unknown, the existing information relying on data from commercial fisheries. Available data refers to areas where fisherman expect to have higher catches of the species, resulting in fishing locations that are not selected randomly but preferentially. The BSF captures in Portuguese waters were previously modelled, taking the sampling preferentiality into account, using a Bayesian approach and INLA methodology, considering stochastic partial differential equations (SPDE) for geostatistical data, jointly with a Log-Cox point process model. Based on this work, the aim of this study is to construct a new survey design to improve the BSF capture estimates and to analyse the effect of preferential sampling on the choice of new sampling locations and its influence in the sampling design choice. Within this approach, different design classes are investigated, namely random, simple inhibitory and adaptive geostatistical sampling designs, regarding the problem of spatial prediction, in order to achieve the optimal BSF design towards the objective of the analysis.

Keywords INLA · Geostatistics · Preferential sampling · Sampling design

---

P. Simões (✉) · A. Monteiro · I. Natário
NOVA MATH - Center for Mathematics and Applications (CMA), NOVA University of Lisbon, Lisbon, Portugal
e-mail: pc.simoes@campus.fct.unl.pt

P. Simões
Military Academy Research Center - Military University Institute (CINAMIL), Lisbon, Portugal

M. L. Carvalho · I. Figueiredo
Centre of Statistics and its Applications (CEAUL), Faculty of Sciences of the University of Lisbon, Lisbon, Portugal

I. Figueiredo
Portuguese Institute for Sea and Atmosphere (IPMA), Caparica, Portugal

I. Natário
Department of Mathematics, NOVA School of Science and Technology, Caparica, Portugal

R. Bispo et al. (eds.), *Recent Developments in Statistics and Data Science*, Springer Proceedings in Mathematics & Statistics 398,
https://doi.org/10.1007/978-3-031-12766-3_11

1 Introduction

Preserving species and habitats depends on a large scale of knowing where they occur. In order to map, the distribution of plants and animals is usually carried out field surveys, but despite this the full distribution of species often remains unknown as field surveys cannot cover the entire region or area considered. Improving knowledge about biodiversity and species abundance has become a scientific and societal important issue. On the Portuguese coast, the spatial distribution and abundance of the highly appreciated species black scabbardfish (BSF) is mostly unknown, relying mainly on information from commercial fisheries. Recent advances in statistics (and computing) presently allow a comprehensive mapping of the species spatial distribution and abundance using species distribution modelling. This approach is being widely used in ecology, at a terrestrial and maritime level, for management and conservation purposes, standing out the spatial models, in particular the geostatistical models. The main objective is to predict where a species is likely to be present in unsampled locations, using available information about the species occurrence and about environmental covariates in a finite number of locations. Standard geostatistical methodology assumes that sampling locations are stochastically independent over the observed region and sometimes such assumption may be unrealistic. If the sampling process that determines the data locations and the species observations are not independent, i.e. sampling locations are deliberately chosen in areas where the values of the species of interest are thought likely to be (low or high depending on the problem), which is referred to as preferential sampling [1], standard geostatistical methods yield biased results. The chosen species observation sites should be accounted for in the modelling process of the preferentially sampled data. Therefore, abundance estimation using standard geostatistical methods is not the most appropriate approach. Since commercial fishing takes place where fisherman expects to find the species, leading to the choice of sampling locations that are not random but preferentially selected, a species distribution modelling that address this question to the black scabbardfish is required. Considering the previous work [2], which has performed species distribution modelling of BSF captures using geostatistical methods that has taken preferentiality into account, different design classes are outlined to reach the most suitable sampling design for BSF species.

2 Methods

2.1 Geostatistical Model Under Preferential Sampling

The preferential sampling model is considered as a two part model that share information [3], first in terms of the observed locations $(s_1, ..., s_n)$, assumed to come from a non-homogeneous Poisson process with intensity $\lambda(\boldsymbol{s})$. The intensity function measures the average number of events per unit of area based on the point pattern that is responsible for the occurrence of the events, in the considered region. A Log-Gaussian Cox Process (LGCP) is assumed for this. Under this assumption it is possible to model the log intensity of the Cox process, a Poisson process with diversified intensity, with a Gaussian process that captures the spatial effect. Secondly the species characteristic (abundance/captures) y is assumed to follow an exponential family distribution, whose mean is related with the spatial term using a link function $g(.)$, being the spatial term shared with the LGCP. To allow differences in scale between the abundances/captures and the LGCP, a scale parameter (β) is considered in the spatial term [3]. Inference can be made using INLA (Integrated Nested Laplace Approximation), under the new approach considering stochastic partial differential equations (SPDE) models for geostatistical data. This alternative uses an approximate stochastic weak solution of a Stochastic Partial Differential Equation that is a continuous Gaussian field with a Matérn covariance structure [4, 5]. This approximation given by the finite element approach enables to deal with non-regular areas allowing flexibility on the choice of the required mesh of the study region.

The model is then given by (without covariates):

$$\begin{aligned} &Y_i|S \sim Normal(\mu_i, \tau^2)\\ &Y_i|(S, \boldsymbol{X} = \boldsymbol{x})] = \beta_0^y + \beta S(x_i) + e_i\\ &\boldsymbol{e} \sim N(0, \tau^2) \qquad (1)\\ &\\ &\lambda_i = \exp(\beta_0^{pp} + S(x_i)) \end{aligned}$$

where the observed locations $(x_1, ..., x_n)$ come from a non-homogeneous Poisson process with intensity λ_i, a Log-Gaussian Cox Process (LGCP) is assumed for $X|S$, β_0^{pp} is the correspondent intercept, $S(x_i)$ spatial effect of the model, where the observed locations are modelled by a LGCP, $i = 1, ..., n$ (index of i-location).

The response, Y_i, belongs to the exponential family distribution, $S(x)$ is a stationary Gaussian Process with mean zero, variance σ^2, and a Matérn correlation (correlation shape parameter fixed $k = 1.5$, correlation range ϕ and nugget variance τ^2), $S(x) \sim N(0, \Sigma)$, with

$$\begin{aligned} &\rho(u) = Corr(S(x), S(x')), u = \|x - x'\|,\\ &\rho(u, \phi, \kappa) = \{2^{k-1}\Gamma(k)\}^{-1}(\tfrac{u}{\phi})^k K_k(\tfrac{u}{\phi})), \end{aligned} \qquad (2)$$

where $\phi > 0$ is a scale parameter that controls the rate at which correlation decays with increasing distance, $K_k(.)$ is a modified Bessel function of order $k > 0$, and $S(x)$ is m times mean square differentiable if $k > m$, being the correspondent vector of parameters given by $\theta = (\beta_0^{pp}, \beta, \beta_0^y, \tau^2, \phi, k, \sigma^2)$ [6].

In terms of the referred scale parameter β on the shared random field effect, if $\beta > 0$ the response values tend to be higher where there are more observations, if $\beta < 0$ the response values are lower where there are more observations and in the case that $\beta = 0$ corresponds to non-preferentially sampling [6, 7].

2.2 Sampling Designs

The sampling design problem assuming an underlying stochastic process with a stationary covariance structure, a common assumption on geostatistical applications, is considered in this section and different design classes are presented, namely simple inhibitory and adaptive geostatistical sampling designs.

Inhibitory Design Chipeta [8] and Chipeta et al. [9] address the problem of choosing spatial designs for investigating an unobserved spatial phenomenon, S, in terms of spatial prediction, while taking into account the need to estimate covariance structure. They propose a class of inhibitory sampling designs for accurate spatial prediction with estimated covariance model parameters [8, 9].

An inhibitory design consists of a random design that generates spatially regular configurations points in order to deliver efficient mapping of the complete surface $S(X)$, over the region of interest, including two specific classes, the simple inhibitory design (SI) and the inhibitory design with close pairs (ICP).

Simple inhibitory designs - $SI(n, \delta)$ A simple inhibitory design belonging to a class of non-adaptive sampling design, for accurate spatial prediction with estimated covariance model parameters, consists of n locations chosen at random in domain D, with the constrain that no two locations are at a distance of less than some value δ. It is considered that all designs X that meet the inhibitory constrain are equally likely to be picked. Notation $SI(n, \delta)$ is used for different designs with fixed sample size n and varying δ.

This class of designs considers the average prediction variance (APV) as performance criterion:

$$APV = \int_S Var\{S(x)|Y\}dx. \tag{3}$$

For fixed sample size n, region D, and an assumed geostatistical model (with a specific numerical value for its vector of parameters θ), the algorithm is numerically optimized to determine the combination that minimize the design criterion (APV).

The proportion of the total region covered by n non-overlapping disks of diameter δ is defined as the packing density of the design, $\rho = \frac{n\pi\delta^2}{4|D|}$.

The formal constructions of an $SI(n, \delta)$ design on a region D proceeds as follows [8, 9]:

1. Draw a sample of locations x_i, $i = 1, ..., n$ completely at random in D;
2. Set $i = 1$;
3. Calculate the minimum, d_{min} of the distances from x_i to all other x_j in the current sample;
4. If $d_{min} \geq \delta$, increase i by 1 and return to step 3 if $i \leq n$, otherwise stop;
5. If $d_{min} < \delta$, replace x_i by a new location drawn completely at random in D and return to step 3.

Adaptative Geostatistical Design An adaptive design strategy purposely built to deliver efficient mapping of the complete surface $S(x)$, within a model-based geostatistics framework and considering a design criterion that ensures that data are collected only from locations that will deliver useful additional information of the study region is also proposed by Chipeta et al. [10]. This class of adaptive designs allows to define new sampled locations, defined single or in batches, or over time that depends on information obtained from previous designs in order to optimize data collection and identify critical areas where interventions can have substantial impact on the purpose of analysis.

Adaptive sampling enables efficient identification of hotspots for which data are collected over a period of time and later sampling locations can depend on data collected from earlier locations. According to Chipeta [8] and Chipeta et al. [10]: " this kind of design is well suited to spatial mapping studies in low resource settings" where uniformly precise mapping may be expensive and the priority often identifies critical areas where interventions can have the greatest impact.

An adaptive design strategy proceeds as follows [8, 10]:

1. Specify the finite set, X^* say, of n^* potential sampling locations $x_i \in D$; (Any point $x \in D$ may be a potential sampling location, in which case we take X^* to be a finely spaced regular lattice to cover D)
2. Use a non-adaptive design to choose an initial set of sample locations, $X_0 = \{x_i \in D : i = 1, ..., n_0\}$;
3. Use the corresponding data Y_0 to estimate the parameters of an **assumed geostatistical model**;
4. Specify **a criterion for the addition** of one or more new sample locations to form an enlarged set $X_0 \cup X_1$.
5. Repeat steps 3 and 4 with augmented data Y_1 at the points in X_1;
6. Stop when the required number of points has been sampled, a required performance criterion has been achieved or no more potential sampling points are available.

In step 2, any initial design can be considered, in addition to a suitable addition criterion in step 4, it is also necessary to choose the number and locations of points in the initial design X_0, and the number to be added at each subsequent stage, batch b.

For the present study, a simple inhibitory design, $SI(n_0, \delta)$, is used to obtain the earlier locations $x_1, ..., x_{n_0}$, and the batch adaptive sampling will be sets of $b > 1$ locations chosen, with each set $(x_{n_1+1}, ..., x_{n_1+b})$ depend on data from earlier n_1 locations.

The prediction variance, $PV(x)$, is considered as the selection design criterion. For the predictive target $T = S(x)$ at a particular location x, given an initial set of sampling locations $X_0 = (x_1, ..., x_{n_0})$, the available set of additional sampling locations are $A_0 = X^* \setminus X_0$. For each $x \in A_0$ the prediction variance, $PV(x)$, is $Var(T|Y_0) = Var(S(x)|Y_0)$. For example, one or more new sample locations would be the elements of X^* with the largest values of $PV(x)$ amongst all points not already included in X_0 [8, 10].

Notation $AD(n_0, n, \delta, b)$ is used with fixed initial sample size n_0, with the constrain that any two locations are at a distance of less than some value δ, with a batch of b new locations in order to obtain the final proposed design of n locations.

3 Results

3.1 BSF Data

The data considered in this study were provided by the Portuguese Institute of Sea and Atmosphere (IPMA). It is a comprehensive data set of geo-referenced captures of black scabbard fish from commercial fisheries, along the Portuguese coast, between 2002 and 2013. Since fishing takes place where fisherman expects to find large amount of this species, preferential sampling should be accounted. Several other variables have also been registered along with the captures as, for example, the speed, the vessel tonnage and identification, and also the depth at which the capture has been made.

A subset of the original data was taken for this data analysis: the fishing area with latitude minor than 39.3°, captures that have occurred from September to February for the years between 2009 and 2013, resulting in a total set of 732 observations. The locations of the data are displayed in Fig. 1.

Original data follows approximately a Gamma distribution, $BSF \sim Gamma$, a Box-Cox transformation of BSF data was carried out, according with the expression $Y = \frac{BSF^{\lambda}-1}{\lambda}$, with $\lambda = \frac{1}{2}$, so that the response follows approximately a Normal distribution, $Y = 2\sqrt{BSF} - 2 \sim Normal$.

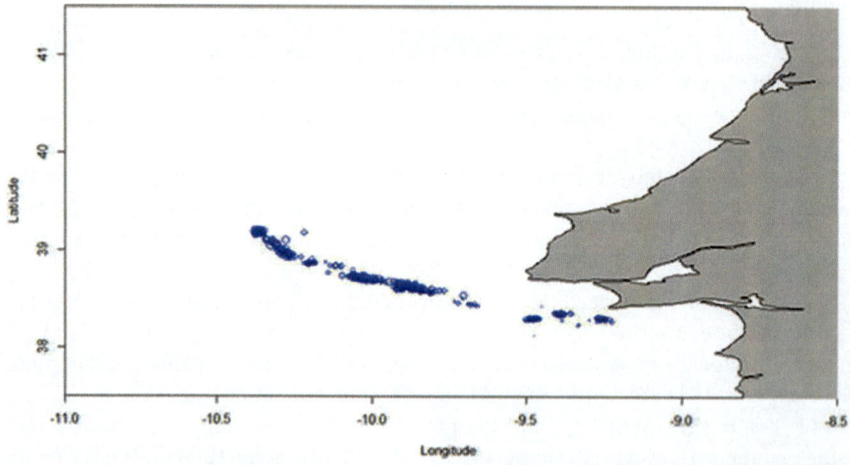

Fig. 1 BSF data locations

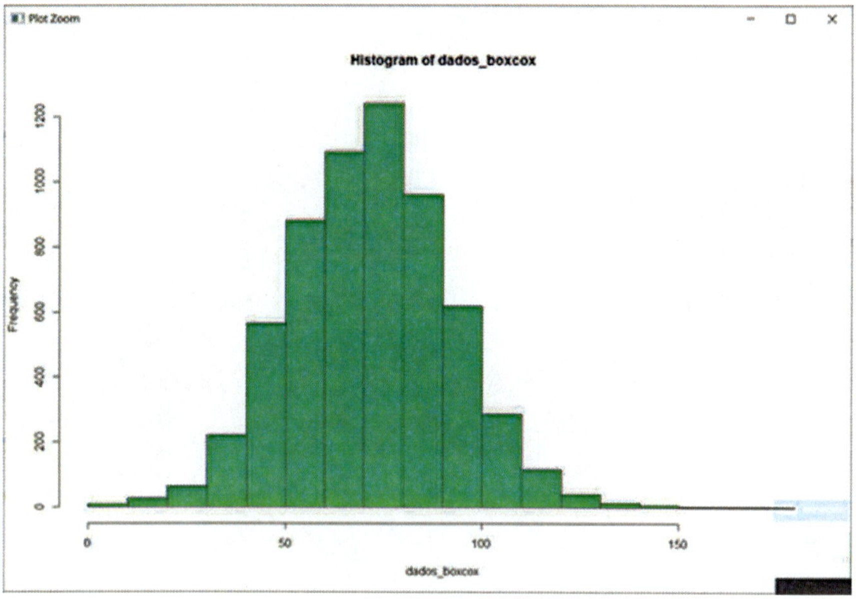

Fig. 2 Box-Cox transformation of BSF data

The transformed variable, Y, as a minimum value of 16.22, a first quartil of 56.14, median value of 68.80, the 3rd quartil of 80.53 with a maximum value of 121.74 and mean 69.02 (see Fig. 2).

3.2 Model Fitting Under Preferential Sampling

This section performs species distribution modelling that address the question of the sampling preferentiality for black scabbardfish, since commercial fishing takes place where fisherman expects to find the species, leading to the choice of sampling locations that are not random but preferentially selected.

The BSF captures in Portuguese waters were previously modelled, taking the sampling preferentiality into account, using a Bayesian approach and INLA methodology, considering stochastic partial differential equations (SPDE) for geostatistical data jointly with a Log-Cox point process (LGCP) model [2].

For appropriate inference of the geostatistical model under preferential sampling using the SPDE approach, the first step is the triangulation of the considered spatial domain by building a mesh that covers the study region, D, the constrained refined Delaunay triangulation. The SPDE approach for point pattern defines the model at the nodes of the mesh, in order to fit the LGCP model, these points are considered as integration points. Figure 3 shows the considered mesh and corresponding integration points.

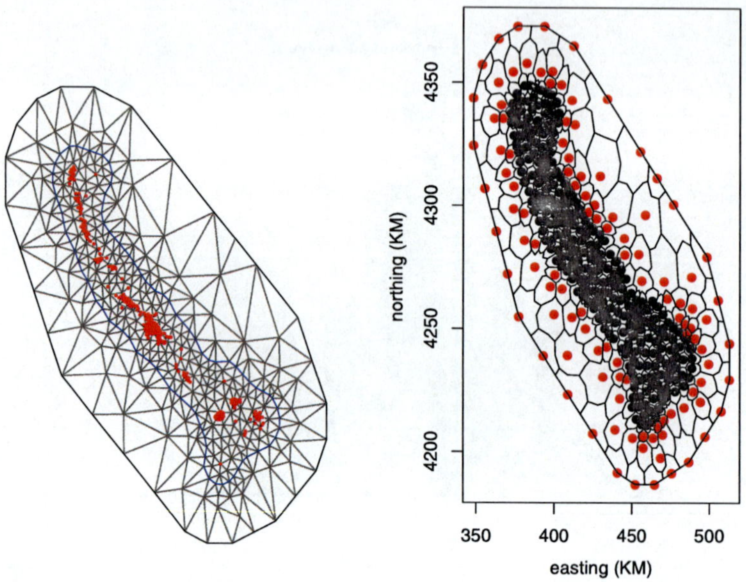

Fig. 3 Considered Mesh for BSF data

The preferential sampling model, in terms of the response, for the i-th spatial point location, the observation Y_i is modelled as

$$Y_i \sim N(\eta_i, \sigma_e^2), \quad i = 1, .., n,$$

where n is the total number of fishing hauls, σ_e^2 is the nugget effect. The response mean is defined as

$$\eta_i = \beta_0^y + \beta S_i + e_i,$$

where $e \sim N(0, \sigma_e^2)$.

S_i is the i-realization of the latent Gaussian Field (GF) $S(x)$ with Matérn covariance function shared with the LGCP and scaled by β. $S(x) = \sum_{g=1}^{G} A_{ig} \widetilde{S}_g$, where $\widetilde{S}_g$ are zero mean Gaussian distributed weights; A_{ig} is the generic element of the sparse $n \times G$ matrix A that maps the GMRF $\widetilde{S}$ from the triangulation vertices of a mesh to the n locations $(x_1, ..., x_n)$ [6, 7, 11].

The observed locations $(x_1, ..., x_n)$ come from a non-homogeneous Poisson process with intensity λ_i, a Log-Gaussian Cox Process (LGCP) is assumed for $X|S$, β_0^{pp} is the correspondent intercept.

It was considered in the point process with intensity λ_i the covariate depth (D), having

$$\lambda_i = \exp(\beta_0^{pp} + \beta_1 D_i + S_i),$$

Table 1 Parameter estimates for BSF preferential model

Parameter	Mean	Sd	0.025	0.0975
β_0^{pp}	−10.710	2.781	−17.360	−6.389
β_1	−0.002	0.001	−0.003	−0.001
β_0^{y}	62.253	2.681	55.749	66.193
Precision of Gaussian observations	0.003	0.000	0.003	0.004
Range (r) of spatial field	39.128	12.268	20.852	68.441
Stdev (σ) of spatial field	3.784	1.316	1.916	7.006
β	1.237	0.237	0.764	1.698

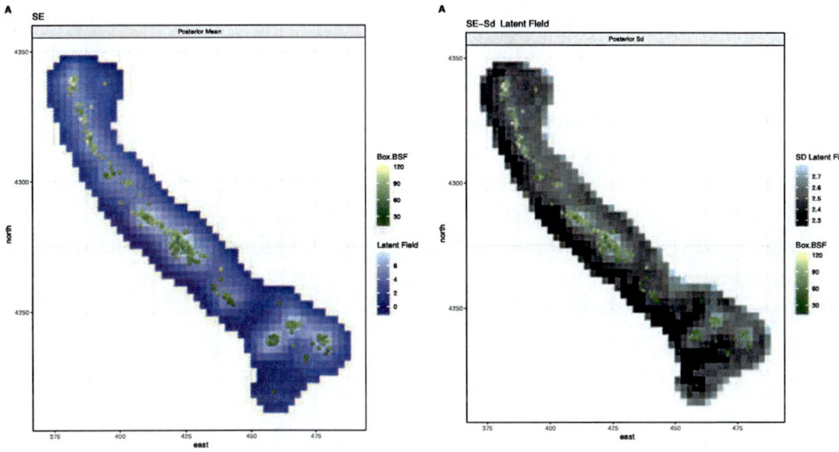

Fig. 4 Posterior predicted mean of the spatial effect in the BSF preferential model

considering penalized complexity priors (PC Priors) for the range r and for the the marginal standard deviation σ (of the spatial effect) [11],

$$P[r < 30] = 0.2,$$

$$P[\sigma > 10] = 0.01.$$

Parameter estimates for the selected model (BSF preferential model) are summarized in Table 1, and the corresponding posterior predicted mean and standard deviation of the spatial effect are represented in Fig. 4. This model has an estimated value of β of **1.237**, so $\beta > 0$ the response values are **higher** where there is **more** observation locations.

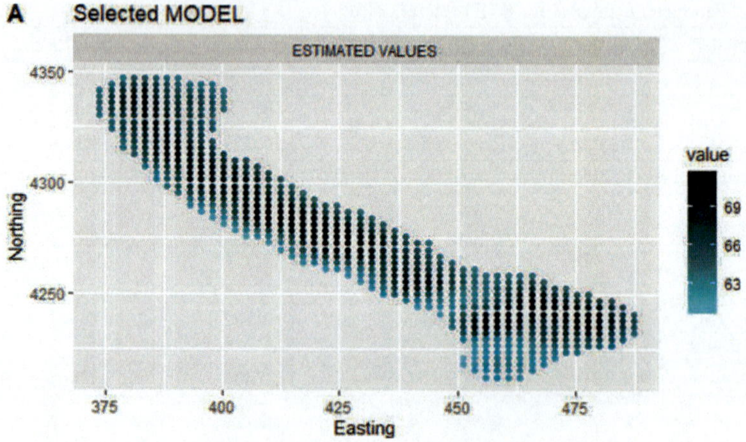

Fig. 5 BSF captures estimates at considered unobserved potential sampling locations

The construction of a new survey design, for the BSF captures estimates, requires predictions to be made at considered unobserved locations, named as potential sampling locations. These locations are obtained through the triangulation of the considered spatial domain, taking into account the chosen mesh. The estimated values for Y in the $N = 612$ spatial prediction coordinates (potential sampling locations) are represented in Fig. 5.

3.3 Sampling Designs for Black Scabbardfish

The proposed design strategies are implemented in order to achieve the optimal BSF sampling design under preferential sampling, and are presented in this section. The first stage involves deciding on the initial sampling design, a non-adaptive design. It was considered BSF simple inhibitory design, $SI(45, 2)$, that consists of $n = 45$ locations chosen at random in D, from N = 612 spatial prediction coordinates (potential sampling locations), with the constrain that no two locations are at a distance of less than 2 km. It as a packing density of $\rho = \frac{n\pi\delta^2}{4|D|} = 0.03$, with $|D| = 4241.124$, and an APV = 6.13 (see Fig. 6). Once data have been collected from sample locations in the chosen design the second stage is to analyse the data in order to reestimate model parameters, within our assumed geostatistical model without preferentiality, where $\eta_i = \beta_0^y + \beta_1 D_i + S_i + e_i$ is the correspondence response mean.

In Fig. 7 are represented the correspondent posterior predicted mean and standard deviation of the spatial effect, for BSF Simple Inhibitory Design new model fitting. Note that the minimum mean square error predictor of T for any given design X

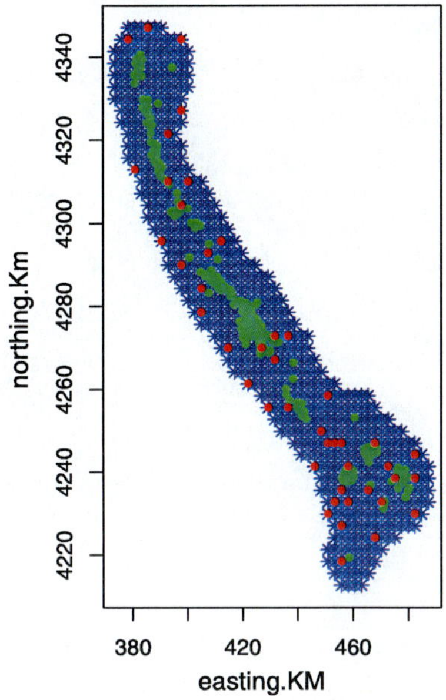

Fig. 6 BSF simple inhibitory design, $SI(45, 2)$. Green points denote BSF data locations

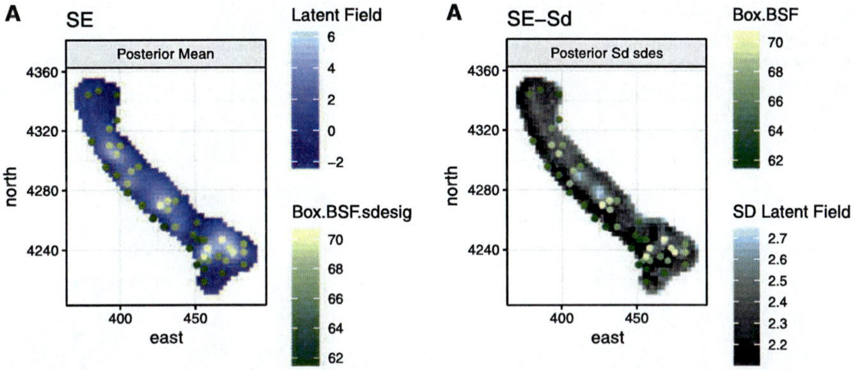

Fig. 7 Posterior predicted mean and standard deviation of the spatial effect, for BSF Simple Inhibitory Design new model fitting under $SI(45, 2)$

in D, $MSE(\widehat{T})$, with T a predictive target, where $\widehat{T} = E[T|Y; X]$ is considered as a generic measure of predictive accuracy of a design X. The selected design as an MSE $= 3.67$.

The third stage consists in to predict all unobserved potential sampling locations, considering the non-adaptative design $SI(45, 2)$, using the geostatistical model without preferential sampling. The estimated values are represented in Fig. 8.

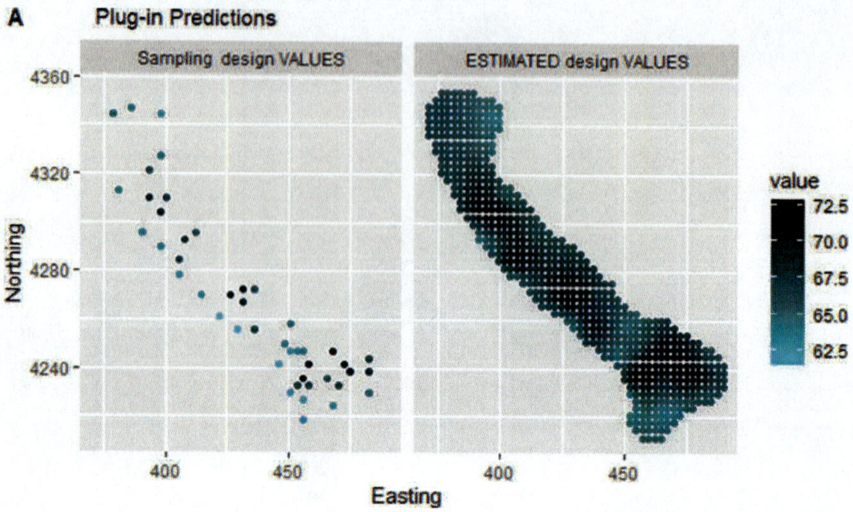

Fig. 8 BSF simple inhibitory design $SI(45, 2)$ predictions for potential sampling locations; Green points denote BSF data locations

Fig. 9 BSF final design proposal, the black dots ($n_0 = 45$) denote the initial sampling locations and the red dots ($b = 15$) the adaptive sampling locations

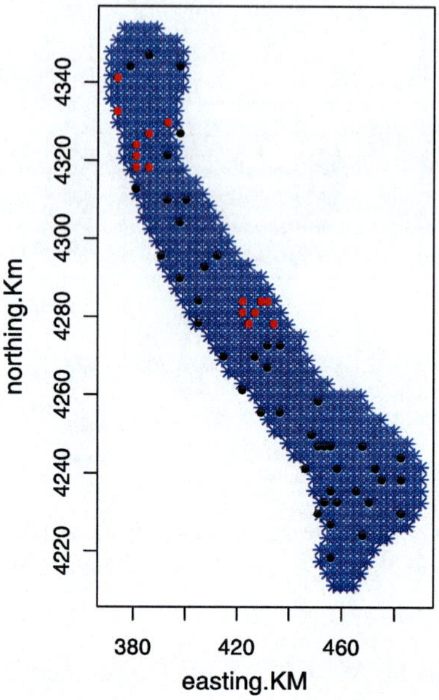

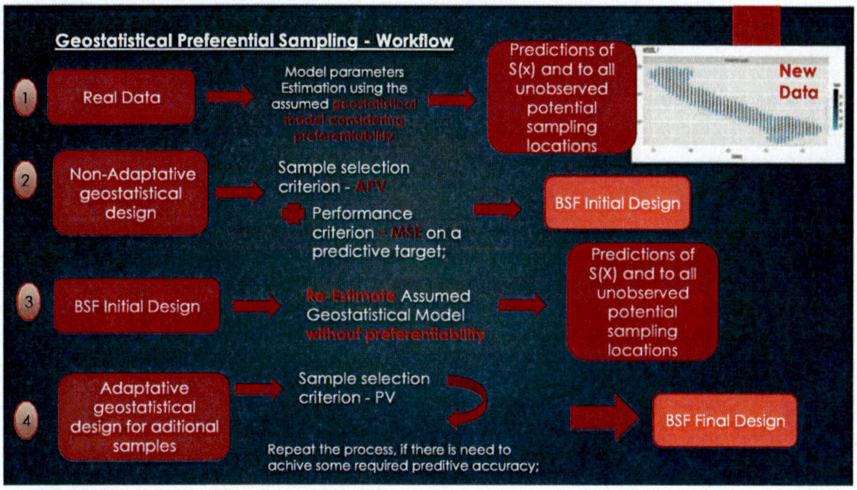

Fig. 10 BSF sampling design workflow

The fourth stage is the implementation of adaptive sampling if there is a need for additional samples to achieve the required predictive accuracy. BSF adaptative geostatistical design, $AD(45, 60, 2, 15)$, has been considered with $n_0 = 45, n = 60$, $b = 15, \delta = 2$, and a corresponding $\rho = 0.04$ and APV $= 6.12$. The constrain that no two locations are at a distance of less than 2 km was kept. The first final design proposal is produced and represented in Fig. 9, black dots ($n_0 = 45$) are the initial sampling locations and the red dots ($b = 15$) are adaptive sampling locations added after analysing data from the initial design.

In order to resume the proposed steps, a scheme of the workflow is presented in Fig. 10.

4 Discussion

Regarding the problem of constructing a new survey design to improve the BSF capture estimates, this study takes a first approach/proposal for implementing a BSF sampling design. The previously modelling of BSF captures in Portuguese waters is taken into account. BSF captures were modelled using a Bayesian approach and INLA methodology, considering stochastic partial differential equations (SPDE) for geostatistical data jointly with a Log-Cox point process model, taking the sampling preferentiality into account.

Different design classes are investigated, namely simple inhibitory and adaptive geostatistical sampling designs. Regarding the problem of spatial prediction, the proposed approach involves repeated estimation and prediction stages. Several sampling rounds can be implemented allowing for spatial constraints to change at each stage. Required inputs include predictions at considered unobserved potential sampling locations and a sample selection criterion.

In terms of generating adaptive sample locations, given the initial or existing sample locations (usually a simple inhibitory design), the prediction variance criterion is used to determine new locations that can be added to the existing sample in an adaptive manner. In this stage, is also important to explore several issues in a future work, namely the selection of the initial sampling locations n_0 of the design, and the number of locations to be added, at each subsequent stage (batch b), or even to explore other possible values for the constrain that no two locations are at a distance of less than some value δ.

A measure to choose between different initial and final proposed designs is also necessary. This paper presents one first possible combination of choices, for proposed sampling methodology, however others can be implemented and compared with each other. Developing a comparative study of alternative combinations of sampling designs choices may constitute the next phase in the present analysis, in achieving the ideal design for BSF species.

With regard to the question of understanding the effect of preferential sampling in determining new sampling locations and its effect in the BSF sampling design, it is necessary to consider other initial available modelling options of BSF captures assumed model (taking preferentiality into account). For example, the covariable group of tonnage could be considered in the modelling approaches. On the other hand, it is necessary to investigate the assumed geostatistical model for BSF captures (not taking preferentiality into account) for predictions at unobserved potential sampling locations. This will enable to compare and evaluate the effect of preferential sampling and its influence in the sampling design choice as well as the corresponding impact on its performance criteria.

Other important issues in this study, for future approach, will be to carry out the development of a new survey design to improve the BSF capture estimates without BSF transformation. The sampling design problem, under preferential sampling, for BSF captures should be also addressed considering Gamma distribution.

It is considered that this first approach is an important step towards solving the problem of the need to build mathematical/statistical models that take into account the problem of preferentiality, making it possible to produce maps of abundance that are more consistent and less biased, that will allow the responsible institutions to rely on concrete data to define more precise quotas, ensuring the sustainability of commercial fisheries and protecting the biodiversity of species that are of high interest for consumption.

Acknowledgements This work is funded by national funds through the FCT - Fundação para a Ciência e a Tecnologia, I.P., under the scope of the projects PREFERENTIAL, PTDC/MAT-STA/28243/2017; UIDB/00297/2020 and UIDP/00297/2020 (Center for Mathematics and Applications); and UIDB/00006/2020 and UIDP/00006/2020 (CEAUL).

References

1. Diggle, P.J., Menezes, R., li Su, T.: Geostatistical inference under preferential sampling. J. R. Stat. Soc. Ser. C **59**, 191–232 (2010)
2. André, L.M., Figueiredo, I., Carvalho, M.L., Simões, P., Natário, I.: Spatial modelling of black scabbardfish fishery under preferential sampling of the portuguese coast. In: Computational Science and Its Applications—ICCSA 2020 (2020)
3. Martínez-Minaya, J., Cameletti, M., Conesa, D., Pennino, M.G.: Species distribution modeling: a statistical review with focus in spatio-temporal issues. Stoch. Environ. Res. Risk Assess. **32**, 3227–3244 (2018)
4. Lindgren, F., Rue, H., Lindström, J.: An explicit link between Gaussian fields and Gaussian Markov random fields: the stochastic partial differential equation approach. J. R. Stat. Soc. Ser. B **73**(4), 423–498 (2011)
5. Rue, H., Martino, S., Chopin, N.: Approximate Bayesian inference for latent Gaussian models by using integrated nested Laplace approximations. J. R. Stat. Soc. Ser. B **71**(2), 319–392 (2009)
6. Krainski, E., Gómez-Rubio, V., Bakka, H., Lenzi, A., Castro-Camilo, D., et al.: Advanced Spatial Modeling with Stochastic Partial Differential Equations Using R and INLA. Chapman and Hall/CRC, Boca Raton, FL (2018)
7. Blangiardo, M., Cameletti, M., Baio, G., Rue, H.: Spatial and spatio-temporal models with R-INLA. Spat. Spatio-temporal Epidemiol. **7**, 39–55 (2013)
8. Chipeta, M.: Geostatistical design and analysis for estimating local variations in malaria disease burden. Ph.D. thesis, Lancaster University, UK (2016)
9. Chipeta, M., Terlouw, D., Phiri, K., Diggle, P.: Inhibitory geostatistical designs for spatial prediction taking account of uncertain covariance structure. Environmetrics **28**, e2425 (2016)
10. Chipeta, M., Terlouw, D.J., Phiri, K.S., Diggle, P.J.: Adaptive geostatistical design and analysis for prevalence surveys. Spat. Stat. **15**, 70–84 (2016)
11. André, L.M., Figueiredo, I., Carvalho, M.L., Simões, P., Natário, I.: Spatial modelling of black scabbardfish fishery off the portuguese coast. In: Computational Science and Its Applications—ICCSA 2020, pp. 332–344. Springer, New York (2020)

Modeling Residential Adoption of Solar Photovoltaic Systems

Carolina Goldstein, José Miguel Espinosa, and Regina Bispo

Abstract The world is on an urgent transition to renewable energies. Photovoltaic (PV) solar energy is the most viable green energy source to be produced at the domestic level, allowing every individual to contribute. Understanding the factors that influence the adoption of domestic solar energy, how it changes throughout the country and how spatial dependent factors contribute to the promotion of this technology is of the utmost importance to stimulate adoption. As to this day, to the best of my knowledge, these are not yet known. This study aims to contribute to channeling efforts to where adoption is more likely, ultimately accelerating Portugal's energy transition. Hence, the goal of this study is to build a spatial model that estimates for each spatial unit in Portugal the probability of individuals adopting domestic PV systems. The study uses data related to past solar PV installations as well as socioeconomic and demographic data from public sources. An exploratory spatial analysis including the study of spatial correlation across municipalities confirmed the importance of spatial considerations. Three dependent variables were considered sequentially: installations (binary), number of panels installed (discrete), and installed power (continuous). To model the latter, it being the main focus of the study, eight models were compared: linear regression (OLS), spatial lag (SAR), spatial error (SEM), Kelejian-Prucha (GSM), spatial lag of the explanatory variables (SLX), spatial Durbin (SDM), spatial Durbin error (SDEM), and Manski models. It was concluded that socioeconomic factors do spill over to neighbor locations and in

C. Goldstein (✉)
MSc in Analytics and Big Data Engineering, Department of Computer Science and Department of Mathematics, NOVA School of Science and Technology, NOVA University of Lisbon, Campus de Caparica, 2829-516 Caparica, Portugal
e-mail: c.goldstein@campus.fct.unl.pt

J. M. Espinosa
Tech Garage, IT & Digital Department. Galp Energia, SGPS, S.A., 1600-209 Lisboa, Portugal

R. Bispo
NOVAMATH Center for Mathematics and Applications, Department of Mathematics, NOVA School of Science and Technology, NOVA University of Lisbon, Campus de Caparica, 2829-516 Caparica, Portugal
e-mail: r.bispo@fct.unl.pt

R. Bispo et al. (eds.), *Recent Developments in Statistics and Data Science*, Springer Proceedings in Mathematics & Statistics 398,
https://doi.org/10.1007/978-3-031-12766-3_12

that way influence solar PV adoption, but also that unobserved characteristics result in similar decisions in nearby municipalities. The SDEM was found to be best to fit the data and a final map representing the likelihood of adoption across the different municipalities in Portugal was produced according to its estimations.

Keywords PV system adoption · Social effects · Spatial modeling · Technology diffusion

1 Introduction

Rethinking the use of energy stemming from fossil sources and transitioning to renewable energies is increasingly becoming a necessity. Photovoltaic (PV) energy, attained through the installation of solar panels, is the most viable of being produced at the level of the individual consumer for domestic use. There are companies developing highly advanced technologies to identify the energetic potential of homes and to install these solar panels. However, inquiring about potential customers without knowing their predisposition ends up wasting many resources.

The overall goal of this project is the construction of a spatial model that estimates for each spatial unit, with the finest possible granularity, the probability of adopting domestic solar PV systems. In doing so, companies will be able to better channel their selling efforts to locations where adherence is more likely, ultimately accelerating Portugal's transition to renewable energies.

More specifically, using data related to past solar panel installations, the first goal is to describe the geographical distribution of the current installations across Portugal. Furthermore, using socioeconomic and demographic data from public sources, the goal is to cross this information and characterize each region, in order to understand the factors that may explain the decision of installing solar panels. The ultimate goal is to build a map representing the adoption likelihood for each spatial unit.

This study is structured as follows: in the first section the topic is put into context and the goals of the project are defined. The motivations for this work are also presented in this chapter, as well as a review of the literature on similar problems. In Sect. 2 the available data that are to be used are presented, along with their description, characterization, and preprocessing. This section also presents the statistical methods to be used, both to perform an initial exploratory analysis and to build different model specifications, while explaining the logic that resulted in the presented decisions. In Sect. 3, the results of the exploratory analysis and the different regression models are shown and described. In Sect. 4, the results are discussed and conclusions are presented.

1.1 Decision-Making in PV Technology Adoption

Schelly [1] explores the decision-making process of individuals regarding energy technology adoption through interviews with domestic PV panel owners and indicates three models to explain adoption: environmental motivations, economic rationality, and social spillover. Richter [2] studied the diffusion of solar PV technology in the United Kingdom through a panel model with time-varying fixed effects and found that higher educated neighborhoods installed more PV systems than neighborhoods with, on average, lower educated populations. The author also found a correlation between the number of systems installed in an area and the number installed three months later. Hence, Richter [2] concludes that higher educated neighborhoods may be more inclined to promote the spread of technology within their neighborhoods. Bollinger and Gillingham [3], who studied the diffusion of solar PV panels in California with a similar panel model, also found significant evidence that the decision to install PV systems may be influenced by the neighbors' previous decision to install. Graziano and Gillingham [4] examined the diffusion of this technology in Connecticut in a similar way and found that demographic and socioeconomic variables significantly influenced PV adoption and that higher numbers of previously installed systems also significantly increased the number of later adoptions nearby. Schelly and Letzelter [5] examined the decision factors that influence the adoption of residential solar electric power systems in upstate New York through questionnaire data and found that environmental motivations are slightly more important than economics. As Richter [2] points out, spatial econometric methods could allow the study of social effects across borders, recognizing the study of spillover only within the neighborhood as a limitation of her model. Baginski and Weber [6] use spatial econometric models to study the spread of PV systems over space and the factors that drive the regional uptake in Germany to conclude that spatial dependence is a relevant factor for explaining regional clusters of PV adoption and that spatial spillover is not mainly driven by social imitation but by unobserved regional characteristics. High values for solar radiation, the share of detached houses, electricity demand, and inverse population density of a region favor the PV uptake. Predicting that also in the case of this study, the demographic and socioeconomic factors as well as built environment associated with each region will be key to mapping the country's regions and identifying which are more likely to be receptive to domestic solar panels, these variables were extracted from publicly available sources to test how they fit the data. The approach of Baginski and Weber [6] will be closely followed, adding a predictive component using the results found to build a map representing the likelihood of adoption, making it more directly usable by decision-makers in the field.

Most studies that try to explain the factors influencing PV system adoption use the number of PV systems as the target variable to be explained [2–4, 7, e.g.]. Some, as in the case of Rode and Weber [8], use a variation of this discrete variable, like the number of PV installations per building and number of PV installations per owner-occupied household, transforming the target variable into a ratio and therefore essentially continuous. Others, like Baginski and Weber [6] and Schaffer and Brun

[9], use the PV installed capacity (in kw), which is a continuous variable. Naturally, the methods used in each approach will also differ accordingly. In the case of this study, there are three variables that could be used as target variables, namely *Total Price*, *Installed Power* and *Number of Panels*, since all represent the size of PV system installations. Hence, and since the installed capacity has been used by other authors, this study will entail both the analysis of *Installed Power* and *Number of Panels*. Thus analyzing both a continuous and a discrete variable.

Baginski and Weber [6] focus on the spatial diffusion of PV systems using spatial econometric models and considering both exogenous and endogenous spatial interactions. To follow this recommendation, this study will first perform a spatial exploratory analysis. Many spatial analysis authors refer to Tobler's first law of geography, which states that areas closer together are more similar than those further apart (*"the first law of geography: everything is related to everything else, but near things are more related than distant things."* [10]). For that reason, most spatial analysis start by exploring spatial correlation, which implies the correlation among the same variable from different locations.

Spatial dependence is commonly made operational by some measure of spatial autocorrelation, which depend on the specification or estimation of a set of weights describing spatial relationships. To describe possible spatial relationships between locations, one must first define what accounts for neighbors of said locations. Some typical examples of criteria that could be used to define neighbors were described by Anselin [11], namely first-order contiguity and critical distance thresholds. Part of assigning neighbors involves applying a measure of weighting to indicate the extent to which the information from an area's neighbors impacts on the observed estimate for that area. This is commonly summarized in a spatial weights matrix.

2 Material and Methods

2.1 *Data Characterization and Preprocessing*

There are two important data sets to consider for the construction of the models. The main data set contains details from 441 domestic solar panel installations done in Portugal between the end of June and November of 2020, provided by a company that specializes in such installations. The second data set involves demographic and socioeconomic variables extracted from *Instituto Nacional de Estatística (INE:* www.ine.pt). These variables were downloaded as isolated data sets and then aggregated by geographical location. The selection of the variables was based on the factors found in the literature to influence the decision to install solar panels. These were then subjected to a correlation analysis to select the final list.

The available variables regarding the solar PV installations, their type, and their meaning are described in Table 1.

Table 1 Description of the variables regarding solar PV installations

Variable	Type	Description
Date	Categorical	Date of the installation
Postal code	Categorical	Postal code of the house of installation
Number of panels	Numerical	Number of panels installed
Installed power	Numerical	Power installed, in kwh

Data preprocessing tasks included both data exclusion and variable creation. The data exclusion task involved removing some values that do not make sense and are likely to be database mistakes. The geographical aspect of the data is very important to pursue the goals of this paper. Hence, since the only variable containing geographic information in the dataset is *Postal Code*, this information was expanded to include *Locality*, *Municipality*, *District*, *NUTSII*, and *NUTSIII*, creating these 5 new variables. *NUTS* refers to the Nomenclature of Territorial Units for Statistics, and it is a standard for referencing subdivisions of European countries. *NUTSI* represents major socioeconomic regions, which corresponds to three regions in Portugal. *NUTSII* refers to basic regions for the application of regional policies and is made up of seven regions in Portugal, five if the islands are excluded. *NUTSIII* represents smaller regions and corresponds to 25 regions in Portugal, 23 of these in continental Portugal.

The list of selected explanatory variables and their description can be seen in Table 2. A summary of descriptive statistics can be seen in Table 4 (Table 3).

From the initial set of 45 variables that have data at the municipality level, these 13 were selected based primarily on correlation analysis.

2.2 Data Modeling

Spatial Weights Matrix Spatial weights represent geographic relationships between the different units in a spatially referenced dataset, usually in the form of a spatial weights matrix. This is defined as a $n \times n$ positive matrix W with elements w_{ij} at location pairs i, j $(i \neq j; i, j = 1, ..., n)$ for n locations. An element w_{ij} is the weight for each pair of locations, which is assigned by some rules that define the spatial relations between the locations.

There are several ways to define this matrix, commonly based on contiguity. A pair of spatial units is said to be contiguous if they share a common border. Rook contiguity constructs a weight object from a collection of polygons that share at least one edge. Queen contiguity is a more inclusive notion of contiguity, since it requires a pair of polygons to share one or more vertices.

Table 2 Description of explanatory variables

Variable	Description
Population	Number of people who live in each municipality
Purchase power	Purchase power per person who lives in each municipality
Gross income Gini	Gini coefficient calculated per taxable persons
Gross income	Gross income per person who lives in each municipality
Subsidies	Number of people who receive government subsidies per person who lives in each municipality
Rental agreements	Number of rental agreements per person who lives in each municipality
Energy consumption	Domestic consumption of electrical energy per consumer (kWh/consumer), where consumed energy might have been produced by hydroelectric, nuclear or thermal conventional centrals or also wave, mares, wind or solar energy
Votes in the most voted	Percentage of votes in the most voted in elections for the Assembly of the Republic
Abstention	Percentage of abstention in the elections for the Assembly of the Republic
Temperature	Average temperature in the last available year
Art exhibitions	Number of art gallery exhibitions per person who lives in each municipality
Family housing	Number of classic family housing
Habitation buildings	Number of habitation buildings

Table 3 Results for the spatial dependence tests in the OLS model

Test	Statistic	P-value
Moran (residuals)	0.0856	0.002021
LMerr	5.5948	0.01801
LMlag	1.4397	0.2302
RLMerr	6.1968	0.0128
RLMlag	2.0417	0.153
SARMA	7.6365	0.02197

Since there is very little information available about what type of relation would make a municipality in Portugal influence one more than another and to make the least number of assumptions, a k-nearest neighbors matrix will be chosen and k decided based on the most common number of neighbors a municipality has in Portugal (discovered through rook and queen contiguity).

Spatial Correlation An important part of spatial analysis is the particular analysis of spatial correlation. Popular options for area-level data that will be considered include Moran's I, Geary's C, Gettis and Ord's G and the Localized Indicators of

Table 4 Summary description of explanatory variables

Variable	Count	Mean	RSD[4] (%)	Min	Median	Max
Population	278	35247.69	57526.42	1634	14608	509515
Purchase power	278	80.51	18.68	55.32	77.21	219.63
Gross income Gini	272	26.89	2.34	21.10	26.70	37.20
Gross income	278	7608.82	1726.30	4352.00	7384.50	19574.00
Subsidies	278	0.03	0.01	0.01	0.03	0.13
Rental agreements	182	0.006	0.003	0.002	0.006	0.016
Energy consumption	278	2082.81	712.62	1026.00	2082.15	10393.00
Votes in the most voted	278	40.64	4.58	31.20	40.10	61.50
Abstention	278	47.35	5.79	30.40	46.50	66.20
Temperature	278	15.43	1.37	11.70	15.40	18.00
Art exhibitions	278	0.0002	0.0002	0.0000	0.0001	0.0018
Family housing	278	0.74	0.26	0.39	0.70	2.95
Habitation buildings	278	0.60	0.27	0.07	0.58	1.61

Spatial Association (LISA). It is important to be attentive of the distinction between global and localized correlation. Some methods study global clustering (like Moran's I), which assesses spatial correlation throughout the entire study region. Localized correlation is also called local clustering or hot-spot analysis and includes methods such as LISA.

To model adoption of solar PV systems across Portugal, this study will start by estimating a binary dependent variable, namely whether there are PV installations in a certain region or not. Taking this a step further, a discrete dependent variable will be modeled, specifically the number of panels installed in each region. Finally we will focus more attentively on modeling a continuous dependent variable, namely the installed power.

For all the following models in this chapter, this notation is used:

- n is the number of observations;
- K is the number of explanatory variables;
- $\mathbf{Y}$ is a $n \times 1$ vector of observations on the dependent variable;
- X is a $n \times K$ matrix of observations on the explanatory variables with an associated vector of regression coefficients $\boldsymbol{\beta}$ $(K \times 1)$;
- W is the spatial weights matrix $(n \times n)$;

- WY denotes the endogenous interactions among the dependent variable associated with the spatial autoregressive parameter ρ, which measures the effect of spatial lag on this variable;
- WX denotes the exogenous interactions among the independent variables associated with a vector of regression coefficients γ $(K \times 1)$;
- Wu denotes interactions among the residuals of spatial units, associated with the spatial autocorrelation parameter λ;
- ε represents an independently identically normally distributed error term vector with zero mean and constant variance ($\varepsilon \sim N_n\left(0, \sigma^2 I_n\right)$);
- α represents the models' intercept.

Binary Dependent Variable To model the binary dependent variable *Installation*, the probit model will be used, as it is typically privileged in econometrics.

This is a particular type of binary regression model that ultimately allows to classify the observations based on their predicted probabilities. Considering the generalized linear model framework, the probit model uses a probit link function and will be estimated using maximum likelihood. This is represented by the following equation

$$\mathrm{P}(\mathbf{Y} = \mathbf{1} \mid X) = \Phi\,(X\boldsymbol{\beta}) \tag{1}$$

where $\mathbf{Y}$ is a vector of the binary outcome, $\mathbf{1}$ is a vector of ones, Φ is the cumulative distribution function of the standard normal distribution, and $\boldsymbol{\beta}$ is the vector of parameters β estimated by maximum likelihood.

To introduce a spatial component in this analysis, a Bayesian Estimation of Spatial Probit Models will be used. The Bayesian estimation of the spatial autoregressive probit model (SAR Probit model) is described by

$$\mathbf{Y} = \rho W\mathbf{Y} + X\boldsymbol{\beta} + \varepsilon \tag{2}$$

with notation as previously described. Note that ρ is the scalar parameter that describes the strength of spatial dependence in the sample of observations.

The prior distributions are $\beta \sim N(c, T)$ and $\rho \sim Beta(a_1, a_2)$, where c is the mean value of β, T is the variance of β, while a_1 and a_2 are shape parameters.

In general the coefficients of any probit regression cannot be interpreted directly. The marginal effects of the regressors should be considered partial derivatives. Additionally, in the case of the SAR Probit model, the direct, indirect, and total effects are to be considered. A change in one explanatory variable x_{ki} for location i ($i = 1, \ldots, n$) will not only affect the observations y_i directly (this is considered the direct impact), but this change can also affect the observations in locations nearby y_j (which is the indirect impact). Let $S_k(W)$ be the matrix $(n \times n)$ of impacts from location i to location j for explanatory variable x_k, defined as

$$S_k(W) = \frac{dE[\mathbf{Y} \mid x_k]}{dx_k} = \phi((I_n - \rho W)^{-1} I_n \bar{x}_k \beta_k) * (I_n - \rho W)^{-1} I_n \beta_k \tag{3}$$

where $\bar{x}_k$ denotes the mean value of variable x_k and β_k the parameter estimate for this variable.

Then the direct impact of a change in x_{ki} on y_i can be described as $S_k(W)_{ii}$ and the indirect impact from observation x_{kj} on y_i as $S_k(W)_{ij}$ $(i \neq j)$. Hence, the average direct impact of k can be calculated as the average of the diagonal elements. The average total impact is the mean of the row sum, and the average indirect impacts can be calculated as the difference between average total impacts and average direct impacts.

Discrete Dependent Variable To model the Number of Panels installed across the municipalities, linear regressions were considered and estimated by OLS. The following models will be used

$$\mathbf{Y} = X\boldsymbol{\beta} + \varepsilon \tag{4}$$

$$\mathbf{Y} = X\boldsymbol{\beta} + WX\boldsymbol{\gamma} + \varepsilon. \tag{5}$$

Equation 4 describes the linear regression estimated by OLS (referred to as OLS Model in Sect. 3), while Eq. 5 describes the SLX Model, which includes the spatially lagged explanatory variables, weighted by the spatial weights matrix.

Continuous Target Variable This study will take a general-to-specific approach, as suggested by Baginski and Weber [6], thus starting with a simple non-spatial linear regression and successively adding different spatial interaction effects. Still using OLS estimation, the model will be expanded with the spatial lag of the explanatory variables (SLX). The model will then be expanded with a spatially lagged dependent variable, thus estimating the spatial lag or spatial autoregressive model (SAR). The spatial error model (SEM) is also specified, incorporating spatial autoregressive process in the error term. Then, estimating a spatial durbin model (SDM) can be appropriate, where the SAR model is expanded with spatially lagged explanatory variables, as it seems reasonable to think that spatially correlated variables are probably omitted. For the same reason, the spatial durbin error model (SDEM) will also be estimated and compared. Finally, because the underlying spatial process is often unclear, all three spatial effects will be combined in the most general model, the Manski model. Here it is important to take into consideration that one of the components has to be removed for the spatial coefficients to be properly interpreted and distinguished [12].

It has been shown in LeSage and Pace [13] that a valid way to interpret the β coefficients in spatial econometric models is partial derivative interpretations of the impacts. The direct impact is the change in one location associated with the explanatory variable that affects that same region. The indirect effect is the potential effect that this explanatory variable has on all other regions it affects. The sum of both is the total effect. These impact measures are valid for models including a spatially lagged variable, thus in OLS and SEM the indirect effects are zero.

The first OLS estimation is the same as described for the discrete dependent variable in Eq. 4. Six different statistics for spatial dependence will be run to test for residual spatial dependence of the OLS regression:

- Moran's I test for residual spatial autocorrelation;
- simple LM test for error dependence (LMerr);
- simple LM test for a missing spatially lagged dependent variable (LMlag);
- variants of these robust to the presence of the other:
  - test for error dependence in the possible presence of a missing lagged dependent variable (RLMerr);
  - test for a missing spatially lagged dependent variable in the possible presence of error dependence (RLMlag);
- portmanteau test (SARMA, in fact LMerr + RLMlag).

The most straightforward way to include spatial dependence in a regression is by considering not only an explanatory variable, but also its spatial lag. This implies estimating the SLX model, described by Eq. 5.

The spatial lag model (SAR) introduces a spatial lag of the dependent variable, as seen in the following equation

$$\mathbf{Y} = \rho W \mathbf{Y} + X\beta + \varepsilon. \tag{6}$$

This model violates the exogeneity assumption, crucial for OLS to work and therefore a maximum likelihood estimation will be used.

The spatial error model (SEM) includes a spatial lag in the error term of the equation, resulting in the following term

$$\begin{aligned} \mathbf{Y} &= X\beta + \mathbf{u} \\ \mathbf{u} &= \lambda W \mathbf{u} + \varepsilon. \end{aligned} \tag{7}$$

As this specification violates the assumptions about the error term in a classical OLS model, a maximum likelihood will be used.

The spatial Durbin error model (SDEM) includes a spatial lag in the error term of the equation and the spatial lag of explanatory variables, resulting in

$$\begin{aligned} \mathbf{Y} &= X\beta + WX\gamma + \mathbf{u} \\ \mathbf{u} &= \lambda W \mathbf{u} + \varepsilon. \end{aligned} \tag{8}$$

The spatial Durbin model (SDM) includes the spatial lag of the dependent variable and of the explanatory variables, resulting in

$$\mathbf{Y} = \rho W \mathbf{Y} + X\beta + WX\gamma + \varepsilon. \tag{9}$$

The Kelejian-Prucha model (GSM) includes the spatial lag of the dependent variable and in the error term of the equation, resulting in

$$\begin{aligned} \mathbf{Y} &= \rho W \mathbf{Y} + X\beta + \mathbf{u} \\ \mathbf{u} &= \lambda W \mathbf{u} + \varepsilon. \end{aligned} \tag{10}$$

The Manski model is the most general model and includes the spatial lag of the dependent variable, in the error term of the equation and of the explanatory variables, resulting in

$$\begin{aligned} \mathbf{Y} &= \rho W\mathbf{Y} + X\beta + WX\gamma + \mathbf{u} \\ \mathbf{u} &= \lambda W\mathbf{u} + \varepsilon. \end{aligned} \tag{11}$$

Model Selection In this study, AIC will be the main criteria used to select the best model. To do model diagnosis, residual plots will be produced for all the regressions. Some important aspects when analyzing the regression results estimated by OLS are the t and F statistics. To test for heteroskedasticity, the Breusch-Pagan test will be used. To compare different models, the Nagelkerke pseudo R-squared will be used.

Ultimately, this study sets out to build a spatial model that estimates, for each spatial unit in Portugal, the probability of adopting domestic solar PV systems. Hence, a map will be produced where each region has a value, in a scale that ranges from 0 to 1, representing the probability of a solar installation being adopted. This may be achieved by dividing the predicted value of Installed Power for each region by the total predicted value for the country.

3 Results

3.1 *Exploratory Analysis*

Dependent Variables Firstly, a general exploratory analysis is important to understand the distribution of the dependent variables. Bar plots and histograms were built to achieve this, as well as simple tables with descriptive statistics and maps to visualize their geographical distribution.

As mentioned before, there are three variables that will be considered to be dependent throughout this study. Installation is a binary variable that is 1 when a municipality has at least one installation. Number of Panels is a discrete variable that represents the total sum of panels. Installed Power is a continuous variable that contains the sum of installed power (in kwh). Since the patterns found in the variables Number of Panels and Installed Power are very similar, the graphs for Number of Panels are presented only in the Appendix. Indeed the similarity can be seen in the scatter plot of Fig. 7.

Most installations have 3 panels installed and half the installations have 4 or less panels, but the number of panels can vary between 1 and 22. The installed power ranges from 0.3 to 7.5, with half of the installations having around 1.4kwh or less. Both variables present a positive skewness at installation level, as can be seen in Figs. 1a and 8.

At municipality level, around 63% of regions have solar PV installations, hence the total number of panels and installed power show a large positive skewness and zero-inflation, as shown in Figs. 1b and 9 as well as Table 5.

Figure 2 shows that in general, the municipalities that do not have solar PV installations are mainly in the interior part of Portugal. The regions that do show some installations vary a lot in size, described by the Number of Panels and capacity, represented by the Installed Power. The biggest installations can be found in coastal

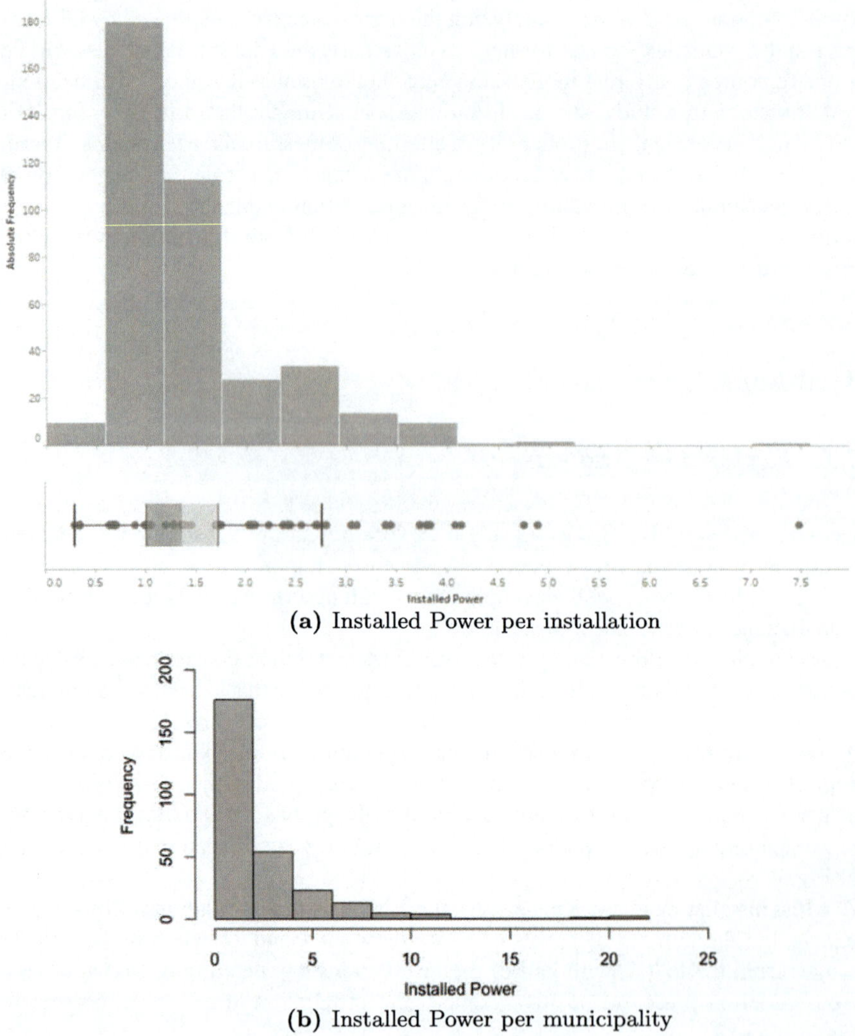

Fig. 1 Distribution of installed power

Table 5 Summary description of numerical dependent variables

Variable	Count	Mean	RSD[5] (%)	Min	Median	Max
Number of panels	278	6.892	144.8758	0	3	65
Installed power (in kw)	278	2.057	148.9829	0.0	1.020	21.16

[5]Relative Standard Deviation or Coefficient of Variation

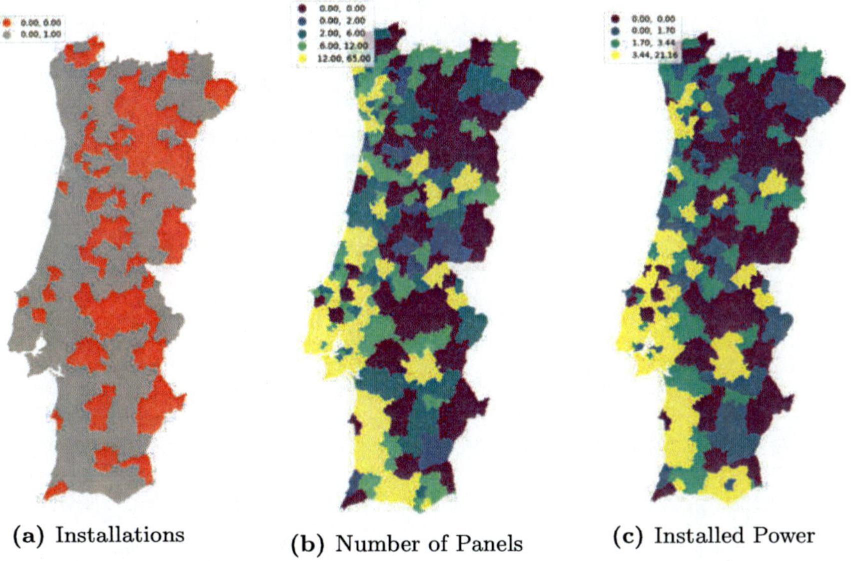

Fig. 2 Choropleth maps of dependent variables

Portugal, especially in the center and south regions, but also some in the north around the city of Porto (Figs. 3, 4, 5, 6, 7, 8 and 9).

Spatial Weights Matrix In this subsection, the choice of the weights matrix is presented. In this case, the queen and rook weights matrix attribute to all locations the same neighbors. Since the grid is not regular, there is no "edge" case and so both matrices are being the same. Figure 10a shows the contiguity relationships represented by the centroids of each municipality and edges connecting them. Figure 10b shows that the minimum number of neighbors in this case is 1, while one municipality has 10 rook neighbors. The most common number of neighbors is 5.

Instead of having to assume that contiguity will affect more than distance or vice-versa, a simple approach is applied by using k-nearest neighbors weights matrix and choosing $k = 5$, which is the mode of the number of neighbors.

Spatial Correlation The Moran Plot shows the relation between a variable and its spatial lag. To help with the interpretation, a linear fit, which represents the best linear

Fig. 3 Moran's I

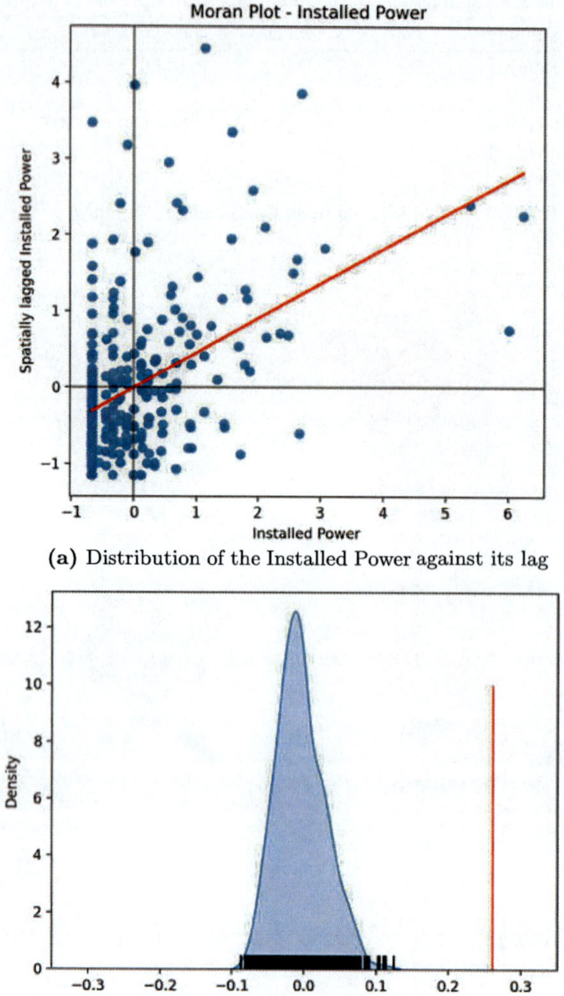

(a) Distribution of the Installed Power against its lag

(b) Distribution of simulated Moran's I statistics for Installed Power and vertical line showing the estimated value (in red)

fit to the scatter plot is included. The slope of this line is the value of the Moran's I statistic. Figures 3a and 11 show the plots for the dependent variables. The plots display positive relationships between both variables, which is associated with the presence of positive spatial autocorrelation, meaning that similar values tend to be located close to each other.

To test whether this is statistically significant, a simulation was run with 999 permutations and the distribution of these values is shown in Figs. 3b and 12. It

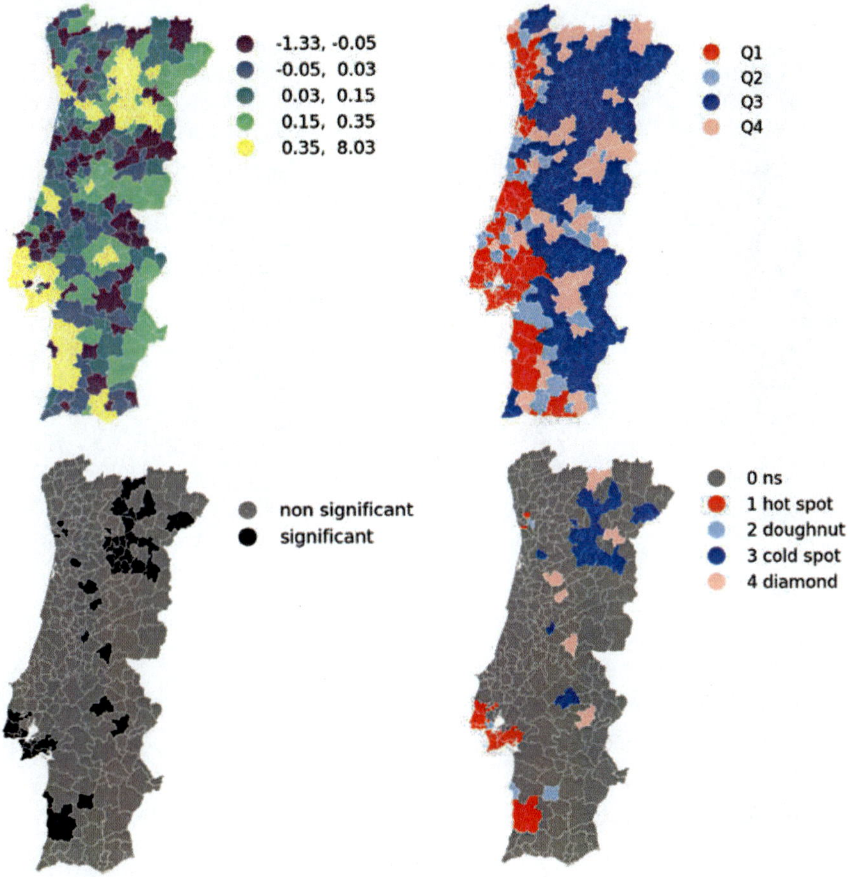

Fig. 4 LISA statistics for Installed Power across municipalities

corresponds to a kernel density estimation plot and a rug showing all of the simulated points, as well as a vertical line denoting the observed value of the statistic. It shows that it is not likely that the pattern came from a spatially random process, allowing for the conclusion that there is indeed spatial autocorrelation in the dataset.

Geary's C statistic is in line with Moran's I, as a value lower than 1 indicates that neighboring observations are similar. Geary's C simulated p-value is also 0.001. Gettis and Ord's G requires a binary spatial weights matrix with ones for all points defined as being within a certain distance of any given location, so that a different weights matrix was used to calculate this statistic. To ensure that every municipality has at least one neighbor, the minimum distance band was calculated. This needs to be at least around 31km for this data. Using this d results in the value of 0.0597 for the G statistic and the pseudo p-value of 0.001, which also suggests a clear departure from the hypothesis of no concentration. These values are summarized in Table 6.

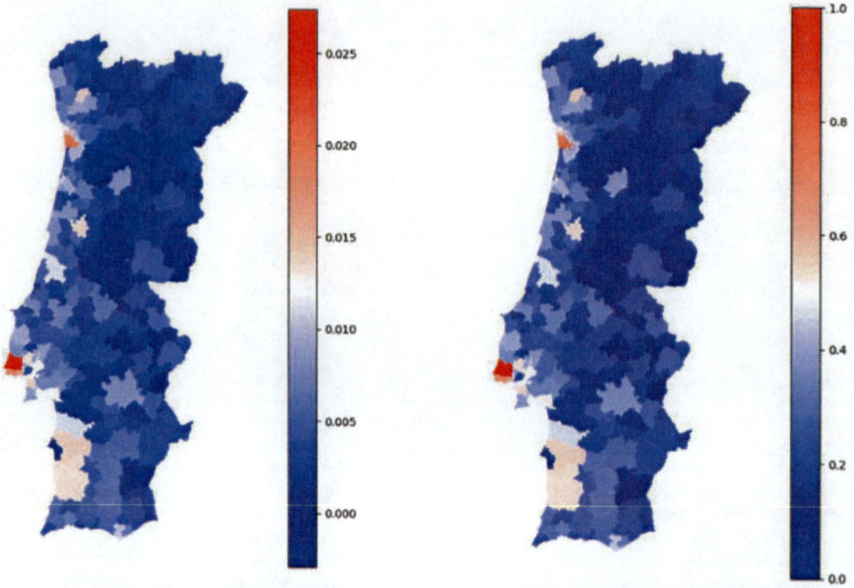

(a) Likelihood map (b) Normalized Likelihood map

Fig. 5 Likelihood maps

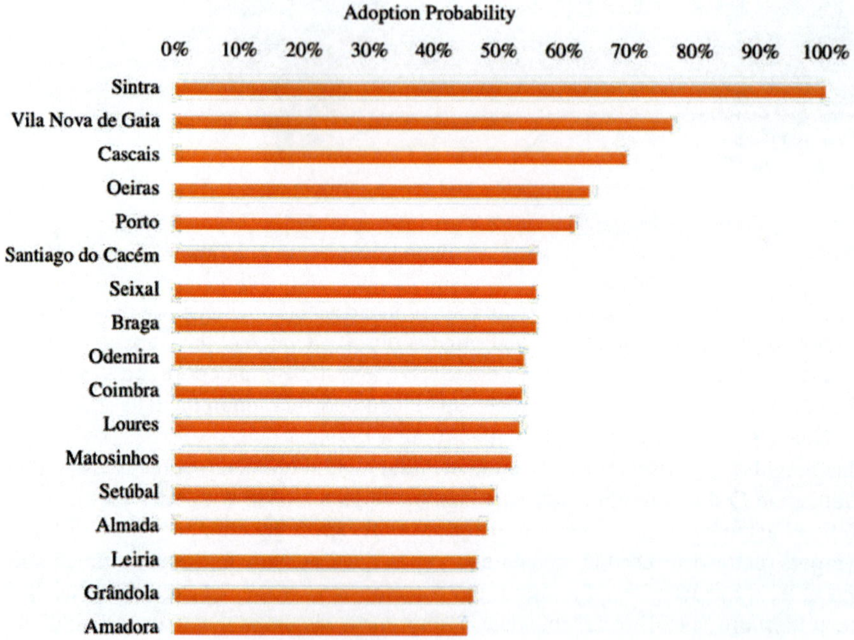

Fig. 6 Adoption probability per municipality

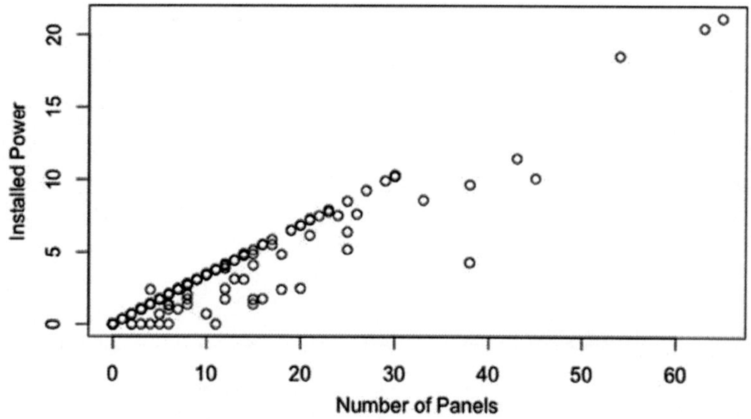

Fig. 7 Number of panels against installed power

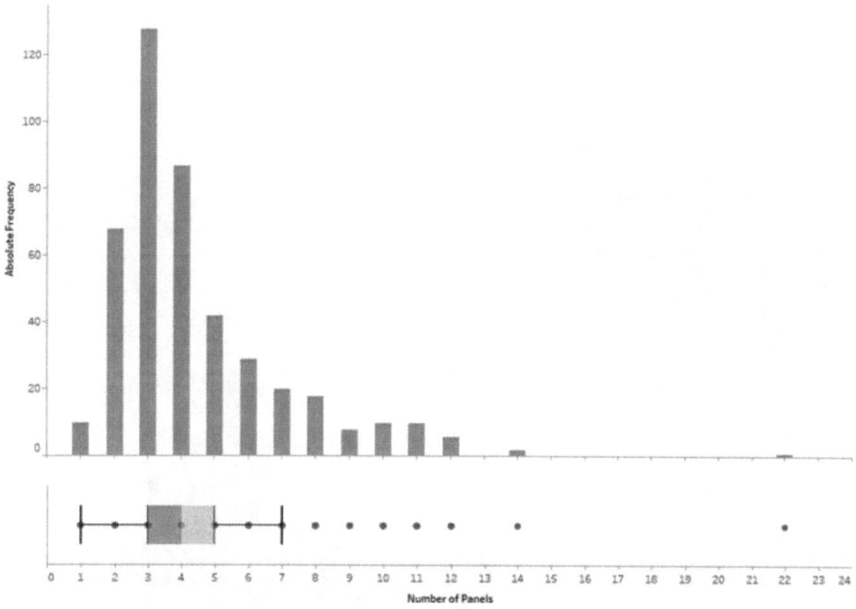

Fig. 8 Distribution of the number of panels per installation

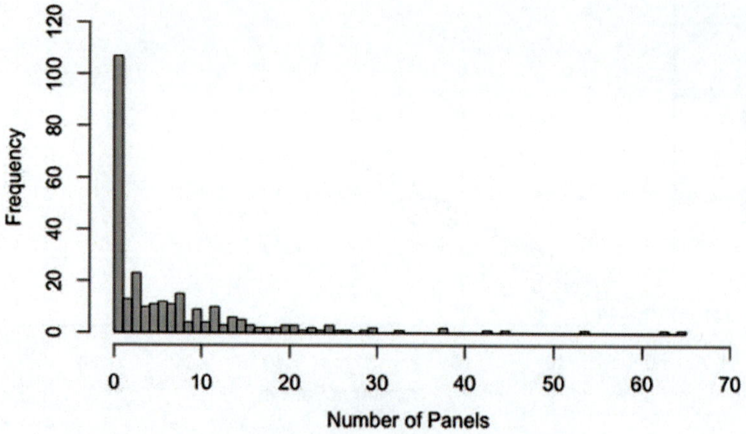

Fig. 9 Distribution of number of panels per municipality

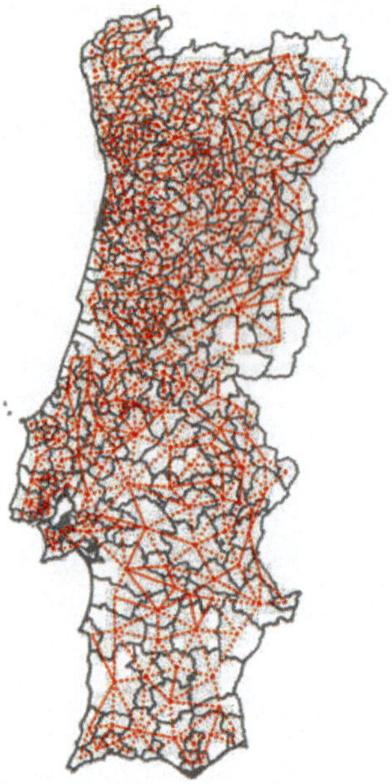

(a) Centroids and edges used in rook and queen weights matrix

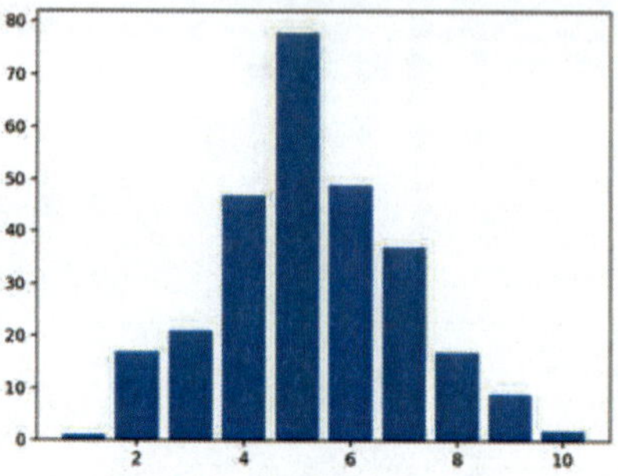

(b) Histogram number of neighbors in the rook and queen weights matrix

Fig. 10 Rook and Queen contiguity in Portuguese municipalities

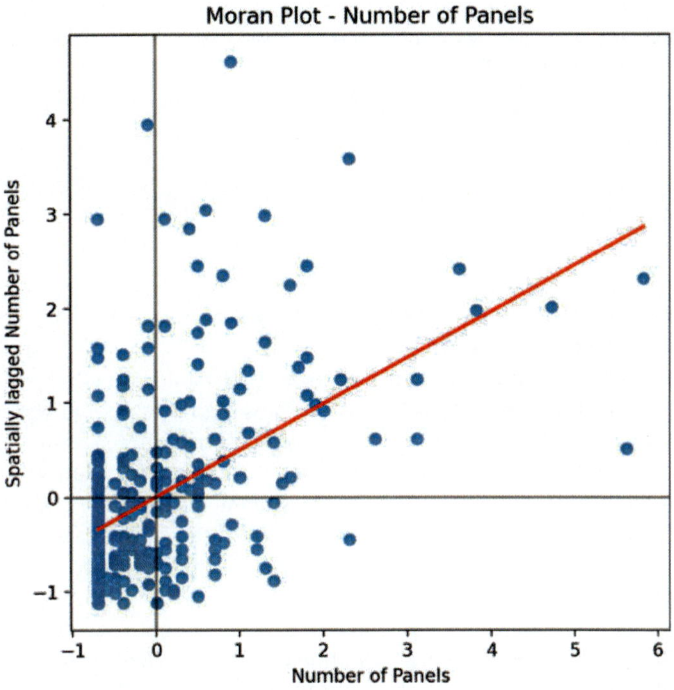

Fig. 11 Distribution of the number of panels against its lag

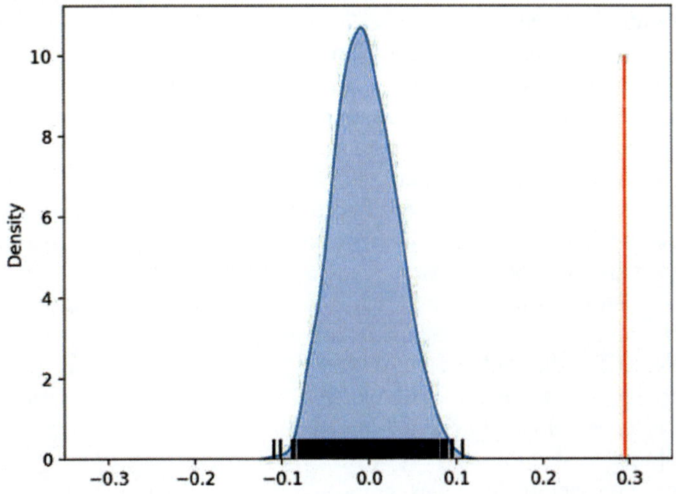

Fig. 12 Distribution of simulated Moran's I statistics for number of panels and vertical line showing the estimated value (in red)

Table 6 Results of global spatial correlation statistics for variables Number of Panels and Installed Power with respective pseudo p-values in brackets

	Number of panels	Installed power
Moran I	0.2951 (0.001)	0.2610 (0.001)
Geary's C	0.6455 (0.001)	0.6758 (0.001)
Getis and Ord's G	0.0597 (0.001)	0.0583 (0.001)

Figure 4 shows four plots that bring the different perspectives of the results for LISA for Installed Power together.

The upper-left map shows the result for local spatial autocorrelation represented by the LISA statistics. The municipalities that show high local spatial correlation in Installed Power are represented in yellow. There are some differences in the municipalities with high local spatial correlation when it comes to the Number of Panels, as can be seen in Fig. 13, namely there are less municipalities in the north of Portugal with this characteristic. The upper-right maps show the location of the LISA statistic in the quadrant of the Moran scatter plot. Comparing these two maps one can see that the positive association in the north interior part of Portugal is due to low adoption in these municipalities, while in the coastal south part of Portugal the positive association is due to the high adoption of solar PV. However, it is important to introduce the underlying statistical significance of the local values when analyzing this. Positive forms of local spatial autocorrelation are of two types: significant HH (high-high) clustering, i.e., hot spots, or LL (low-low) clustering, i.e., cold spots. Locations with significant but negative local autocorrelation are either doughnuts (low value is neighbored by locations with high values) or diamonds (high value is neighbored by locations with low values). In the last map, in bright red are the locations with an unusual concentration of high installed power surrounded also by similar locations. In light red there are the first type of spatial outliers, areas that have high installed power despite being surrounded by areas with low values. These correspond to some areas in the interior of Portugal. In darker blue one can see the spatial clusters of low power. In light blue there is another type of spatial outlier, areas with low installed power nearby areas with high.

The core idea of LISA statistics is to identify cases in which the comparison between the value of an observation and the average of its neighbors is either more similar (HH, LL) or dissimilar (HL, LH) than one would expect from chance. Figures 14 and 15 show the distribution of LISA values for the dependent variables, indicating a skewed distribution due to the dominance of the positive forms of spatial association.

The maps representing the values for the G statistics, which can be seen in Fig. 16, show similar results to LISA.

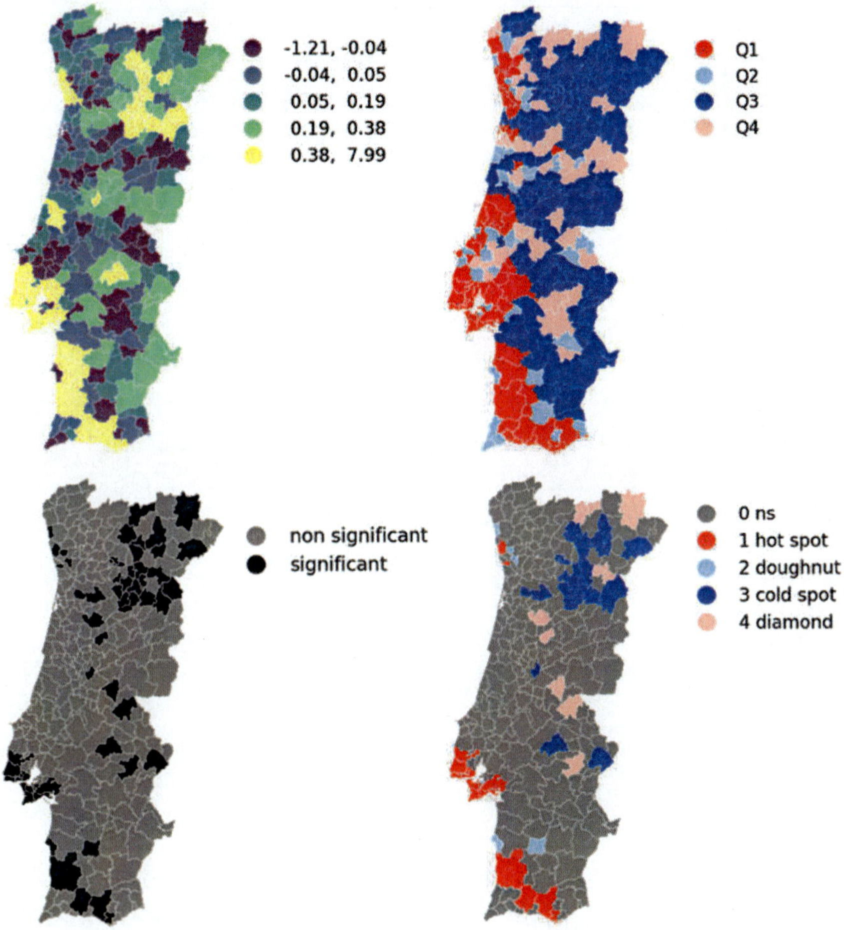

Fig. 13 LISA statistics for number of panels across municipalities

3.2 Models

Binary Target Variable In this section, the results of the non-spatial and the SAR Probit models to estimate the adoption of Installations are presented. A summary of these results is shown in Table 7.

The variables Purchase Power, Subsidies, Rental Agreements, Gross income Gini coefficient, Votes in the most voted, Family housing, and Abstention were not significant to explain whether a certain municipality adopts solar PV installations. Table 7 shows that all of the fitted models' coefficients are statistically significant. The exception lies in the SAR Probit model's spatial lag coefficient rho, thus indicating that

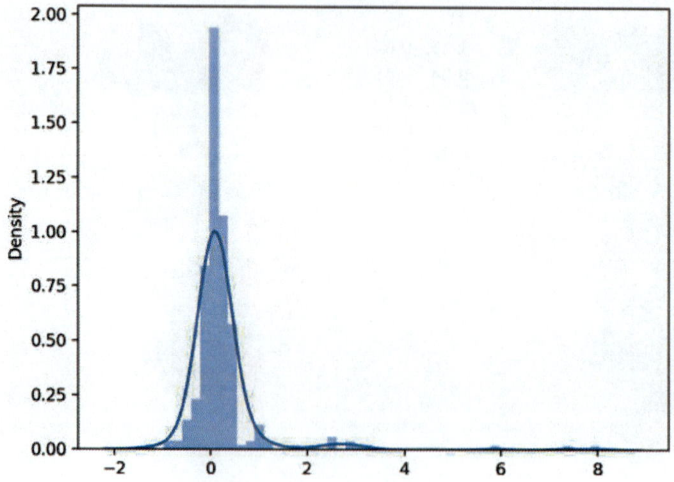

Fig. 14 Distribution of LISA values for the installed power

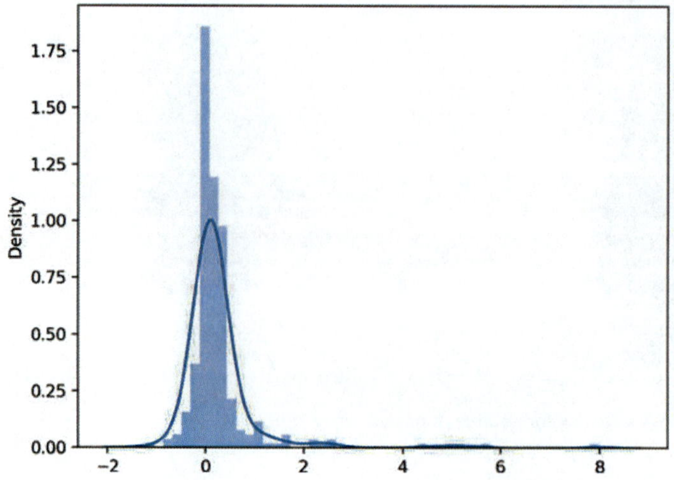

Fig. 15 Distribution of LISA values for the number of panels

the decision to adopt PV installations in one location does not seem to directly affect this decision in other locations. Regarding the log-likelihood statistics shown at the end of Table 7, they seem to show a negligible difference between the Probit and the SAR Probit model.

When considering the marginal effects presented in Table 8, one can see that while Population, Temperature, and Gross Income contribute positively to the probability of installing PV systems, Energy Consumption, Art Exhibitions, and Housing buildings seem to have a negative contribution. Regarding the SAR Probit marginal effects,

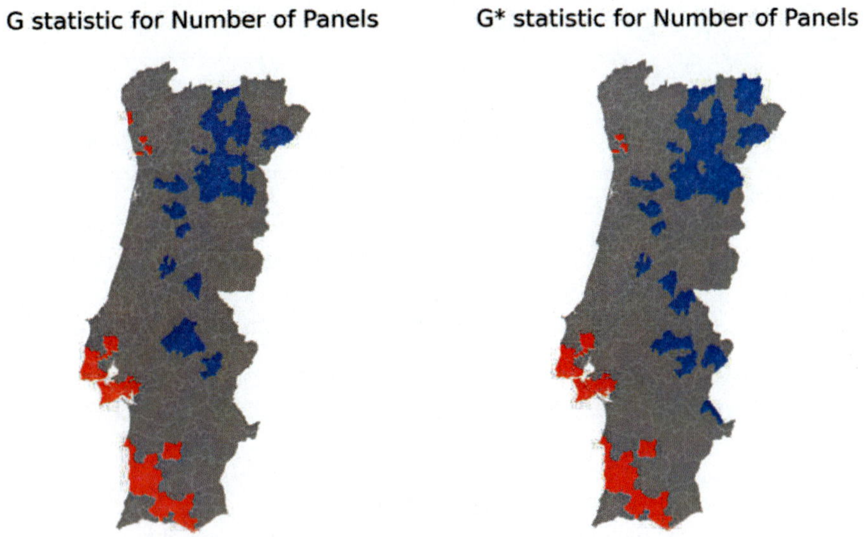

Fig. 16 Distribution of G statistic values for the number of panels

Table 7 Summary of the installation (binary) model (SE between brackets)

	Probit	SAR Probit
(Intercept)	−2.779**	−2.835**
	(1.150)	(1.262)
Population	0.00002**	0.00002**
	(0.00001)	(0.00001)
Energy consumption	−0.0003*	−0.0004**
	(0.0002)	(0.0002)
Temperature	0.166**	0.181**
	(0.082)	(0.085)
Art exhibitions	−10.674**	−11.660**
	(5.416)	(5.686)
Gross income	0.0002**	0.0002**
	(0.0001)	(0.0001)
Housing buildings	−0.011**	−0.012**
	(0.005)	(0.006)
rho		−0.026
		(0.132)
AIC	280.806	283.2535
BIC	306.1991	312.2745
Log likelihood	−133.403	−133.6267
Note:	*p<0.1; **p<0.05; ***p<0.01	

Table 8 Marginal effects

	Probit	SAR Probit		
		Direct	Indirect	Total
Population	0.000005	0.000002	−0.000001	0.000002
Energy consumption	−0.000094	−0.000201	−0.000026	−0.000207
Temperature	0.045030	0.010450	−0.012240	0.009950
Art exhibitions	−2.902000	−5.627000	−0.728900	−5.725000
Gross income	0.000065	0.000024	−0.000016	0.000023
Housing buildings	−0.002939	−0.005602	−0.000640	−0.005565

it is clear that the direct effects are larger in the case of every explanatory variable, except for temperature. The direct effect of Temperature in the probability to install is positive, while the indirect effect is negative in a similar magnitude.

Discrete Target Variable In this section, the results of the OLS and SLX models to estimate the Number of Panels are presented. A summary of these results is shown in Table 9.

The variables Purchase Power and Rental agreements are not included in either of the models, together with the spatially lagged variables Population, Rental Agreements, Gross Income Gini, Housing Buildings, Votes in the most voted, and Abstention. When comparing both models, one can see that the introduction of the spatially lagged variables improves the fit, as the adjusted R^2 increases by 0.032. Both models estimate that the Number of Panels increases when Population, Gross Income, Housing buildings, and Abstention increase. Both estimate that the dependent variable decreases when Energy Consumption, Art exhibitions, Votes in the most voted, and Family housing increase. Subsidies and Temperature are not present in the SLX model, but are statistically significant in the OLS model and their lagged variant is also present in the SLX model. This means that although the temperature and subsidies received in each municipality do not seem to influence the number of solar panels acquired in the same municipality, their values contribute to explain the variance of this phenomenon in neighboring municipalities. While the lagged temperature has a positive influence on the number of panels in neighboring municipalities, lagged subsidies result in the opposite behavior, although the latter is not statistically significant. The value of the Gini coefficient of gross income is not considered relevant for the OLS, but it is statistically significant at a 90% significance level in the SLX model. Spatially lagged Purchase Power also seems to negatively influence the number of Panels acquired in neighboring locations, even though the Purchase Power of a certain location does not explain the number of panels in the same location. Energy consumption, Gross income, Family housing, and Art exhibitions, all seem to influence the total number of panels in both the locations they relate to and their neighbors, although spatially lagged Art exhibitions are not statistically significant.

Table 9 Summary of the number of panels models

	OLS	SLX
(Intercept)	−24.894***	−14.345***
	(9.033)	(3.645)
Population	0.0001***	0.00004***
	(0.00001)	(0.00000)
Energy consumption	−0.002***	−0.001***
	(0.001)	(0.0002)
Subsidies	1.275***	
	(0.436)	
Temperature	1.210***	
	(0.402)	
Art exhibitions	−48.850**	−15.889**
	(23.676)	(7.229)
Gross income Gini coefficient		0.161*
		(0.082)
Gross income	0.002***	0.0003*
	(0.0004)	(0.0002)
Votes in the most voted	−0.233**	−0.060*
	(0.110)	(0.033)
Housing buildings	0.179***	0.062***
	(0.044)	(0.013)
Family housing	−0.207***	−0.077***
	(0.036)	(0.011)
Abstention	0.260***	0.060**
	(0.087)	(0.028)
L. Purchase Power		−0.132***
		(0.043)
L. Energy consumption		0.003***
		(0.001)
L. Subsidies		−0.369
		(0.231)
L. Temperature		0.478**
		(0.188)
L. Art exhibitions		−23.992
		(15.767)
L. Gross income		0.001**
		(0.0005)
L. Family housing		0.038***
		(0.013)
R^2	0.4924	0.533
Adjusted R^2	0.473	0.505
Residual Std. Error	7.246	2.156
F Statistic	25.902***	18.655***
AIC	1902.82	1234.495
Log likelihood	−939.41	−599.2476
Note:	*p<0.1; **p<0.05; ***p<0.01	

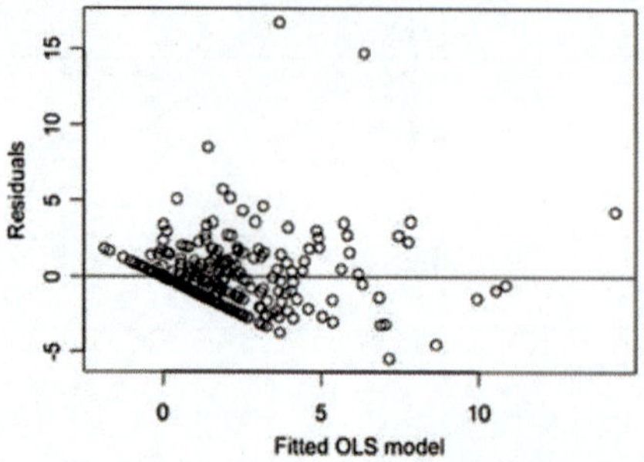

(a) Distribution of the fitted values of the OLS regression against the residuals

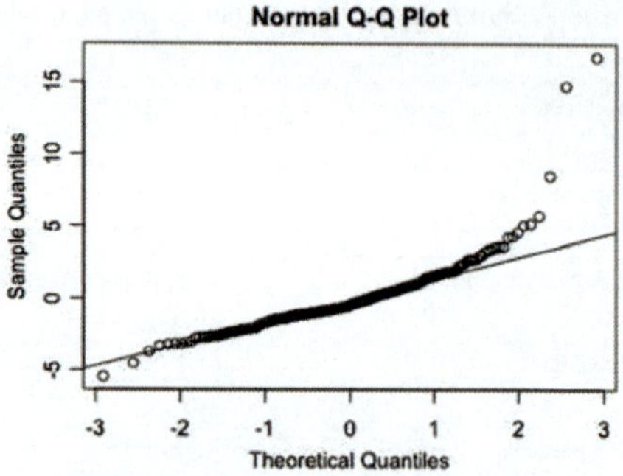

(b) Q-Q plot from OLS regression residuals

Fig. 17 Residuals of the OLS regression

Gross income in a certain location has a positive influence on the number of panels in this same location as well as its numbers, while Energy Consumption and Family housing have opposite effects when comparing their influence on their location and its neighbors.

Continuous Target Variable In this section, the results of the OLS, SAR, SEM, GSM, SLX, SDM, SDEM, and Manski models to estimate the Installed Power are presented. Summaries of these results are shown in Tables 10 and 11.

To analyze these results, it is important to firstly analyze the residuals of the regressions and inspect the chance of heteroscedasticity as well as normality of the residuals. Analyzing Fig. 17a the residuals seem to be heteroscedastic. Looking at the Q-Q plot in Fig. 17b, the residuals tend to stray from the line near the tails, especially the right tail, which can indicate that they are not normally distributed.

Spatial autocorrelation is at least partly the suspected cause of some heteroscedasticity and non-normality found in the residuals, thus the results for spatial dependence tests in the OLS residuals were produced and can be found in Table 3. Moran's I value for global spatial autocorrelation in the residuals of the estimated model of 0.09 is statistically significant, indicating that spatial autocorrelation seems indeed to exist in the residuals of this regression. Both statistics that test for spatial error dependence (LMerr and RLMerr) are statistically significant at a 95% significance level, as well as the portmanteau test (SARMA). On the other hand, test statistics LMlag and RLMlag, which test for a missing spatially dependent variable, are not statistically significant. This seems to indicate that there is in fact spatial dependence in the residuals, but the cause is rather the spatial error dependence and not so much a spatially lagged dependent variable.

An analysis of the residuals of the other regressions, namely SAR, SEM, GSM, SLX, SDM, SDEM, and Manski, shown in the Appendix in Figs. 18, 19, 20, 21, 22, 23, and 24 reveals that their distributions remain very similar despite the different model specifications.

Table 10 Summary of the installed power models

	OLS	SAR	SEM	GSM
(Intercept)	−8.248***	−7.649***	−7.268**	−7.300**
	(2.821)	(2.781)	(3.190)	(3.434)
Population	0.00003***	0.00003***	0.00004***	0.00004***
	(0.00000)	(0.00000)	(0.00000)	(0.00000)
Energy consumption	−0.001**	−0.001**	−0.001***	−0.001***
	(0.0002)	(0.0002)	(0.0002)	(0.0002)
Temperature	0.442***	0.410***	0.432***	0.456***
	(0.120)	(0.121)	(0.142)	(0.161)
Art exhibitions	−16.745**	−16.050**	−14.229**	−0.135*
	(7.430)	(7.269)	(7.242)	(7.172)
Gross income	0.001***	0.001***	0.001***	0.001***
	(0.0001)	(0.0001)	(0.0001)	(0.0001)
Votes in the most voted	−0.068**	−0.068**	−0.065*	−0.063*
	(0.035)	(0.034)	(0.034)	(0.034)
Housing buildings	0.068***	0.068***	0.069***	0.068***
	(0.013)	(0.013)	(0.013)	(0.013)
Family housing	−0.079***	−0.078***	−0.084***	−0.087***
	(0.011)	(0.011)	(0.011)	(0.011)
Abstention	0.081***	0.080***	0.081***	0.080***
	(0.027)	(0.026)	(0.029)	(0.030)
Rho		0.10802		-0.15075
		(0.079751)		(0.14566)
Lambda			0.28883***	0.40034***
			(0.084845)	(0.12999)
R^2	0.4668			
Adjusted R^2	0.449			
Residual Std. Error	2.274 (df = 268)			
F Statistic	26.072*** (df = 9; 268)			
Nagelkerke Pseudo R^2		0.470	0.480	0.483
AIC	1257.633	1258.062	1252.472	1253.096
BIC	1297.536	1301.593	1296.004	1300.255
Log likelihood	−617.8163	−617.031	−614.236	−613.548
σ^2		4.949	4.787	4.6737
Wald Test (df = 1)		1.835	11.589***	160.61***
LR Test (df = 1)		1.571	7.160***	8.5366**
Breusch Pagan	14.162	14.624	15.836*	15.685*
Note:	*p<0.1; **p<0.05; ***p<0.01			

Table 11 Results Installed Power with spatially lagged explanatory variables

	SLX	SDM	SDEM	Manski
(Intercept)	−14.345***	−10.865***	−12.184***	-8.3895**
	(3.645)	(3.415)	(3.896)	(3.7336)
Population	0.00004***	0.00004***	0.00004***	0.00004***
	(0.00000)	(0.00000)	(0.00000)	(0.00000)
Energy consumption	−0.001***	−0.001***	−0.001***	-0.001***
	(0.0002)	(0.0002)	(0.0002)	(0.0002)
Art exhibitions	−15.889**	−16.293**	−14.632**	−12.267*
	(7.229)	(6.938)	(6.894)	(6.614)
Gross income Gini	0.161*	0.144*	0.166**	0.153*
	(0.082)	(0.079)	(0.083)	(0.084)
Gross income	0.0003*	0.0003*	0.0003*	0.0003**
	(0.0002)	(0.0002)	(0.0002)	(0.0002)
Votes in the most voted	−0.060*	−0.063*	−0.060*	-0.054*
	(0.033)	(0.032)	(0.032)	(0.032)
Housing buildings	0.062***	0.061***	0.066***	0.068***
	(0.013)	(0.013)	(0.013)	(0.013)
Family housing	−0.077***	−0.078***	−0.080***	-0.082***
	(0.011)	(0.011)	(0.011)	(0.011)
Abstention	0.060**	0.060**	0.061**	0.047
	(0.028)	(0.027)	(0.029)	(0.031)
L. Purchase Power	−0.132***	−0.146***	−0.157***	−0.185***
	(0.043)	(0.041)	(0.044)	(0.049)
L. Energy consumption	0.003***	0.002***	0.003***	0.003***
	(0.001)	(0.001)	(0.001)	(0.001)
L. Subsidies	−0.369			
	(0.231)			
L. Temperature	0.478**	0.306*	0.295	
	(0.188)	(0.164)	(0.203)	
L. Rental agreements				3.251*
				(1.910)
L. Art exhibitions	−23.992			
	(15.767)			
L. Gross income	0.001**	0.001***	0.001***	0.002***
	(0.0005)	(0.0004)	(0.0005)	(0.0005)
L. Family housing	0.038***	0.032***	0.024*	
	(0.013)	(0.012)	(0.013)	
Rho		0.20689**		−0.29091*
		(0.085)		(0.1604)
Lambda			0.28517***	0.55031***
			(0.085074)	(0.11073)

(continued)

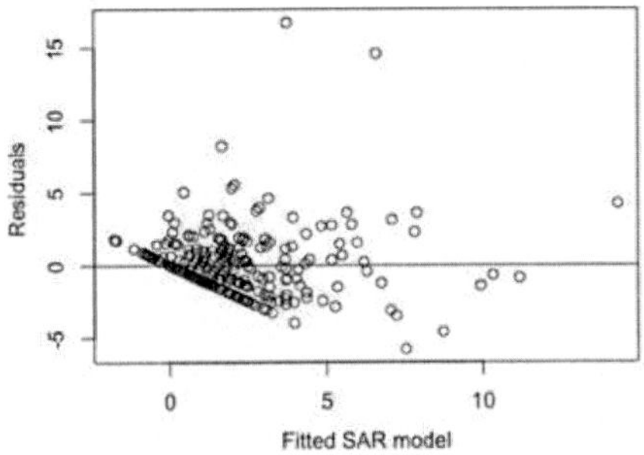

(a) Distribution of the fitted values of the SAR regression against the residuals

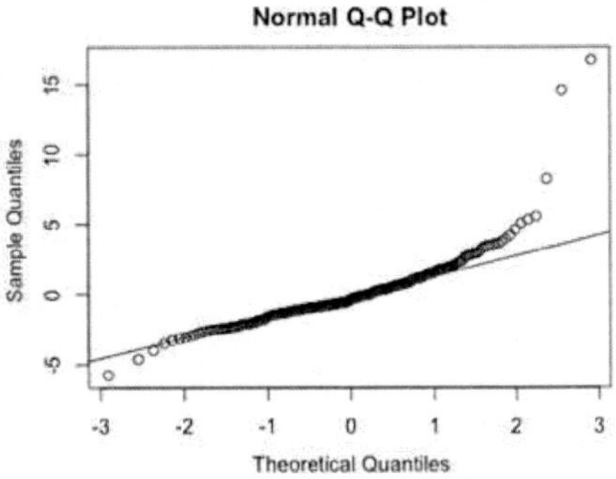

(b) Q-Q plot from SAR regression residuals

Fig. 18 Residuals of the SAR regression

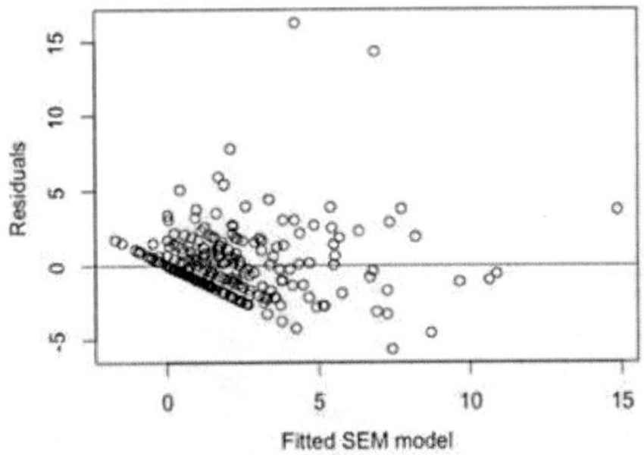

(a) Distribution of the fitted values of the SEM regression against the residuals

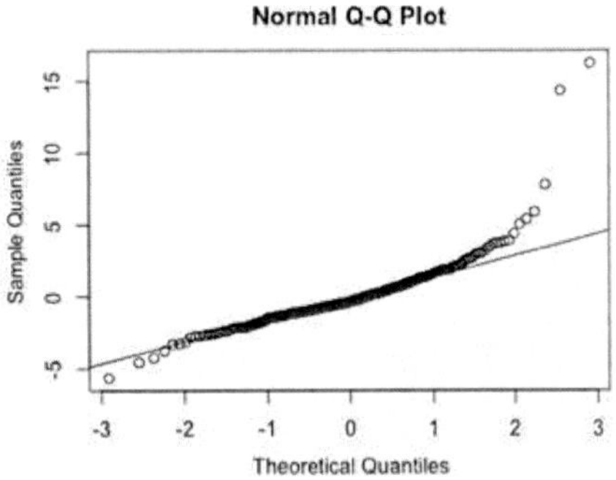

(b) Q-Q plot from SEM regression residuals

Fig. 19 Residuals of the SEM regression

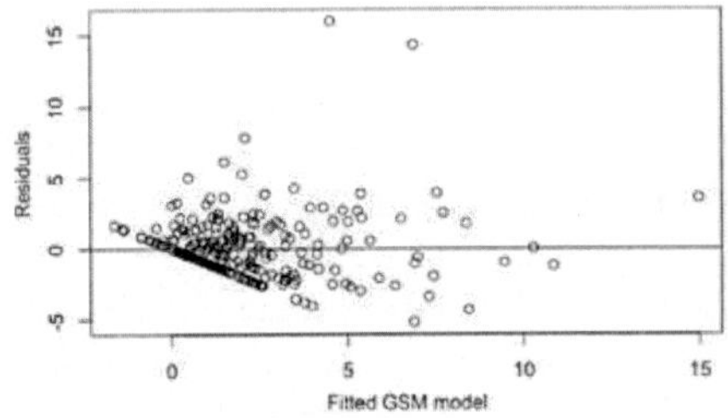

(a) Distribution of the fitted values of the GSM regression against the residuals

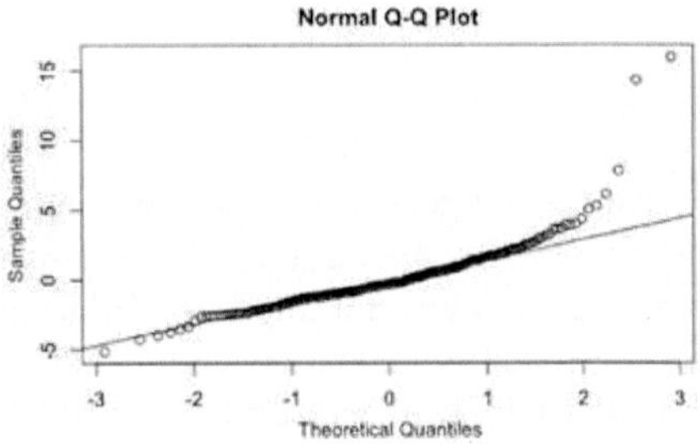

(b) Q-Q plot from GSM regression residuals

Fig. 20 Residuals of the GSM regression

Table 11 (continued)

	SLX	SDM	SDEM	Manski
R^2	0.534			
Adjusted R^2	0.505			
Residual Std. Error	2.156			
F Statistic	18.65***			
Nagelkerke Pseudo R^2		0.5317	0.5397	0.54044
AIC	1234.495	1233.565	1228.771	1228.324
BIC	1299.792	1295.235	1290.441	1289.994
Log likelihood	-599.248	−599.783	−597.386	−597.162
σ^2		4.359	4.242	3.984
Wald Test (df = 1)		4.128**	11.236***	238.26***
LR Test (df = 1)		3.244*	8.038***	173.08***
Breusch Pagan	32.139***	31.411***	32.088***	32.922***
Note:	*p<0.1; **p<0.05; ***p<0.01			

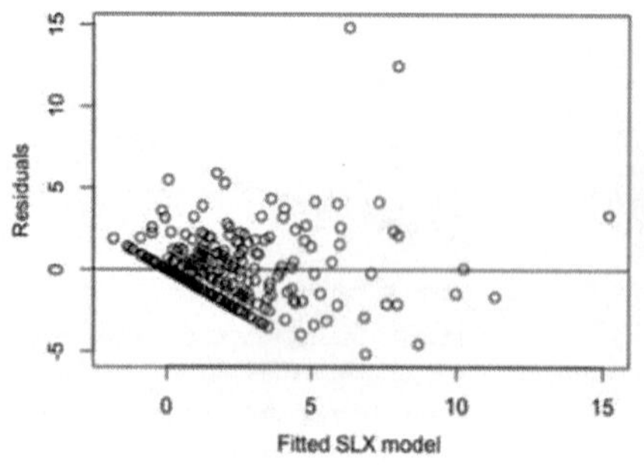

(a) Distribution of the fitted values of the SLX regression against the residuals

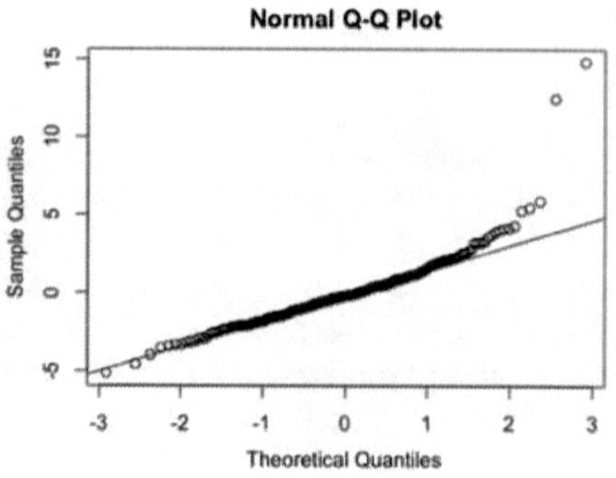

(b) Q-Q plot from SLX regression residuals

Fig. 21 Residuals of the SLX regression

All models that include a spatial term seem to produce a better fit, considering the Pseudo R-squared, than the non-spatial OLS estimation. The SAR regression produces only a slight improvement from the OLS estimation, and the ρ coefficient for the spatially lagged dependent variable is not statistically significant. Hence it seems that the Installed Power in one municipality does not affect the Installed Power in its neighbors directly. On the other hand, the λ coefficient for the spatial dependence in the error is positive and statistically significant. This indicates that similar unobserved characteristics result in similar decisions regarding Installed Power in nearby municipalities. This may be the result of a concentration of solar initiatives, local PV supplier activities, marketing campaigns or even other socioeconomic and demographic variables that were not taken into account. It is interesting to notice that

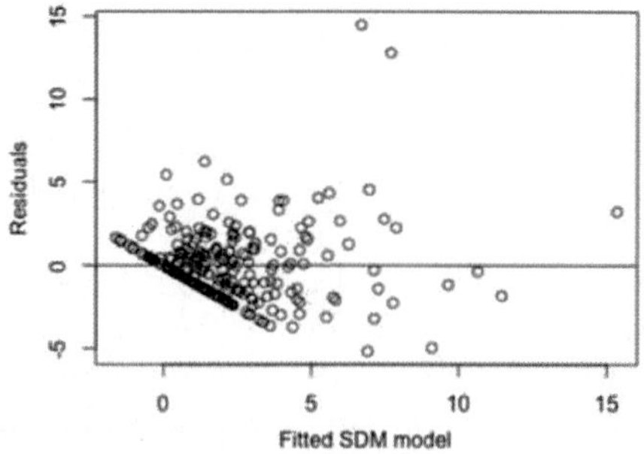

(a) Distribution of the fitted values of the SDM regression against the residuals

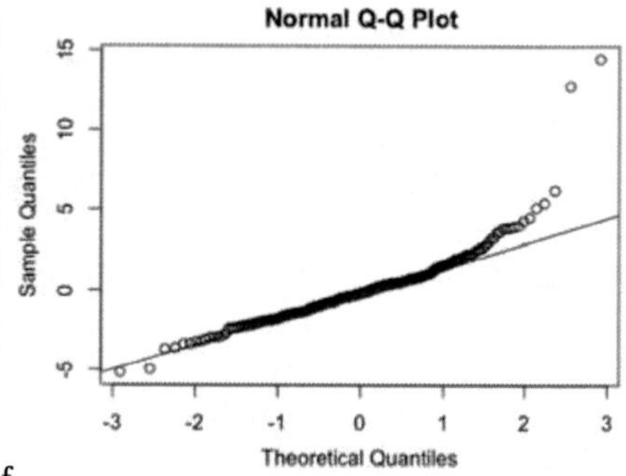

(b) Q-Q plot from SDM regression residuals

Fig. 22 Residuals of the SDM regression

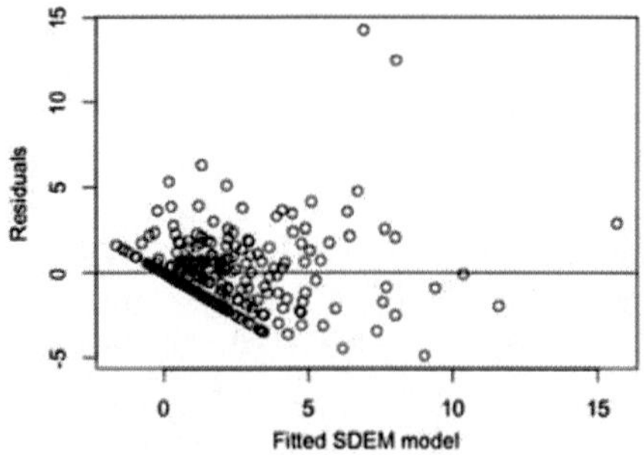

(a) Distribution of the fitted values of the SDEM regression against the residuals

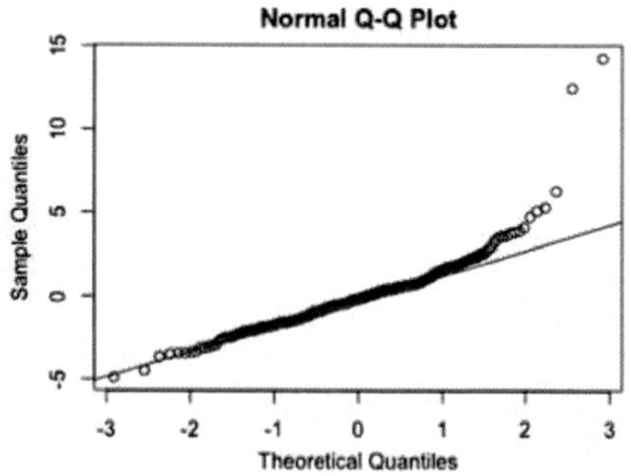

(b) Q-Q plot from SDEM regression residuals

Fig. 23 Residuals of the SDEM regression

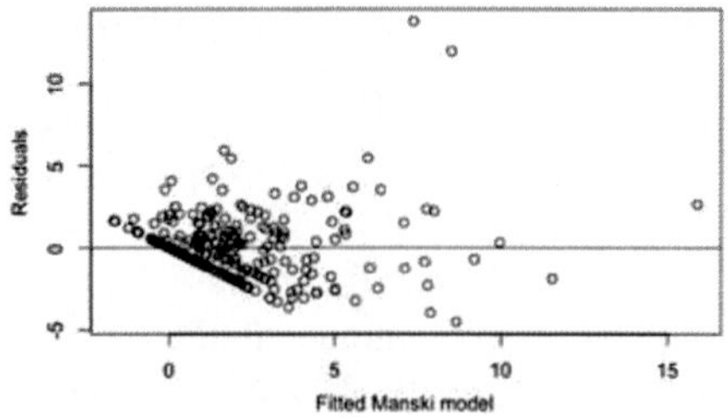

(a) Distribution of the fitted values of the Manski regression against the residuals

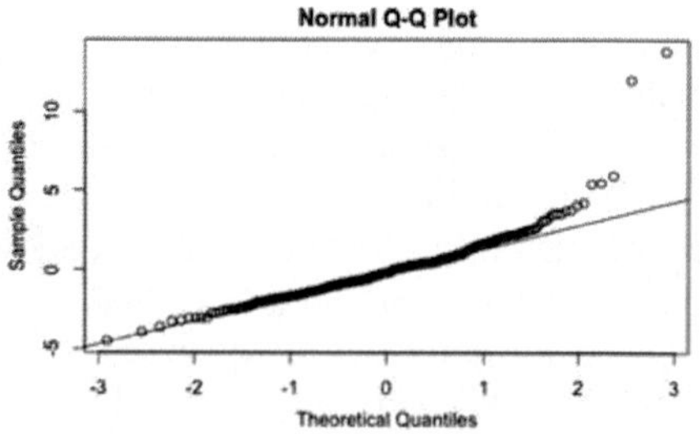

(b) Q-Q plot from Manski regression residuals

Fig. 24 Residuals of the Manski regression

the λ coefficient is higher and still statistically significant at 99% significance level for the GSM model. This means that although the spatially lagged dependent variable by itself does not seem to help to model the data, it increases the influence of the spatial component in the error term. The model fit, however, measured by the pseudo R-squared increases only slightly when compared to the SEM model. These four models include the same explanatory variables and all excluded the variables Purchase Power, Temperature, Subsidies, Rental Agreements, and Gross Income Gini. All of the remaining variables are statistically significant, meaning that they contribute to explain Installed Power. Population, Temperature, Gross Income, Housing buildings, and Abstention provide a positive contribution towards Installed Power, so that when their values increase, so does the chosen Installed Power. On the other hand when Energy consumption, Art exhibitions, Votes in the most voted, or Family housing increases, the Installed Power decreases.

When adding some of the explanatory variables with a spatial lag to the OLS model (SLX model), the adjusted R-squared increases when compared to the four previous models and many of these variables are significant, showing that indeed some characteristics of neighbor municipalities seem to influence Installed Power. As was the case when lagged explanatory variables were not considered, including a spatially lagged dependent variable (SDM) improves the fit slightly. It is further improved when instead a spatially dependent error term is considered (SDEM) and even more when both spatial components are included (Manski). In the SDM, however, ρ is statistically significant at a 95%, which did not happen in SAR, meaning that when the spatial lag of explanatory variables is considered, the Installed Power in nearby municipalities seems to influence the Installed Power of an individual municipality directly. In SDEM λ also has a positive statistically significant influence on the Installed Power. Similar to the case without lagged explanatory variables, the λ coefficient increases when the spatially lagged dependent variable is added (Manski). However, the coefficient of this variable, ρ, becomes negative with a similar magnitude (0.2 and -0.3), impacting the Installed Power in the opposite way when comparing to the SDM.

The Breusch-Pagan test reveals the presence of heteroscedasticity, by rejecting the null hypothesis of homoscedasticity, in residuals of SEM, GSM, and all models that include lagged explanatory variables.

As to the β estimates, they generally do not change drastically in magnitude when comparing OLS to spatial models, what also indicates that the spatial association does not account for a great part of the model.

As mentioned in Sect. 2.2, to analyze in a more precise way the influence of each explanatory variable in models with a spatial autoregressive component (SAR, GSM, SDM, Manski), a distinction should be made between direct and indirect impacts. These can be found in the Appendix in Tables 12, 13, 14, and 15, but such a detailed analysis was considered out of the scope of this study.

Likelihood of Adoption Distribution Map The likelihood of adoption distribution map, which represents the estimated probability of PV solar installations being adopted in a certain municipality, was produced with the predicted values for Installed

Power of the SDEM regression. The estimated value for the Installed Power for each region was divided by the total estimated value. The resulting map and its normalized version can be seen in Fig. 5.

The municipalities that have a probability higher than 50% of adopting PV systems belong mainly to five clusters. Sintra being the municipality with the highest probability is also surrounded by other municipalities with high adoption probability, namely Cascais, Oeiras, Seixal, and Loures. On the north of Portugal, there is another cluster containing Vila Nova de Gaia, Porto, and Matosinhos. In the south, there is another cluster made up from Santiago do Cacém and Odemira. Furthermore, there are two municipalities that are isolated that form their own single clusters, namely Braga and Coimbra. Hence, these are the municipalities towards which selling efforts should be focused.

Table 12 Impacts SAR model

	Direct	Indirect	Total
Population	0.00003	0.000004	0.00005
Energy consumption	−0.0006	−0.0001	−0.0006
Temperature	0.4112	0.0489	0.4601
Art exhibitions	−16.0826	−1.9114	−17.9939
Gross income	0.0006	0.0001	0.0006
Votes in the most voted	−0.069	−0.008	−0.0767
Housing buildings	0.0681	0.0081	0.0762
Family housing	−0.0782	−0.0093	−0.0875
Abstention	0.0802	0.0095	0.0897

Table 13 Impacts GSM model

	Direct	Indirect	Total
Population	0.000038	−0.000005	0.000033
Energy consumption	−0.000783	0.000105	−0.000678
Temperature	0.457296	−0.061306	0.395990
Art exhibitions	−13.55226	1.816842	−11.73542
Gross income	0.000564	0.000076	0.000488
Votes in the most voted	−0.062910	−0.084338	−0.054476
Housing buildings	0.068347	−0.009163	0.059184
Family housing	−0.087023	0.011666	−0.075356
Abstention	0.080357	−0.010773	0.069584

Table 14 Impacts SDM model

	Direct	Indirect	Total
Population	0.000036	0.000007	0.000043
Energy consumption	−0.000772	−0.000514	−0.000924
Art exhibitions	−16.37473	−3.209359	−19.58409
Gross income Gini	0.1444413	0.028310	0.1727511
Gross income	0.000287	0.000056	0.000343
Votes in the most voted	−0.063155	−0.012378	−0.075532
Housing buildings	0.061716	0.012096	0.073812
Family housing	−0.078398	−0.015366	−0.093763
Abstention	0.059877	0.011736	0.071612
L. Purchase Power	−0.146840	−0.028780	−0.175620
L. Energy consumption	0.002395	0.000469	0.002865
L. Temperature	0.307829	0.060333	0.368161
L. Gross income	0.001155	0.000226	0.001381
L. Family housing	0.031831	0.006239	0.038070

Table 15 Impacts Manski model

	Direct	Indirect	Total
Population	0.000038	−0.000009	0.000029
Energy consumption	−0.000630	0.000148	−0.000482
Art exhibitions	−12.42235	2.920080	−9.502266
Gross income Gini	0.154449	−0.036306	0.118143
Gross income	0.000336	−0.000079	0.000257
Votes in the most voted	−0.054868	0.012898	−0.041971
Housing buildings	0.069294	−0.016289	0.053005
Family housing	−0.082595	0.019415	−0.063179
Abstention	0.047514	−0.011169	0.036345
L. Purchase Power	−0.187175	0.043999	−0.143176
L. Energy consumption	0.003149	−0.000740	0.002409
L. Rental agreement	3.292395	−0.773932	2.518463
L. Gross Income	0.001714	−0.000403	0.001311

4 Conclusions and Discussion

In this study, the problem of modeling the adoption of domestic solar PV systems was addressed. To do so, related data as well as socioeconomic and demographic data from each municipality was gathered. After the conclusion was reached that spatial correlation was present in the data, several models were run to try to model this behavior. Adoption was considered using three variables, namely simply whether each municipality had any installation at all, how many panels were installed and the installed power.

The purchase power and rental agreements of each municipality do not seem to add explanatory value to any of the models. Rental agreements, on the other hand, were inserted in the model to identify municipalities where many people own their house and can in fact decide on adoption of solar PV systems. For that reason, it was unanticipated. Energy consumption per capita seems to have a negative influence on the installed power, which was also not anticipated. It does, interestingly, seem to have a positive significant influence on neighboring municipalities. Temperature, as expected, has a positive significant influence on the installed power in neighboring municipalities. Municipalities that have less votes in the most voted party for government tend to have more solar power installed. One interpretation could be that these municipalities have larger environmental concerns and this is usually not represented in the most voted parties. Abstention has a positive influence, which was not expected. Intuitively one would think that more education results in less abstention and education was shown to be a positive influence on solar panel adoption.

Art exhibitions seem to be the major predictor for PV adoption, but this is most likely due to unobserved characteristics. Art exhibitions are only available on highly urban areas and these do not have high PV systems adoption rates, as apartment buildings are more common. As expected, gross income has a positive influence on adoption. A higher income naturally allows families to have space in their budget for environmentally conscious products. This positive relationship between economic status and PV installations is also reinforced by the negative influence that having a high rate of subsidies beneficiaries exerts on installed power in some model specifications. Another variable that refers to this economic factor is the Gini coefficient of gross income. Here a greater income inequality results in an increase in installed power, which is likely related to the fact that municipalities with a large total gross income result in a large Gini coefficient. Number of housing buildings has a positive influence on installed power, whereas one could have expected that an increase in housing buildings would diminish PV installations. Family housing on the other hand has a positive influence, both directly and indirectly through spatial lag, which intuitively makes sense.

The SDEM model, which considers spatially correlated explanatory variables and spatial effects in the error component is the final selected model, which means that the spatial lag is negligible. Thus, the total installed power that the population in a particular municipality in Portugal chooses to adopt does not seem to be directly dependent on the installed power of neighbor municipalities. Rather, it seems directly and indirectly dependent on some observed demographic and socioeconomic variables of its neighbors, as well as unobserved characteristics (not controlled).

Considering the adoption likelihood map in Fig. 5, the focus should primarily go to Sintra. Other municipalities with high adoption likelihood can be seen in Fig. 6. When deciding on where to allocate efforts to promote solar adoption, following this order of municipalities should be optimal to accelerate Portugal's transition to renewable energies.

Acknowledgements This work is funded by national funds through the FCT—Fundação para a Ciência e a Tecnologia, I.P., under the scope of the projects UIDB/00297/2020 and UIDP/00297/2020 (Center for Mathematics and Applications).

Appendix: Complementary Figures and Tables

See Figs. 7, 8, 9, 10, 11, 12, 13, 14, 15, 16, 17, 18, 19, 20, 21, 22, 23 and 24. Tables 4, 5, 6, 7, 8, 9, 10, 11, 12, 13, 14 and 15.

References

1. Schelly, C.: Residential solar electricity adoption: what motivates, and what matters? A case study of early adopters. Energy Res. Soc. Sci. **2**, 183–191 (2014)
2. Richter, L. -L.: Social effects in the diffusion of solar photovoltaic technology in the UK. Technical Report CWPE 1357 & EPRG 1332, Cambridge Working Papers in Economics (2013)
3. Bollinger, B., Gillingham, K.: Peer effects in the diffusion of solar photovoltaic panels. Mark. Sci. **31**(6), 900–912 (2012)
4. Graziano, M., Gillingham, K.: Spatial patterns of solar photovoltaic system adoption: the influence of neighbors and the built environment. J. Econ. Geogr. **15**(4), 815–839 (2014)
5. Schelly, C., Letzelter, J.C.: Examining the key drivers of residential solar adoption in upstate New York. Sustainability **12**(6), 2552 (2020)
6. Baginski, J.P., Weber, C.: Coherent estimations for residential photovoltaic uptake in Germany including spatial spillover effects. HEMF Working Paper 02/2019, Essen (2019)
7. Müller, S., Rode, J.: The adoption of photovoltaic systems in wiesbaden, Germany. Econ. Innov. New Technol. **22**(5), 519–535 (2013)
8. Rode, J., Weber, A.: Does localized imitation drive technology adoption? a case study on rooftop photovoltaic systems in Germany. J. Environ. Econ. Manag. **78**, 38–48 (2016)
9. Schaffer, A.J., Brun, S.: Beyond the sun—socioeconomic drivers of the adoption of small-scale photovoltaic installations in Germany. Energy Res. Soc. Sci. **10**, 220–227 (2015)
10. Tobler, W.R.: A computer movie simulating urban growth in the Detroit region. Econ. Geogr. **46**, 234–240 (1970)
11. Anselin, L.: Local indicators of spatial association–LISA. Geogr. Anal. **27**(2), 93–115 (1995)
12. Elhorst, J.P.: Applied spatial econometrics: raising the bar. Spat. Econ. Anal. **5**(1), 9–28 (2010)
13. LeSage, J., Pace, R.K.: Limited dependent variable spatial models. In: Introduction to Spatial Econometrics, pp. 279–320. Chapman and Hall/CRC, Boca Raton, FL (2009)

Comparison of Semiparametric Approaches to Two-Way ANOVA in the Presence of Heteroscedasticity

Dulce G. Pereira and Anabela Afonso

Abstract Factorial analysis of variance designs is commonly used in several fields like biology, ecology and social sciences. However, in practice, the underlying assumptions, normality and homoscedasticity, are easily violated. In recent years, several alternative tests were proposed to relax these assumptions, the Wald-type statistics and the ANOVA-type statistics, and tests based on the permutation of observations. Few studies are focusing on the performance of the permutation tests in the presence of heterogeneity. This work intends to contribute to this last analysis. A simulation study is carried out, considering balanced designs, with an equal number of factor levels and several types of discrete distributions with different degrees of dispersion.

Keywords Interaction · Permutation tests · Robustness · Wald statistics

1 Introduction

Factorial Analysis of variance (ANOVA) is used to compare the mean of several sets of data and is based on the assumptions: (i) normality of error distribution, (ii) homoscedasticity and (iii) independence of residuals. But, in practice, these assumptions are easily violated. Moreover, for categorical data, parametric ANOVA may not be appropriate due to the non-metric nature of the data.

Several authors have proposed nonparametric tests, which are based on the rank transform and aligned rank of the observations [1–4, e.g.]. However, simply replacing observations by their ranks and using the same sampling distributions as for the

D. G. Pereira (✉) · A. Afonso
Research Centre for Mathematics and Applications, University of Évora, Évora, Portugal
e-mail: dgsp@uevora.pt

A. Afonso
e-mail: aafonso@uevora.pt

Department of Mathematics, School of Sciences and Technology, University of Évora, Évora, Portugal

R. Bispo et al. (eds.), *Recent Developments in Statistics and Data Science*,
Springer Proceedings in Mathematics & Statistics 398,
https://doi.org/10.1007/978-3-031-12766-3_13

parametric counterpart is generally not a valid approach [5]. The hypothesis tested by the nonparametric tests, in general, are not the same as those of the parametric F-test [6].

In the late 1990s, two semiparametric approaches were proposed that allow relaxing homoscedasticity assumptions: the Wald-Type Statistics (WTS) and ANOVA-Type Statistics (ATS) [7]. While the ATS assumes that the data has a normal distribution, the WTS does not require such assumption but has the big disadvantage that for small and moderate sample sizes the test tends to be liberal [7]. Reviews about these tests are available in Hahn and Salmaso [8] and Pauly et al. [9].

In recent years, permutation-based tests have gained much attention because they do not require the normality assumption and can be used with small samples. In addition, they can be used with discrete and ordinal data used quite often in many fields, e.g. social sciences, biology and ecology. The most popular permutation tests for factorial designs are the Constrained Synchronized Permutation (CSP), the Unconstrained Synchronized Permutation (USP) [10, 11] and the Wald-Type Permutation Statistic (WTPS) [9]. Salmaso [11] carried out a simulation study with synchronized permutations tests, which shows that, for small sample sizes, the power of these tests is close to that of parametric counterparts based on normality of errors. However, there are few studies about their performance in the presence of heteroscedasticity.

In the literature, one can find several studies on these tests with continuous error distributions [7–9, 11, 12, e.g.], but not with discrete distributions. However, unlike continuous scales, in the discrete scale, equal observations (ties) occur with positive probabilities. Thus, it seems relevant to study whether the performance of these tests is affected by the presence of tied observations, in particular for small sample sizes. In this paper, we intend to contribute to filling this gap in the analysis.

This paper aims to study and compare the Type I error rate and power of classical ANOVA with the alternative approaches ATS, WTS, WTPS, CSP and USP, which are designed to address the same hypotheses. Discrete data, with different degrees of dispersion, were simulated to investigate the impact of tied observations. Homoscedastic and heteroscedastic balanced designs are considered.

2 Statistical Model and Hypotheses

The general two-way completely randomized factorial balanced design is described by the effects model:

$$Y_{ijk} = \mu + \alpha_i + \beta_j + \gamma_{ij} + \varepsilon_{ijk}, \qquad \begin{cases} i = 1, \ldots, a; \\ j = 1, \ldots, b; \\ k = 1, \ldots, n, \end{cases} \tag{1}$$

where μ is the global mean effect, α_i is the effect of level i of factor A, β_j is the effect of level j of factor B, γ_{ij} is the effect of the interaction between the level i of factor A and level j of factor B and ϵ_{ijk} is the random error. The global number of observations is $N = abn$.

All the effects are assumed to be fixed, consequently, the conditions are fulfilled: $\sum_{i=1}^{a} \alpha_i = 0, \sum_{j=1}^{b} \beta_j = 0$ and $\sum_{i=1}^{a} \gamma_{ij} = \sum_{j=1}^{b} \gamma_{ij} = 0$ [13]. The null hypotheses of the no-main effect of factor A, the no-main effect of factor B and the no interaction effect between factors A and B are:

- $H_0^{\mu}(A) : \alpha_i = 0$, for all i,
- $H_0^{\mu}(B) : \beta_j = 0$, for all j and
- $H_0^{\mu}(AB) : \gamma_{ij} = 0$, for all i, j.

These null hypotheses can be written in terms of contrasts as:

- $H_0^{\mu}(A) : \boldsymbol{C}_A \boldsymbol{\mu} = 0$,
- $H_0^{\mu}(B) : \boldsymbol{C}_B \boldsymbol{\mu} = 0$,
- $H_0^{\mu}(AB) : \boldsymbol{C}_{AB} \boldsymbol{\mu} = 0$,

where $\boldsymbol{\mu} = (\mu_{11}, \ldots, \mu_{1b}, \ldots, \mu_{a1}, \ldots, \mu_{ab})', \mu_{ij} = E(Y_{ijk}) = \mu + \alpha_i + \beta_j + \gamma_{ij}$, and $\boldsymbol{C}_L$ the contrast matrix, with $L = A, B, AB$.

3 Compared Methods

This paper compares the classical ANOVA and the alternative methods ATS, WTS, CSP, USP and WTPS. The performance of these methods is evaluated for homoscedastic and heteroscedastic balanced designs, considering several types of discrete distributions and different degrees of dispersion.

3.1 Wald-Type Statistic (WTS)

WTS was developed by Brunner et al. [7]. The WTS is asymptotically exact in the general factorial design for $N \to \infty$, even in the case of heteroscedastic and nonnormal errors.

The statistic of this test is

$$W_N(L) = N\overline{\boldsymbol{Y}}_{.}'\boldsymbol{C}_L' \left(\boldsymbol{C}_L \boldsymbol{S}_N \boldsymbol{C}_L'\right)^{+} \boldsymbol{C}_L \overline{\boldsymbol{Y}}_{.} \overset{\circ}{\sim} \chi^2_{rank(\boldsymbol{C}_L)}, \tag{2}$$

where

$$\overline{\boldsymbol{Y}}_{.} = (\overline{Y}_{11}, \ldots, \overline{Y}_{ab})' \tag{3}$$

is the vector of the sample means $\overline{Y}_{ij.} = \frac{1}{n}\sum_{k=1}^{n} Y_{ijk}$,

$$S_N = \frac{N}{n} diag(s_{11}^2, \ldots, s_{ab}^2) \tag{4}$$

the diagonal matrix of the sample variances $s_{ij}^2 = \frac{1}{n-1}\sum_{k=1}^{n}(Y_{ijk} - \overline{Y}_{ij.})^2$ and M^+ denotes the Moore–Penrose inverse of matrix M.

This test is asymptotically exact and requires large sample sizes to keep the nominal Type I error level.

3.2 ANOVA-Type Statistic (ATS)

ATS was proposed by Brunner et al. [7]. The ATS relies on the assumption of normally distributed error terms, and it is an approximate test.

The statistic of this test is defined by

$$F_N(L) = \frac{N}{trace\,(\boldsymbol{T}_L\boldsymbol{S}_N)}\overline{\boldsymbol{Y}}_.'\boldsymbol{T}_L\overline{\boldsymbol{Y}}_. \mathrel{\overset{\circ}{\frown}} f_{df_1,df_2}, \tag{5}$$

with

$$df_1 = \frac{(trace\,(\boldsymbol{T}_L\boldsymbol{S}_N))^2}{trace\,\left((\boldsymbol{T}_L\boldsymbol{S}_N)^2\right)} \quad \text{and} \quad df_2 = \frac{(trace\,(\boldsymbol{T}_L\boldsymbol{S}_N))^2}{trace\,\left(\boldsymbol{D}_{T_L}^2\boldsymbol{S}_N^2\boldsymbol{\Lambda}_{ab}\right)}, \tag{6}$$

where $\boldsymbol{T}_L = \boldsymbol{C}_L'\left(\boldsymbol{C}_L\boldsymbol{C}_L'\right)^+\boldsymbol{C}_L$ is projection matrix, $\boldsymbol{D}_{T_L}$ the diagonal matrix of the diagonal elements of $\boldsymbol{T}_L$, $\boldsymbol{\Lambda}_{ab} = \frac{1}{n-1}\boldsymbol{I}_{ab}$, $\boldsymbol{I}_{ab}$ the $a \times b$-dimensional identity matrix and $\overline{\boldsymbol{Y}}_.$ and $\boldsymbol{S}_N$ as defined in expression (4).

The ATS tends to behave conservatively in the case of small sample sizes, being more conservative for skewed distributions [9].

3.3 Permutation Tests

The permutation tests are computationally intensive and distribution-free procedures. Under the assumption of exchangeability, the permutation tests are exact, i.e. the Type I error of the test is exactly equal to the preassigned significance level [9]. The assumption of exchangeability means that the joint distribution of the observations is invariant under the permutations of the observations, i.e. the order in which they are collected [14]. Basso et al. [12] proposed the use of synchronized permutations to test for main effects and interaction together. Pauly et al. [9] proposed a permutation test (WTPS) which can be used in cases with heteroscedastic error variances (i.e., not exchangeable) being asymptotically exact.

Synchronized Permutation Tests In synchronized permutation tests, values are permuted between two levels of a factor, keeping the level of the remaining factors in the model constant and exchanging the same number of units within each pair of the considered blocks [12].

Let $T^*_{is|j} = T^*_{ij} - T^*_{sj}$ and $T^*_{jh|i} = T^*_{ij} - T^*_{ih}$, where

$$T^*_{ij} = \sum_{k=1}^{n} Y^*_{ijk}, \tag{7}$$

and Y^*_{ijk} denotes the permutation value of Y_{ijk}, of the block $A_i B_j$, according to some permutation scheme.

The proposed test statistics in the two-way design are given by

- Main effect A:

$$T^*_A = \sum_{i=1}^{a} \sum_{s>i} \left(\sum_{j=1}^{b} T^*_{is|j} \right)^2, \tag{8}$$

- Main effect B:

$$T^*_B = \sum_{j=1}^{b} \sum_{h>j} \left(\sum_{i=1}^{a} T^*_{jh|i} \right)^2, \tag{9}$$

- Interaction effect AB:

$$T^*_{AB} = \sum_{i=1}^{a} \sum_{s>i} \sum_{j=1}^{b} \sum_{h>j} \left(T^*_{is|j} - T^*_{is|h}\right)^2 + \sum_{j=1}^{b} \sum_{h>j} \sum_{i=1}^{a} \sum_{s>i} \left(T^*_{jh|i} - T^*_{jh|s}\right)^2. \tag{10}$$

The effects not of interest are eliminated by the synchronization and are not present in the test statistic of the effect of interest. When testing the main effect A, observations are permuted within the blocks constructed by the levels of the factor B, i.e. $A_i B_j$ and $A_s B_j$. When testing the B main effect, observations are permuted within the blocks constructed by the A factor levels, i.e. $A_i B_j$ and $A_i B_h$ [15]. When testing the interaction the test statistic is composed of two parts: (i) the first part is obtained from permutations involving factor A; and (ii) the second part is obtained from permutations involving factor B [12].

P-value is calculated as the proportion of permutations for which test statistics values of permuted data sets are greater or equal to the test statistic value for the original data set.

There are two ways to obtain a synchronized permutation: constrained and unconstrained [10, 11].

Constrained Synchronized Permutation (CSP) CSP consists of applying the same permutation in all pairs of blocks, i.e. exchanged units must be in the same original position within each block. In balanced designs, if the number of replicates n is too small, CSP could give a minimum achieved significance level higher than the desired Type I error [12].

Unconstrained Synchronized Permutation (USP) In the USP, exchanged units may not be in the same original position within each block. The only requirement is that the number of exchanges is the same. USP is computationally more intensive compared to CSP. Basso et al. [12] refer that the difference between these two tests quickly decreases with the growth of the number of replicates available. Therefore, the authors recommend using the USP when n is small (say $n \leq 3$).

Wald-Type Permutation Statistic (WTPS) Pauly et al. [9] proposed a permutation procedure (WTPS) based on the Wald-Type Statistic (WTS). The proposed test is exact under the exchangeability condition and is asymptotically exact and consistent in the presence of heteroscedasticity.

The WTPS is based on the permutation of data $Y^* = (Y^*_{111}, \ldots, Y^*_{abn})'$ within the whole data set. Under the hypothesis $H_0^{\mu}(L) : \boldsymbol{C}_L \boldsymbol{\mu} = 0$, the test statistics are [9]:

$$W_N^*(L) = N(\overline{\boldsymbol{Y}}^*_{\cdot})' \boldsymbol{C}_L' \left(\boldsymbol{C}_L \boldsymbol{S}_N^* \boldsymbol{C}_L'\right)^+ \boldsymbol{C}_L \overline{\boldsymbol{Y}}^*_{\cdot} \mathrel{\overset{\circ}{\frown}} \chi^2_{rank(\boldsymbol{C}_L)}, \tag{11}$$

where $\overline{\boldsymbol{Y}}^*_{\cdot} = \left(\overline{Y}^*_{11.}, \ldots, \overline{Y}^*_{ab.}\right)'$ denote the vector with the permuted means $\overline{Y}^*_{ij.} = \frac{1}{n}\sum_{k=1}^{n} Y^*_{ijk}$ and $\boldsymbol{S}_N^* = \frac{N}{n}.diag\left(s_{11}^{*2}, \ldots, s_{ab}^{*2}\right)'$ is the matrix with the permuted sample variances $s_{ij}^{*2} = \frac{1}{n-1}\sum_{k=1}^{n}\left(Y^*_{ijk} - \overline{Y}^*_{ij.}\right)^2$.

WTPS was constructed without the assumption of equal sample sizes, equal variances and a particular distribution of the errors. In general, the test does not perform satisfactorily well for extremely skewed and heteroscedastic distributions, in particular when the larger sample has a smaller variance [16].

4 Simulation

A simulation study was carried out to evaluate the performance of the testing procedures presented in Sect. 3, i.e. the Type I error and power of these tests. The simulation experiments were performed in the R programming language, version 3.6.3 [17]. For ATS, WTS and WTPS tests, we used the functions implemented in the R package GFD [16]. For CSP and USP, we used the R functions available at http://static.gest.unipd.it/salmaso/web.

Type I error rates and power of the tests were assessed under the following effect conditions (models):

M1. all effects null (i.e. null model): $\alpha_i = 0$; $\beta_j = 0$; $\gamma_{ij} = 0$,

M2. the main effect A nonnull and all other effects null, considering $\alpha_i = 0.25\sigma$, 0.5σ, 1σ; $\beta_j = 0$; $\gamma_{ij} = 0$,

M3. the main effects A and B nonnull and the interaction effect AB null, considering $\alpha_i = \beta_j = 0.25\sigma, 0.5\sigma, 1\sigma$; $\gamma_{ij} = 0$,

M4. the interaction effect AB nonnull, and both main effects null, considering $\alpha_i = \beta_j = 0$; $\gamma_{ij} = 0.25\sigma, 0.5\sigma, 1\sigma$,
M5. the main effect A and the interaction effect AB nonnull, and main effect B null, considering $\alpha_i = \gamma_{ij} = 0.25\sigma, 0.5\sigma, 1\sigma$ and $\beta_j = 0$,
M6. all effects nonnull (i.e., full model), considering $\alpha_i = \beta_j = \gamma_{ij} = 0.25\sigma, 0.5\sigma, 1\sigma$,

where σ represents the standard deviation of the error distribution.

Balanced design was considered ($n = 3, 5, 10$) with two factors, A and B, with equal number of levels (3×3). The homoscedastic setting was generated from discrete distributions, with different parameters to obtain distinct degrees of dispersion and skewness:

i Positive asymmetric binomial: $B(K; 0.2)$ with $K = 25, 50, 100$;
ii Binomial symmetric: $B(K; 0.5)$ with $K = 10, 20, 40$;
iii Binomial Negative: $BN(K; 0.4)$ with $K = 2, 4, 8$;
iv Poisson: $P(\lambda)$ with $\lambda = 5, 10, 20$; and
v Uniform: $U\{0, \ldots, K\}$ with $K = 10, 20, 40$.

To generate the heteroscedastic setting the following steps were performed:

1. For $i = 1, \ldots, a - 1$ and $j = 1, \ldots, b$ the homogeneous case was generated;
2. For $i = a$ and $j = 1, \ldots, b$, the data was generated from the distributions:

   a. (i) Positive asymmetric binomial: $B(K; 0.2)$ with $K = 13, 25, 50$; (ii) Binomial symmetric: $B(K; 0.5)$ with $K = 5, 10, 20$; (iii) Binomial Negative: $BN(K; 0.4)$ with $N = 1, 2, 4$; (iv) Poisson: $P(\lambda)$ with $\lambda = 2.5, 5, 10$; and (v) Uniform: $U\{0, \ldots, K\}$ with $K = 7, 14, 28$;
   b. To get distributions with the same mean as in the homogeneous case, a constant was added to the values obtained in step 2a. The constants added were (i) $0.1K$; (ii) $0.1K$; (iii) 0.5λ; (iv) $0.5K$; and (v) $0.15K$.

For each distributional scenario configuration, the number of simulations and permutations were $n_{sim} = 1000$ and $n_{per} = 1000$, respectively.

For each of the tests described in the previous section, the empirical distribution was recorded of the p-values and the proportion of repetitions that lead to rejection of the null hypothesis ($\alpha = 0.01, 0.05, 0.1$) in the total number of repetitions. When the null hypothesis is true this proportion gives the empirical Type I error rate, otherwise, gives the empirical power. Bradley's liberal criterium of robustness was adopted to classify the tests [18]. According to this criterium, a test is considered robust if its empirical Type I error rate is within the interval $(0.5\alpha, 1.5\alpha)$, is considered conservative when $\leq 0.5\alpha$ and is liberal when $\geq 1.5\alpha$, where α is the nominal level (i.e. level of significance).

5 Results

Results referring to the error distributions will not be presented, since a different behavior was not found in the various discrete distributions considered in this work.

In the next subsections, only the results for $\alpha = 5\%$ will be presented.

5.1 *Homoscedastic Versus Heteroscedastic Settings*

There are differences in empirical Type I error rates and empirical power between tests, due to the presence/absence of homogeneity (Fig. 1).

All tests that do not meet the Bradley criterium are classified as liberal. There are more liberal tests in the heteroscedastic setting. All tests are liberal in the heteroscedastic setting when the main effect *A* is not present (Fig. 1a).

The USP and WTS tests are the most powerful, but they are almost always liberal. Among the robust tests, ANOVA is the most powerful, followed by WTPS and ATS (Fig. 1b).

5.2 *Effect Size*

The performance of the tests seems to be similar in the homoscedastic and heteroscedastic settings (Fig. 2).

With the increase of the effect size present (0.25σ, 0.5σ, 1σ), the Type I error rate remains virtually unchanged, but the power of the tests increases (Fig. 2).

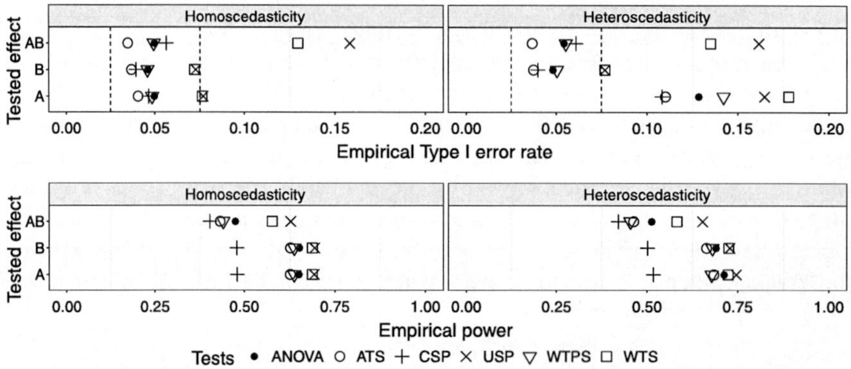

Fig. 1 **a** Empirical Type I error rate and **b** empirical power, of each test, when $\alpha = 5\%$, in the absence and presence of heterogeneity. The dashed vertical lines represent the robustness limits of the Bradley criterium

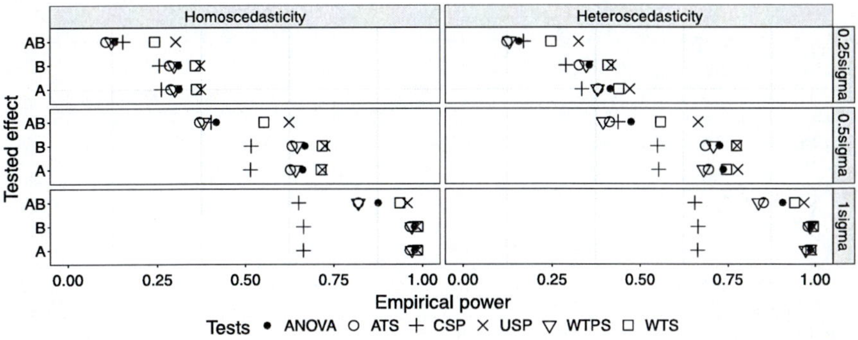

Fig. 2 Empirical power, of each test, when $\alpha = 5\%$, by effect value, in the absence and presence of heterogeneity

5.3 *Model Effect*

The presence of heterogeneity affects the Type I error rate, especially when effect A is not present (Fig. 3).

USP and WTS are not robust to testing for interaction whether or not the main effects are present (models 1–3). In the test for the presence of effect B, both procedures are robust in the homoscedastic setting but are no longer robust in the heteroscedastic setting whether or not the interaction and A effects are present (models 1, 2, 4 and 5).

When heteroscedasticity is introduced, all tests are liberal when testing for the presence of effect A whether or not the interaction and B effects are present (models 1 and 4, Fig. 3a).

In the heterogeneous settings, the tests are more powerful than in the homogenous settings (Fig. 3b).

5.4 *Sample Size Effect*

The behaviour of the tests depends on the number of replicates (Fig. 4).

CSP never rejected the null hypothesis, whenever sample sizes were too small ($n = 3$). Consequently, this test had a zero empirical Type I error rate (Fig. 4a) and power (Fig. 4b). In the test for the presence of interaction, as the sample size increased, CSP changed from being a conservative test to a liberal test, both homogeneous and heterogeneous settings. The difference between CSP and USP rapidly decreases as the sample size increases.

When testing for the presence of main effect A, in all tests there is an increase in the empirical Type I error rate when heteroscedasticity is included in the model, which worsens with the increase in sample size.

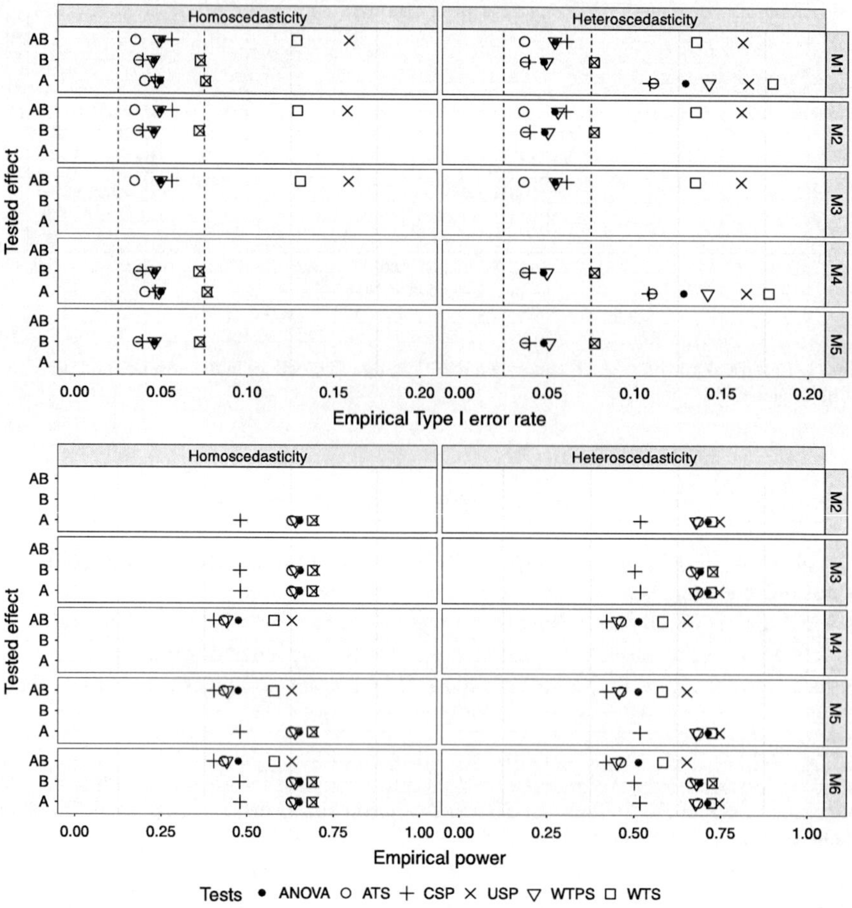

Fig. 3 **a** Empirical Type I error rate and **b** empirical power, of each test, when $\alpha = 5\%$, by model, in the absence and presence of heterogeneity. The dashed vertical lines indicate the robustness bounds of the Bradley criterium

ATS turned out to be conservative when testing for interaction in the case where the sample is too small ($n = 3$). WTS was never robust in testing for interaction, but as the sample size increases, the test seems to approach the desired robustness (Fig. 4a).

The empirical power of the tests increases with sample size, being higher in the heteroscedastic than in the homoscedastic setting (Fig. 4b).

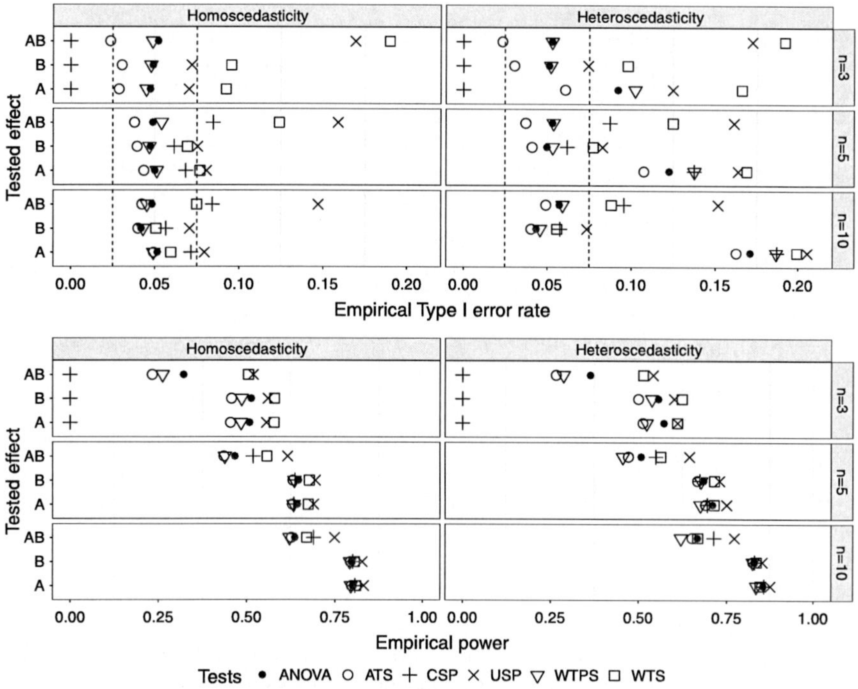

Fig. 4 **a** Empirical Type I error rate, and **b** empirical power, of each test, when $\alpha = 5\%$, by number of replicates n, in the absence and presence of heterogeneity. The dashed vertical lines indicate the robustness bounds of the Bradley criterium

5.5 *Ties Effect*

ATS, WTS and WTPS tests did not always return results, mainly when the number of replicates was too small ($n = 3$). This situation occurred when at least in a given cell $A_i B_j$ the values are all equal (i.e. all observations are tied), which led to a zero variance in that cell. For data generated from discrete distributions, this is more likely to happen when the number of possible outcome values is small.

6 Conclusions

This simulation study showed that the performance of the tests is affected by the presence of heterogeneity in the data, as well as by the present effects (model) and their size, and by the number of replicates in each cell. In addition, it was not possible to obtain results in some tests (ATS, WTS and WTPS) when at least one of the cells had the same value for all observations (i.e. full tied), which leads to zero variances.

Table 1 Summary of test performance as a function of empirical Type I error rate

Tested effect	Setting	Empirical Type I Error Rate	
		Robust tests	Liberal tests
AB	Homoscedastic	ANOVA, WTPS	USP
	Heteroscedastic	ANOVA, WTPS	WTS, USP
A	Homoscedastic	ANOVA, WTPS	–
	Heteroscedastic	–	ANOVA, WTS, WTPS, CSP, USP
B	Homoscedastic & Heteroscedastic	ANOVA, WTPS, ATS	–

This situation is common when data are generated with discrete error distributions, rather than continuous distributions.

Table 1 presents a summary of the general performance of the compared tests as a function of empirical Type I error rate. In the homoscedastic scenario, ANOVA and WTPS tests showed to be robust in all models, sample sizes and size effect. In the presence of heterogeneity, these tests became liberal when testing for the presence of effect A. ANOVA tends to be more powerful than WTPS.

For 2×2 designs, Hahn et al. [15] notice that ATS is slightly conservative for highly skewed distributions, especially in the homogenous setting. For 2×5 designs, Pauly et al. [9] report the same behaviour for this test. In our study, with a 3×3 balanced design, ATS showed to be slightly conservative just when testing interaction and the sample size was too small, in both homogeneous and heterogeneous settings.

The liberalism of WTS, already reported in other studies [9, 15, 16, e.g.], was also observed in the present study.

Despite WTPS overcomes the liberalism of WTP, this test still presents a liberal behaviour when testing the main effect A, in the heterogeneous setting. This liberal behaviour increases with the sample size. For continuous distributions, it was reported in the literature that WTPS tends to be in liberal decisions in the case of skewed distributions and unequal variances [9, 16]. However, liberalism was not as pronounced as the WTS.

In the interaction analysis, the USP test does not maintain the nominal α level, and it is liberal. This is one limitation of this test because despite having high power, it is very liberal.

The CSP test reveals conservative behavior for a small sample size ($n = 3$). In agreement with the results of Hahn et al. [15], the CSP test has, in general, slightly lower power than the other tests, for both homogeneous and heterogeneous settings.

Based on the obtained results, for small samples ($n \leq 10$) and discrete distributions, parametric ANOVA and WTPS had a stable behaviour and, in general, a better performance.

Acknowledgements This work was partially supported by the FCT—Fundação para a Ciência e a Tecnologia, Portugal, under the "UIDB/04674/2020 (CIMA)" project.

References

1. Hodges, J.L., Lehmann, E.L.: Rank methods for combination of independent experiments in analysis of variance. Ann. Math. Stat. **33**(3), 482–497 (1962)
2. Iman, R.L.: A power study of a rank transform for the two-way classification model when interaction may be present. Can. J. Stat. **2**(1–2), 227–239 (1974)
3. Mansouri, H., Chang, G.-H.: A comparative study of some rank tests for interaction. Comput. Stat. Data Anal. **19**(1), 85–96 (1995)
4. Puri, M.L., Sen, P.K.: Nonparametric Methods in General Linear Models. Wiley, New York (1985)
5. Brunner, E., Bathke, A.C., Konietschke, F.: Rank and Pseudo- Rank Procedures for Independent Observations in Factorial Designs-Using R and SAS. Springer, Heidelberg (2019)
6. Brunner, E., Puri, M.L.: Comments on the paper 'Type I error and test power of different tests for testing interaction effects in factorial experiments. In: Mendes, M., Yigit, S. (eds.) Statistica Neerlandica, pp. 1–26 (2013). Statistica Neerlandica **67**(4), 390–396 (2013)
7. Brunner, E., Dette, H., Munk, A.: Box-type approximations in nonparametric factorial designs. J. Am. Stat. Assoc. **92**(440), 1494–1502 (1997)
8. Hahn, S., Salmaso, L.: A comparison of different synchronized permutation approaches to testing effects in two-level two-factor unbalanced ANOVA designs. Stat. Pap. **58**(1), 123–146 (2017)
9. Pauly, M., Brunner, E., Konietschke, F.: Asymptotic permutation tests in general factorial designs. J. R. Stat. Soc.: Ser. B (Stat. Methodol.) **77**(2), 461–473 (2015)
10. Pesarin, F.: Multivariate Permutation Tests: With Applications in Biostatistics. Wiley, Chichester (2001)
11. Salmaso, L.: Synchronized permutation tests in 2^k factorial designs. Commun. Stat.-Theory Methods ISSN **32**(7), 1419–1437 (2003)
12. Basso, D., Chiarandini, M., Salmaso, L.: Synchronized permutation tests in replicated $I \times J$ designs. J. Stat. Plan. Inference **137**(8), 2564–2578 (2007)
13. Montgomery, D.C.: Design and Analysis of Experiments, 8th ed. Wiley, Hoboken (2013)
14. Good, P.I.: Extensions of the concept of exchangeability and their applications. J. Mod. Appl. Stat. Methods **1**(2), 243–247 (2002)
15. Hahn, S., Konietschke, F., Salmaso, L.: A comparison of efficient permutation tests for unbalanced ANOVA in two by two designs-and their behavior under heteroscedasticity. In: Melas, V., Mignani, S., Monari, P., Salmaso, L. (eds.), Topics in Statistical Simulation, pp. 257–269. Springer, New York (2014)
16. Friedrich, S., Konietschke, F., Pauly, M.: `GFD`: an R package for the analysis of general factorial designs. J. Stat. Softw. **79**(1), 1–18 (2017)
17. R Core Team: R: A Language and Environment for Statistical Computing. R Foundation for Statistical Computing, Vienna, Austria (2020)
18. Bradley, J.V.: Robustness? Br. J. Math. Stat. Psychol. **31**(2), 144–152 (1978)

Some Determinants for Road Accidents Severity in the District of Setúbal

Paulo Infante, Anabela Afonso, Gonçalo Jacinto, Leonor Rego, Pedro Nogueira, Marcelo Silva, Vitor Nogueira, José Saias, Paulo Quaresma, Daniel Santos, Patrícia Gois, and Paulo Rebelo Manuel

Abstract In Portugal, the district of Setúbal is among those with the higher number of road accidents with fatal injuries but with fewer accidents. This work analyzes data from road accidents that occurred in the area under the jurisdiction of the Territorial Command of Setúbal, belonging to the Guarda Nacional Republicana, the Portuguese Gendarmerie. A spatial analysis of the accidents was carried out, using the Getis–Ord Gi* statistic to identify hotspots and the Local Moran's I statistic for spatial autocorrelation, which allowed the identification of municipalities with identical profiles for fatalities and serious injuries. With a logistic regression model, we identify some determinants which can explain the existence of serious and/or fatal injuries in road accidents: type of accident, geographical factors, temporal factors, road characteristics, drivers' characteristics, vehicles' features, and victims' characteristics.

P. Infante (✉) · A. Afonso · G. Jacinto · P. R. Manuel
Research Centre for Mathematics and Applications, University of Évora, Évora, Portugal
e-mail: pinfante@uevora.pt

A. Afonso
e-mail: aafonso@uevora.pt

G. Jacinto
e-mail: gjcj@uevora.pt

P. R. Manuel
e-mail: pjsrm@uevora.pt

P. Infante · A. Afonso · G. Jacinto · L. Rego
Department of Mathematics, School of Science and Technology, University of Évora, Évora, Portugal
e-mail: lrego@uevora.pt

P. Nogueira · M. Silva
Institute of Earth Sciences, Pole of the University of Évora, Évora, Portugal

Department of Geosciences, School of Science and Technology, University of Évora, Évora, Portugal
e-mail: pmn@uevora.pt

R. Bispo et al. (eds.), *Recent Developments in Statistics and Data Science*,
Springer Proceedings in Mathematics & Statistics 398,
https://doi.org/10.1007/978-3-031-12766-3_14

Keywords Getis–Ord Gi* · Fatalities and serious injuries · Local Moran's I · Logistic regression · Road accidents

1 Introduction

Road accidents are a problem with repercussions in several dimensions: social, economic, health, justice, and safety. In 2018, the Portuguese Secretary of State for Civil Protection referred that road accidents had an economic and social impact in the country equivalent to 1.2% of Gross Domestic Product (GDP), i.e., 2.3 billion euros [1].

Between 2016 and 2019, the District of Setúbal was one of the Portuguese districts with the most road traffic accidents resulting in fatalities or serious injuries. In 2018, in the area under the jurisdiction of the Guarda Nacional Republicana (GNR), it was the sixth district with the highest number of road traffic accidents in Portugal but was the first in the number of fatalities as a consequence of the road traffic accidents (Table 1). To explain the high number of road traffic accidents with fatalities or serious injuries and to find measures to reduce them, a partnership was established between the Territorial Command of Setúbal of GNR (GNR-TC Setúbal) and the University of Évora, and the Modeling and Prediction of Road Traffic Accidents in the District of Setúbal (MOPREVIS) project was created.

In the last years, several methodological approaches were used to analyze traffic road accidents data [2–8].

In this work, we are mainly interested in identifying the factors for the severity of road accidents, combining Geographical Information System (GIS) and statistical models, and leveraging the ability of GIS to perform complex spatial analyses.

M. Silva
e-mail: marcelogs@uevora.pt

V. Nogueira · J. Saias · P. Quaresma
Algoritmi Research Centre, University of Évora, Évora, Portugal
e-mail: vbn@uevora.pt

J. Saias
e-mail: jsaias@uevora.pt

P. Quaresma
e-mail: pq@uevora.pt

V. Nogueira · J. Saias · P. Quaresma · D. Santos
Department of Informatics, School of Science and Technology, University of Évora, Évora, Portugal
e-mail: dfsantos@uevora.pt

P. Gois
Department of Visual Arts and Design, School of Fine Arts, University of Évora, Évora, Portugal
e-mail: pafg@uevora.pt

Table 1 Top 8 of 18 districts in Continental Portugal in 2018, ranked by number of road accidents and associated fatalities, within the 24 h after the accident and in the areas of GNR jurisdiction

District	Number of road accidents	Number of fatalities
Porto	12646	43
Faro	8181	39
Aveiro	8072	30
Lisbon	7497	17
Braga	7640	25
Setúbal	7249	55
Santarém	5128	32
Leiria	4600	37

GIS was used to geocode the accident data and locations, for visualization of accident data on maps and in the analysis and determination of hotspots [5]. Prasannakumar et al. [8] used the Moran's I index, Getis–Ord Gi*, and Kernel density functions to assess spatial clustering of accidents and spatial density hotspots.

Studies with statistical models try to quantify the effect of the determinants in the frequency and severity of road accidents, forecast future accidents and severities, and evaluate the effectiveness of a specific safety measure [9]. Logistic regression models were used to estimate the influence of accident factors on road crash fatalities [10], and as a classification model to predict accidents [2]. A multinomial logit model and a mixed logit model were used to determine risk factors or fatal cases involving motorcycle fatal accidents based on the number of vehicles involved [11]. Chen and Chen [4] modeled road accident severity comparing the logistic regression with machine learning techniques, namely, decision trees and random forest models. Machine learning methods have been mostly used as prediction tools, while statistical models are more frequently used in crash severity modeling [6]. Casado-Sanz et al. [3] applied a multinomial logit model to find the most important factors for the occurrence of a fatal outcome based on single-vehicle crashes.

There are several examples of modeling road accident severity in Portugal. Ordered probit models were used to predict road accident severity in the municipality of Coimbra [12]. Recently, ordered logistic regression was applied to identify the risk factors associated with the increase of the injury severity of powered two-wheeler riders when involved in a road accident in Portugal [13]. Classification and Regression Trees (CART) method was used to predict the effect of vehicle characteristics on crash severity, in Porto metropolitan area [14].

The objective of this work is to determine the risk factors associated with greater severity in road accidents and hence providing a first step to contribute to solving the problem by providing suggestions to reduce their impact. We use several sources of data on road accidents provided by partner entities of the MOPREVIS project. Initially, a local spatial analysis of road accidents was performed. The Getis–Ord

Gi* statistic allowed the identification of critical points. Moran's I local statistic was used to identify local clusters and local spatial outliers. Based on this analysis, the municipalities were grouped into categories with the same vulnerability for road accidents with serious and/or fatal injuries. Then, to identify some determinants that contribute to the existence of fatalities and/or serious injuries in road traffic accidents, which occurred in the district of Setúbal, a logistic regression model was used.

This paper is organized as follows. In Sect. 2, sources and variables used in the dataset are described as well as the statistical methods used in the paper. In Sect. 3 the main results are presented, including a short exploratory analysis of the dataset, and the logistic regression model obtained. In Sect. 4 the main conclusions are presented.

2 Methods

2.1 Study Area

The district of Setúbal is the eighth largest in Portugal with a land area of 5064 km^2, divided by 13 municipalities and six protected areas. It has 293 km of National Road (EN—*Estrada Nacional*), 219 km of Highway (AE—*Auto Estrada*), 19 km of Principal Itinerary (IP—*Itinerário Principal*), and 90 km of Complementar Itinerary (IC—*Itinerário Complementar*). The GNR-TC Setúbal is responsible for around 96% of this territory.

2.2 Data

Our work analyzes the data collected with the Statistical Bulletin of Road Accidents (BEAV [15]) by GNR-TC Setúbal, with an update of the Autoridade Nacional de Segurança Rodoviária (ANSR) for victims at 30 days, and complemented with meteorological information provided by Instituto Português do Mar e da Atmosfera (IPMA). A first effort was taken to join several datasets provided by the partners of the MOPREVIS project, each with different structures. Since an accident can involve several vehicles, drivers, and victims, the team created several summary measures for these variables by accident. This work uses data from January 1, 2016, to December 31, 2019.

The BEAV is a statistical notation instrument filled in by policy entities whenever they become aware of the occurrence of a road accident. This bulletin collects information about the accident, the vehicles, the drivers, the victims, and the severity outcomes.

ANSR updated the information regarding the victims, including their injuries upon 30 days after the accident. The severity of injuries of the victims of road accidents, within 30 days of the occurrence of the accident, are classified as [15]:

- fatality: victim who dies;
- severe injury: victim whose bodily injury requires hospitalization for more than 24 h and who does not die within 30 days of the accident;
- minor injury: victim whose bodily injury did not require hospitalization, or whose hospitalization has been less than 24 h, and who does not die within 30 days of the accident.

Through IPMA it was possible to obtain meteorological information at the time and place of the accident. Information regarding the temperature, the wind velocity, the volume of precipitation, the humidity, and the temperature. The weather information was collected by the team of the project at the hour preceding and following the time of the accident (when information in the previous hour was not available).

Using these sources, we were able to create a unique dataset with all the information regarding the accident. A list of some of the variables used in our analysis are

- **Variables regarding the accident**: county, accident location, type of accident, type and name of the road, type of roadside, type of lane, road conservation state, the existence of works on the road, the existence of light signals, the existence of pavement marks, the existence and type of damage on the road, existence of nearby health facilities, total and type of victims, driver escaping from the location of the accident, causes of the accident, date and time of the accident.
- **Variables regarding the vehicle**: type of vehicle, class, and category of vehicle, a vehicle with or without a trailer, an accident resulting from a vehicle on fire, tire conditions, the existence of insurance, number of occupants.
- **Variables regarding the driver**: gender, date of birth, alcohol and drugs control, existence and year of driving license, driving time, the occurrence of driving maneuvers, use of safety accessories.
- **Variables regarding the victims**: type of victim, use of safety accessories, injury severity of the victim, if the victim is a pedestrian in circulation, number of deaths within 30 days, number and type of victims.
- **Variables regarding the weather conditions**: precipitation, temperature, humidity, wind speed, the occurrence of hail, and the existence of fog or smoke clouds.

2.3 *Statistical Analysis*

A spatial analysis of the accidents was carried out. The Getis–Ord Gi* statistic was used to identify hotspots and the Local Moran's I_i statistic to measure spatial autocorrelation. Let $X_i, i = 1, \ldots, n$, be a numeric variable X at location i and W_{ij} the spatial weight between locations i and j. The Getis–Ord Gi* values are given by [16] and the local Moran's I_i values are given in [17].

Logistic regression was used to identify some determinants for the existence of fatalities and/or serious injuries, at 30 days, in road accidents in the district of Setúbal.

To fit the logistic model, we followed the methodology proposed by Hosmer and Lemeshow [18]. To obtain a parsimonious multivariate model, only the variables that were significant at 0.05 in the univariate analysis were considered and the interactions were considered significant at 0.001 significance level. The linearity of numerical covariates with logit was assessed by lowess methods and fractional polynomials. Some categories were merged, and the likelihood ratio test was used to evaluate the simplified model against the model where the categories were separated.

3 Results

In the district of Setúbal, between 2016 and 2019, there were 28103 accidents in the area under the jurisdiction of the GNR-TC-Setúbal, which resulted in 8260 victims, being 497 severe injuries and 183 fatal injuries (Table 2).

An exploratory spatial analysis of the data available at BEAV was carried out, which, in addition to the description of the variables and identification of some associations, contributed to assessing the quality of the available data. A series of model maps were produced with the purpose of exporting the information from the database. These maps allowed to visualize and interpret the data to be able to draw some conclusions about the accidents. The main conclusions obtained from both approaches were the following:

- Palmela is the municipality with the highest number of serious accidents, being Alcácer do Sal, Palmela, and Alcochete the municipalities more associated with fatalities and serious injuries;
- Accidents occurring in IC/IP, municipal roads (EM), EN, or bridges are more associated with fatalities and serious injuries;
- Accidents with victims occurred mostly on the roads where the pavement was in a good state of conservation, but on roads where the roadside is not paved there are more accidents with fatalities and serious injuries;

Table 2 Number of accidents and victims, at 30 days, by year in the areas under jurisdiction of GNR-CT Setúbal

	Highest injury	2016	2017	2018	2019	Total
Number of accidents	Fatalities	32	52	54	25	163
	Severe	81	120	99	107	407
	Minor	1212	1370	1415	1439	5436
Number of victims	Fatalities	39	55	63	26	183
	Severe	105	147	125	120	497
	Minor	1709	1932	1961	1978	7580

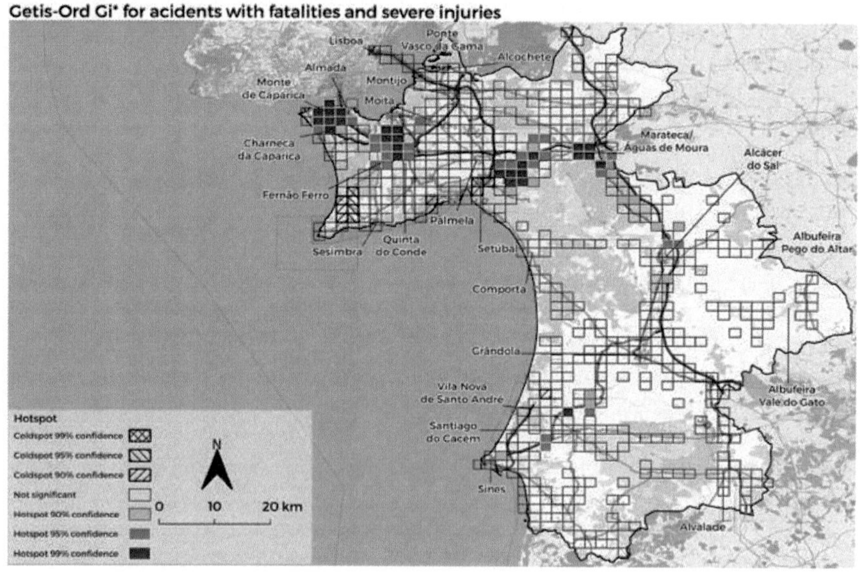

Fig. 1 Getis–Ord Gi* for accidents with fatalities and severe injuries. Areas without squares correspond to regions without data

- An accident where the victims have not used safety accessories has 2.5 higher odds to result in fatalities and serious injuries;
- Accidents where a driver had been driving continuously between 1 and 3 h are more likely to have fatalities and serious injuries;
- An accident involving not just female drivers has 2.5 higher odds to have fatalities and serious injuries;
- On the straight roads, there was a significantly higher percentage of collision accidents and a significantly lower percentage of crash accidents when compared to accidents occurring on curves;
- The majority of accidents that only resulted in damage occur in car parks and on national roads;
- A high number of accidents occur at roundabouts near motorway exits;
- 60% of the accidents occurring on the road are collisions and 75% of the accidents occurring on the limit of the road are collisions.

Using GIS for the spatial analysis we were able to identify four hotspots areas (Fig. 1) with an aggregation of hotspot cells with high levels of confidence in the Northern part of the district, that can be explained, or at least partly, by being located near the access ways to the district, meaning that there are other inherent variables that contribute to the higher concentrations of accidents resulting in serious or fatal injuries.

The concentration of accidents found in the southern half of the district cannot be counted as hotspots per se, since the cells appear in an isolated fashion. Note, however, that these isolated cells gravitate towards the main localities of this section, apart from Grândola, which contains no hotspot cell nearby. The only coldspot found under GNR's jurisdiction is located West of Sesimbra, with no real explanation at the moment.

Having the initial contribution of the exploratory analysis and of the spatial analysis, we proceed to the simple logistic analysis for the existence of severe injuries and/or fatalities in a crash with victims (as recommended by [18])). The variables whose in the univariate test had a p-value less than 0.05 were: municipality, location (outside or inside urban areas), type of road (EN, AE, IC/IP, other roads), type of roadside, type of lane (existence of central road separation), the existence of pavement markings, day of the week, time of the accident, atmospheric factors, average wind intensity (m/s), percentage of male drivers involved in the accident, age of the oldest victim involved in the accident, the median age of the vehicles involved in the accident, age of youngest driver involved, type of vehicles involved in the accident and accident typology. In the multiple logistic regression, some of these variables ceased to be significant.

From the adjusted multiple logistic model with interactions, we can conclude that the determinants for the occurrence of accidents severe injuries and/or fatalities are type of accident, geographical factors (municipality and accident location), temporal factors (day of the week and time of day when the accident occurs), road factors (type of roadside, type of road and type of lane), driver, victims and vehicle factors (% of male drivers, age of drivers involved in the accident, type of the vehicle, age of vehicles and maximum victims age), and associations between the type of the accident and the type of vehicle and between the type of roadside and accident location (Table 3).

The factors that potentiate the existence of serious injuries and/or fatalities in road accidents with victims are:

- **Geographical factors**: the odds of municipalities of Alcochete, Alcácer do Sal and Palmela are 2 times greater than the odds in municipalities of Almada, Moita, Montijo, Sesimbra e Setúbal (OR=1.96; CI_95%:]1.560; 2.462[), and 1.3 times greater than the odds in the municipalities of Santiago do Cacém, Grândola, Sines, Barreiro and Seixal (OR=1.26; CI:]1.006; 1.586[).
- **Temporal factors**: (i) between Thursday and Monday there are 30% higher odds than on the other days of the week (OR=1.30; CI_95%:]1.034; 1.595[); (ii) the odds between 2 and 5 a.m. and between 6 and 7 a.m. are 3 times greater (OR=3.0; CI_95%:]2.390; 3.843[), and the odds between 8 p.m. to 2 a.m, 5 a.m. to 6 a.m. and 7 a.m. to 8 a.m. are almost 2 times greater (OR=1.8; CI_95%:]1.599; 2.122[), than the odds between 8 a.m to 8 p.m.
- **Road characteristics**: (i) accidents occurring on an IC/IP or on an EN have 60% higher odds than those occurring on another type of road (OR=1.6; CI_95%:]1.328; 2.041[); (ii) accidents occurring on a road where the lanes do not have a central separator are 70% more likely of serious injuries and/or fatalities than when there is a central separator (OR=1.7; CI_95%:]1.225; 2.302[); (iii) accidents occurring inside urban areas are almost twice as likely of serious injuries and/or fatalities

Table 3 Logistic regression model for severe injuries and/or fatalities in road accidents with victims. Significant variables of the model and their categories, coefficient estimates, standard errors, and respective *p-values*

Variable	Estimate	Std. Error	*p-value*
Constant	–4.95	0.30	<0.001
Municipality (ref: Alcochete/Alcácer/Palmela)			
Almada/Montijo/Moita/Sesimbra/Setúbal	–0.67	0.12	<0.001
Santiago/Grândola/Sines/Barreiro/Seixal	–0.23	0.12	0.044
Accident location (ref: inside urban area)			
Outside urban area	1.09	0.20	<0.001
Type of accident (ref: collision)			
Trampling	1.61	0.19	<0.001
Crash	0.80	0.16	<0.001
Type of roadside (ref: paved)			
Unpaved or non-existent	0.61	0.16	<0.001
Type of road (ref: AE/bridge or other)			
IC/IP or EN	0.50	0.11	<0.001
Type of lane (ref: without central separator)			
With central separator	–0.52	0.16	0.001
Day of the week (ref: Thursday to Monday)			
Tuesday and Wednesday	–0.25	0.11	0.024
Hour of the day (ref: 8–20 h)			
20–2 h, 5–6 h, 7–8 h	0.61	0.11	<0.001
2–5 h, 6–7 h	1.11	0.19	<0.001
Type of vehicle (ref: light passenger vehicles)			
Motorbikes but not heavy vehicles	1.26	0.14	<0.001
Heavy vehicles	1.39	0.20	<0.001
% of male drivers (ref: <50%)			
$\geq$ 50%	0.84	0.17	<0.001
Median age of vehicle	0.02	0.01	0.009
Maximum victims age	0.02	0.00	<0.001
Age of the youngest driver	–0.01	0.00	<0.001
Type of accident × Type of vehicle			
Trampling × motorbikes but not heavy vehicles	–1.45	0.61	0.017
Crash × motorbikes but not heavy vehicles	–1.08	0.23	<0.001
Trampling × heavy vehicles	–0.25	0.57	0.653
Crash × heavy vehicles	–1.86	0.57	0.001
Type of roadside × Accident location			
Unpaved or non-existent × outside urban area	–0.70	0.22	0.001

than when the roadside is not paved as when it is paved (OR=1.9, CI_95%:]1.366; 2.534[); (iv) accidents that occur on a road with a paved roadside, if they occur outside an urban area, have almost three times the odds of serious injuries and/or fatalities than if they occur inside an urban area (OR=2.9, CI_95%:]1.966; 4.261[);

- **Drivers' characteristics**: (i) accidents in which the majority of drivers involved are male have approximately twice the odds of serious injuries and/or fatalities than accidents in which the majority of drivers are female (OR=2.3; CI_95%:]1.666; 3.253[); (ii) as the age of the youngest driver involved in the accident increases, the odds of serious injuries and/or fatalities decrease (Fig. 2a). For example, an accident where the youngest driver's age is 10 years higher than in another accident has 14% less odds (OR=0.86; CI_95%:]0.797; 0.932[) of having serious injuries and/or deaths, and if this difference is 20 years then it has 26% less odds (OR=0.74; CI_95%:]0.636; 0.869[).
- **Victims' characteristics**: With increasing age of the older victim involved in the accident increases the odds of serious injuries and/or deaths (Fig. 2b). For example, an accident in which the oldest victim is 10 years older than in another accident has 19% higher odds (OR=1.19; CI_95%:]1.120; 1.266[) of having serious injuries and/or deaths, and if this difference is 20 years then it has 42% higher odds (OR=1.42; CI_95%:]1.255; 1.602[).
- **Vehicles' features**: (i) the odds of a crash involving serious injuries and/or deaths increase with the median age of the vehicles involved in the crash (Fig. 3). For example, there are 1.2 times more odds for each 10-year increase in the median age of the vehicles involved in the crash (OR=1.2; CI_95%:]1,049; 1,386[), and 1.5 times more odds for each 20-year increase (OR=1.5; CI_95%:]1,100; 1,921[); (ii) in collision accidents, those involving heavy vehicles have 4 times more odds (OR=4.0; CI_95%:]2.702;5.905[), and those not involving heavy vehicles but involving motorbikes have 3.6 times more odds (OR=3.6; CI_95%:]2.710; 4.740[), relative to accidents involving only light vehicles; (iii) in accidents involving only light vehicles, accidents by trampling have 5 times more odds (OR=5.0;

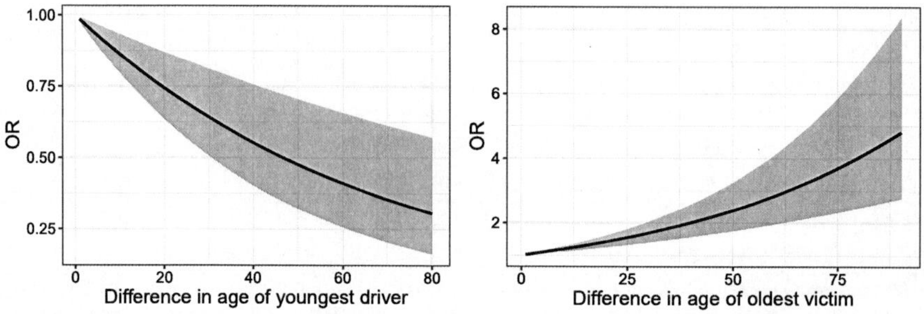

Fig. 2 Odds ratio, and respective 95% confidence interval, for the occurrence of an accident with severe injuries and/or fatalities for different increases in the age of the **a** youngest driver, **b** oldest victim, involved in the accident with victims

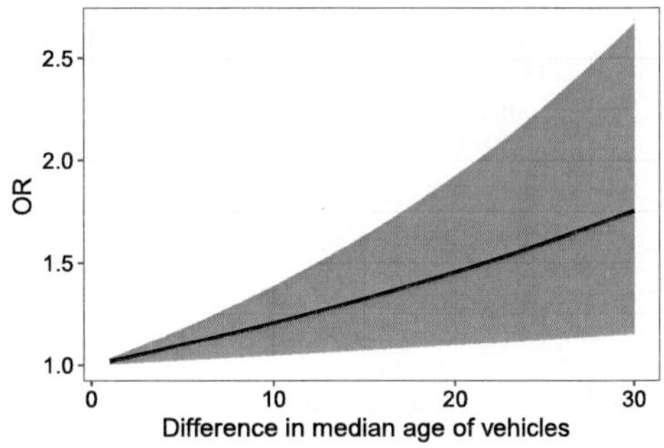

Fig. 3 Odds ratio, and respective 95% confidence interval, for the occurrence of an accident with severe injuries and/or fatalities for different increases in the median age of vehicles involved in the accident with victims

CI_95%:]3.413;7.274[), and those by crashing have about 2 times more odds (OR=2.2; CI_95%:]1.620; 3.010[), than by collision.

4 Conclusions

This work analyzes road accidents that occurred in the area under the jurisdiction of the GNR-CT Setúbal, pooling data from different sources. We used GIS methodology for spatial analysis of the road accidents, and to cluster municipalities by accident vulnerability. Afterward, we fit a logistic regression model to find the determinants for severe injuries and/or fatalities in road accidents in the district of Setúbal.

We have concluded that a greater chance of severe injuries and/or fatalities occur in the municipalities of Alcochete, Alcácer do Sal, and Palmela, between Thursday and Monday, in the periods from 2 a.m. to 5 a.m. and from 6 a.m. to 7 a.m., on an IC/IP or on an EN and on roads outside urban areas and with lanes without a central separator with unpaved or non-existence of roadsides, and when the majority of drivers involved in the accident are male. Accidents with motorbikes, young drivers, and old vehicles also increase the possibilities of severe injuries and/or fatalities.

The main limitation of this work is that it only considers the accidents that occurred under GNR jurisdiction in the district of Setúbal, corresponding to 4888 km^2 (96.5% of the district) covering 417900 habitants (49.2% of the district).

Future work will develop predictive models for the time and place of the accidents. Data from 2020/21, out of the lockdown COVID-19 period, will be used to validate the adjusted models. Finally, a digital decision support tool will be developed to support GNR to make more informed decisions regarding road accident prevention.

Acknowledgements This work was developed under the research project MOPREVIS "FCT DSAIPA/DS/0090/2018" supported by FCT—Fundação para a Ciência e a Tecnologia, under Iniciativa Nacional em Competências Digitais e.2030, Portugal INCoDe.2030. We are also grateful to the partners of this project.

References

1. Lusa: Sinistralidade rodoviária tem impacto económico e social negativo de 1, 2% do PIB—governo (2018). https://www.rtp.pt/noticias/pais/sinistralidade-rodoviaria-tem-impacto-economico-e-social-negativo-de-12-do-pib-governo_n1112193. Accessed 25 Jan 2022
2. Basso, F., Basso, L.J., Bravo, F., Pezoa, R.: Real-time crash prediction in an urban expressway using disaggregated data. Transp. Res. Part C: Emerg. Technol. **86**, 202–219 (2018)
3. Casado-Sanz, N., Guirao, B., Attard, M.: Analysis of the risk factors affecting the severity of traffic accidents on Spanish crosstown roads: the driver's perspective. Sustainability **12**(6) (2020)
4. Chen, M.-M., Chen, M.-C.: Modeling road accident severity with comparisons of logistic regression, decision tree and random forest. Information **11**(5) (2020)
5. Erdogan, S., Yilmaz, I., Baybura, T., Gullu, M.: Geographical information systems aided traffic accident analysis system case study: city of Afyonkarahisar. Accid. Anal. Prev. **40**(1), 174–181 (2008)
6. Iranitalab, A., Khattak, A.: Comparison of four statistical and machine learning methods for crash severity prediction. Accid. Anal. Prev. **108**, 27–36 (2017)
7. Mannering, F.: Temporal instability and the analysis of highway accident data. Anal. Methods Accid. Res. **17**, 1–13 (2018)
8. Prasannakumar, V., Vijith, H., Charutha, R., Geetha, N.: Spatio-temporal clustering of road accidents: GIS based analysis and assessment. Procedia. Soc. Behav. Sci. **21**, 317–325 (2011)
9. Mannering, F.L., Bhat, C.R.: Analytic methods in accident research: methodological frontier and future directions. Anal. Methods Accid. Res. **1**, 1–22 (2014)
10. Al-Ghamdi, A.S.: Using logistic regression to estimate the influence of accident factors on accident severity. Accid. Anal. Prev. **34**(6), 729–741 (2002)
11. Abdul Manan, M.M., Várhelyi, A., Çelik, A.K., Hashim, H.H.: Road characteristics and environment factors associated with motorcycle fatal crashes in Malaysia. IATSS Res. **42**(4), 207–220 (2018)
12. Garrido, R., Bastos, A., de Almeida, A., Elvas, J.P.: Prediction of road accident severity using the ordered probit model. Transp. Res. Procedia **3**, 214–223 (2014)
13. Santos, K., Dias, J.P., Amado, C., Sousa, J., Francisco, P.: Risk factors associated with the increase of injury severity of powered two wheelers road accidents victims in Portugal. Traffic Inj. Prev. **22**(8), 646–650 (2021)
14. Guilhermina, T., Nagui, R., Margarida, C.: Effect of vehicle characteristics on crash severity: Portuguese experience. Inj. Prev. **18**(Suppl 1), A216–A216 (2012)
15. ANSR: Manual de prenchimento. Boletim Estatístico de Acidente de Viação (2013). http://www.ansr.pt/Estatisticas/BEAV/Documents/MANUALPREENCHIMENTOBEAV.pdf. Accessed 24 Nov 2021
16. Getis, A., Ord, J.K.: Local spatial statistics: an overview. In: Longley, P., Batty, M. (eds.) Spatial Analysis: Modelling in a GIS Environment, pp. 261–277. GeoInformation International, Cambridge (1996)
17. Anselin, L.: Local indicators of spatial association–LISA. Geogr. Anal. **27**(2), 93–115 (1995)
18. Hosmer, D.W., Jr., Lemeshow, S., Sturdivant, R.X.: Applied Logistic Regression, vol. 398. Wiley, New Jersey (2013)

Impact of Misclassification and Imperfect Serological Tests in Association Analyses of ME/CFS Applied to COVID-19 Data

João Malato, Luís Graça, and Nuno Sepúlveda

Abstract The diagnosis of ME/CFS is problematic due to the absence of a disease specific biomarker. As such, it is conducted under uncertainty using symptom-based criteria and the exclusion of known diseases. The possibility of misdiagnosing patients reduces the power to detect new and previously identified factors that can be associated with the disease. To investigate this problem, we previously conducted a simulation study to estimate the power of case-control association studies as a function of the misdiagnosed rate. Here we extended this simulation study to the more general situation where there is also the possibility of having misclassification in a binary factor related to a previous exposure to a given infection. Given the suggested link between ME/CFS and past viral infections including SARS-CoV-2 (which causes COVID-19), we performed the simulation study in the specific context of serological testing of this new coronavirus using published data from Portuguese, Spanish and Iranian seroepidemiological studies.

Keywords Myalgic encephalomyelitis/chronic fatigue (ME/CFS) · Misclassification · Power studies · Serology · Simulation

J. Malato (✉) · L. Graça
Faculty of Medicine, Instituto de Medicina Molecular João Lobo Antunes, University of Lisbon, Lisbon, Portugal
e-mail: jmalato@medicina.ulisboa.pt

J. Malato · N. Sepúlveda
CEAUL—Centro de Estatística e Aplicações, University of Lisbon, Lisbon, Portugal

N. Sepúlveda
Faculty of Mathematics and Information Science, Warsaw University of Technology, Warsaw, Poland

R. Bispo et al. (eds.), *Recent Developments in Statistics and Data Science*, Springer Proceedings in Mathematics & Statistics 398,
https://doi.org/10.1007/978-3-031-12766-3_15

1 Background

Myalgic encephalomyelitis/chronic fatigue syndrome (ME/CFS) is one example of a complex disease with uncertainty in its diagnosis [1]. Patients diagnosed with this debilitating disorder manifest heterogeneous symptoms such as unexplained long-lasting fatigue [2], a post-exertional malaise that arises after the slight physical, or mental effort and is not alleviated by rest [3], accompanied by other symptoms. Its prevalence is estimated between 0.4 and 1% depending on the population, affecting more women than men, at a 6:1 ratio [4, 5].

The aetiology of ME/CFS has been proved difficult to determine. Different reported factors such as acute infections, genetic predisposition, or environmental stressors can serve as triggers for the disease onset [6, 7]. Moreover there is no biomarker, or combination of biomarkers, that characterise this heterogeneous disease, which ultimately leave its diagnosis to be mostly done on the basis of specific symptoms and exclusion of other diseases [8]. This further increases the uncertainty surrounding an objective diagnosis, which has resulted in more than 20 symptom-based criteria currently used to clinically diagnose ME/CFS [9]. Despite proposed protocols for criteria standardisation in ME/CFS research [10], distinct studies will inevitably define the cohort of patients differently, potentially with conflicting results [1]. This inherent level of misclassification—non-ME/CFS patients being incorrectly diagnosed as such—amongst ME/CFS cohorts has already been described in a study characterising the genome of suspected patients [11] and should be taken into account in order to minimise the negative effects on association studies [12].

Despite the pathomechanisms of ME/CFS remaining unknown, the disease has been described as having an autoimmune onset [13, 14]. This immune dysregulation often occurs after exposure to an acute viral infection [7, 15, 16], with multiple association studies relating the exposure to viruses as trigger for ME/CFS development [14, 17]. Serological surveys have thus been conducted to better understand the role of distinct viruses in this disease. However, so far there have not been replicable confirmed associations. Possible arguments for this can be the disparate cohorts of (inherently misclassified) suspected ME/CFS patients used and other factors related to study design such as the low sample sizes used [18] or the further stratification of patients into different subtypes [19]. Additionally, the serological tests used to assess exposure/non-exposure to the viruses are based on predetermined and arbitrary cutoff values to determine seropositive individuals [18]. This important but often overlooked aspect can potentially add an additional layer to the misclassification on ME/CFS, with impacts on the studies' reproducibility [20].

Previously, we studied the dissimilarity between different symptom diagnosis criteria and simulated the impacts of misclassification in a single scenario of potential misdiagnosis of suspected patients [12]. In the present paper, we extended the proposed ideas on misclassification and studied its impact on the statistical power of serology hypothetical association studies. More recently, studies have related ME/CFS and the chronic post-viral syndrome developed after infection by the SARS-CoV-2 virus, responsible for the COVID-19 pandemic [21]. Despite the need for more extensive research on this topic, studies have reported that subset of patients following COVID-19 infection can develop a chronic syndrome that fulfils ME/CFS diagnostic criteria [22]. For illustrative purposes we extrapolated on the idea that there is in fact an association between COVID-19 and ME/CFS onset, however mild ($1.25 \leq$ odds ratio ≤ 2.0), and simulated multiple case-control association studies with different sample sizes, using results for seroprevalence surveys from three countries: Portugal [23], Spain [24], and Iran [25]. For each serology study, we hypothesised on the impact of misclassification, also accounting for the estimated levels of sensitivity and specificity.

2 Simulation Study

2.1 Mathematical Formulation of the Problem

Following-up on the reported ideas on misclassification [12], the goal of the proposed hypothetical study was to assess the association of a binary exposure outcome (as exposed versus non-exposed) after a serological survey for COVID-19 with ME/CFS. This was accomplished by comparing a cohort of sampled patients suspected of ME/CFS to a cohort of sampled matched healthy controls. The sampling distribution of the designed case-control study was then, the product of two Binomial distributions given by the number of sampled individuals from the two cohorts, n_0 and n_1, respectively for healthy controls and suspected ME/CFS patients, and the probability of exposure to the virus, θ_0 and θ_1, respectively; with x_0 and x_1 being the observed frequencies of exposed healthy controls and suspected ME/CFS [12]. Altogether, the sampled populations can be summarised by a 2×2 frequency table that presents different outlines depending on the described parameters n_i and θ_i, $i = \{0, 1\}$. Testing the null hypothesis for lack of association to ME/CFS (i.e. $H_0 : \theta_0 = \theta_1$) was done through the Pearson's χ^2 test for independence. After testing, H_0 was rejected if the p-value for the Pearson's χ^2 test was less than the prespecified level of significance of 5%. Through simulation, and by repeating the inference multiple times under the same conditions, the power of the study was estimated as the overall proportion in which H_0 was rejected.

Previously [12], to account for the inherent misclassification as a diluting effect for the detection of a potential association, four assumptions were considered for the ME/CFS cohort: (i) sampled suspected ME/CFS cases can be divided into apparent (false positives) and true positive cases; (ii) the misclassified apparent cases are considered healthy controls, in the sense that they share the same probability of exposure to COVID-19, θ_0; (iii) there is an overall misclassification rate, γ, creating the two distinct possibilities of apparent and true cases within the cohort for suspected cases; and (iv) this misclassification rate is only dependent on the true clinical status of each of the suspected cases. Under the assumption (ii) and the law of total probability, the probability of exposure associated with the suspected cases was written as

$$\theta_1 = \gamma\theta_0 + (1-\gamma)\theta_1^*\,, \tag{1}$$

where θ_1^* is the exposure probability of true ME/CFS cases.

However, this analysis does not account for the sensitivity and specificity of a serology test if the exposure to a given infection is determined this way. Therefore, four additional assumptions were considered for this study, with effects transversal to all data sets: (v) for each serology test performed, individuals can only be classified as seropositive or seronegative—in opposition to serology tests where there are more than two possible outcomes; (vi) the levels of sensitivity, π_{se}, and specificity, π_{sp}, respectively determine the accuracy of a test to identify truly exposed and truly non-exposed individuals; (vii) these parameters related to the performance of the serology test create a category of undetected false positives and false negative for individuals poorly measured by the serology assessment; and (viii) the binary exposure outcomes given by π_{se} and π_{sp} are independent from the assessed cohort. Under these assumptions, the probability of exposure for suspected cases from Eq. (1) can be extended to

$$\theta_1 = \pi_{se}\gamma\theta_0 + (1-\pi_{sp})\gamma(1-\theta_0) + \pi_{se}(1-\gamma)\theta_1^* + (1-\pi_{sp})(1-\gamma)(1-\theta_1^*)\,. \tag{2}$$

Under the eight assumptions, the observable 2×2 frequency table can be augmented, as the cohort for suspected ME/CFS is divided into apparent and true cases based on the misclassification rate, γ, and with sensitivity and specificity, respectively π_{se} and π_{sp}, defining the serology tests' overall accuracy to determine the seropositive (either true positive or false positive) and seronegative (both true and false negative) populations on both cohorts (Table 1).

Notes. Instead of the Pearson's χ^2 test, an analogous investigation could also been proposed using the Fisher's exact test to assess the null hypothesis for lack of association. Equation (2) includes parameters related to the accuracy of serology tests; based on this formulation, one can obtain Eq. (1) by simply assuming $\pi_{se} = \pi_{sp} = 1$.

Table 1 Augmented version of the observable 2×2 frequency table in the case-control association study scenario with possible misclassification of suspected ME/CFS cases (into apparent and true cases) and existence of false positive and false negative serological outcomes observed from serology tests done to assess exposure (confirmed by the true exposure indicator columns, with E for exposed individuals and $\overline{E}$ for non-exposed)

Observed test outcome	True exposure indicator	Controls	Suspected cases	
			(Apparent)	(True)
Seropositive	E	$\pi_{se}\theta_0$	$\pi_{se}\gamma\theta_0$	$\pi_{se}(1-\gamma)\theta_1^*$
	$\overline{E}$	$(1-\pi_{sp})(1-\theta_0)$	$(1-\pi_{sp})\gamma(1-\theta_0)$	$(1-\pi_{sp})(1-\gamma)(1-\theta_1^*)$
Seronegative	E	$(1-\pi_{se})\theta_0$	$(1-\pi_{se})\gamma\theta_0$	$(1-\pi_{se})(1-\gamma)\theta_1^*$
	$\overline{E}$	$\pi_{sp}(1-\theta_0)$	$\pi_{sp}\gamma(1-\theta_0)$	$\pi_{sp}(1-\gamma)(1-\theta_1^*)$

2.2 Parameterisation Using Real-Word Data

As example of real-life application, we looked at data from three distinct seroepidemiologic surveys: Portugal [23], Spain [24], and Iran [25]. The studies occurred between April and August 2020 and applied similar methods of estimation of their populations' seroprevalence. Also, all surveys presented information regarding the sensitivity and specificity estimates for the serology tests performed. The estimated values for the mentioned parameters in each survey are presented in Table 2.

For the purpose of the study, we assumed the existence of an association between exposure to COVID-19 and ME/CFS onset. Despite few evidences thus far due to the novelty of the topic, some studies have mentioned this association based on the idea of immune dysregulation, linking the development of post-COVID-19 chronic symptoms with the autoimmune proposal for ME/CFS [14]. Since there are no biomarkers for ME/CFS diagnosis, we defined the association as a mild relation with three possible values of the overall true odds ratio, $\Delta_T = \{1.25, 1.5, 2\}$. Based on the values of θ_0 from the three surveys and the proposed Δ_T, the probability of exposure on true ME/CFS cases was determined by

$$\theta_1^* = \frac{\theta_0 \Delta_T}{1 + \theta_0 (\Delta_T - 1)} . \qquad (3)$$

2.3 Simulation Structure

The impact of inherent misclassification on the hypothetical case-control association studies was assessed through multiple simulations on different parametric values for θ_0, π_{se}, π_{sp}, in accordance to each serological survey (Table 2), and Δ_T. For each combination of θ_0 and Δ_T, parameters θ_1 and θ_1^* were calculated from Eqs. (2) and (3), respectively. To illustrate how sample sizes also influence the overall power of a study, we performed our simulations considering cohort sample sizes of $n_0 = n_1 = \{100, 250, 500, 1000, 2500, 5000\}$.

To assess the power of rejecting H_0, 10,000 data sets were generated for each value of γ, ranging from 0 (no misclassification) to 1 (no true ME/CFS patients in the cohort for suspected cases) with a lag of 0.01. As previously mentioned, H_0 was

Table 2 Parameter values used in the study, where the probability of exposure to the virus and the sensitivity and specificity of the serology test are given by θ_0, π_{se}, and π_{sp}, respectively

Reference	Country	θ_0	π_{se}	π_{sp}
[23]	Portugal	0.025	0.95	0.98
[24]	Spain	0.050	0.80	0.98
[26]	Iran	0.150	0.75	0.98

rejected at each data set if the p-value from the Pearson's χ^2 test was less than the usual level of significance. Finally, for each parameter set, power was estimated as the proportion of simulated data sets in which H_0 was rejected. All simulations and analyses were done using R statistical software, version 4.1.0 [26], using our own scripts, available upon request.

Notes. For the purpose of study consistency, the estimated seroprevalence values published on the serological surveys were considered as the probability of exposure in the cohort of matched healthy controls, θ_0.

3 Simulation Results

As expected, the estimated power to detect the hypothetical association decreased with misclassification rate (Fig. 1). Looking at the extreme cases, the estimated power was highest when no misclassification was considered and all suspected ME/CFS cases were considered to be true positives ($\gamma = 0$). Irrespective of the scenario, as misclassification increases, the overall power is reduced towards 5% at the opposite most extreme value ($\gamma = 1$)—i.e. the significance level specified for the Pearson's χ^2 test.

Along with gradually increasing the misclassification of suspected patients, the power to detect an association was estimated by varying the values of probability of exposure in healthy controls, θ_0, and sensitivity of the serology test, π_{se}, for each country serological scenario. In all three illustrated scenarios, the specificity was the same and estimated at $\pi_{sp} = 0.98$ (Table 2).

Overall, only sample sizes of $n_i \geq 500$ individuals were able to reach a power of at least 80%—the specified power threshold to identify what can be considered as having acceptable reproducibility level (Table 3). Simulations with larger sample sizes granted a consistency to the reproducibility of the studies, with power remaining above the defined threshold for higher values of misclassification. Similarly, higher values of Δ_T also affected positively the overall power of each study (Table 3).

The Portuguese survey had the smallest estimate for the probability of virus exposure and the highest sensitivity [23]. For this scenario, only higher association values of $\Delta_T = 2$ and cohort sample sizes of 2500 and 5000 reached the power of at least 80%. Under these parametric conditions, the acceptable level of reproducibility was observable at $\gamma \leq 0.45$.

Compared to Portugal's results, the Spain's survey had θ_0 increased and the π_{se} decreased [24]. In this scenario there was an increase on the reproducibility, with more studies surpassing the 80% threshold. Nonetheless, this only occurred for sample sizes of $n_i \geq 1000$.

Lastly, Iran's survey [25] had the highest estimate for θ_0 and lowest estimates for π_{se}. Despite the lower sensitivity, simulations under these parameters had higher power for the same sample sizes than the other two scenarios (Fig. 1 and Table 3).

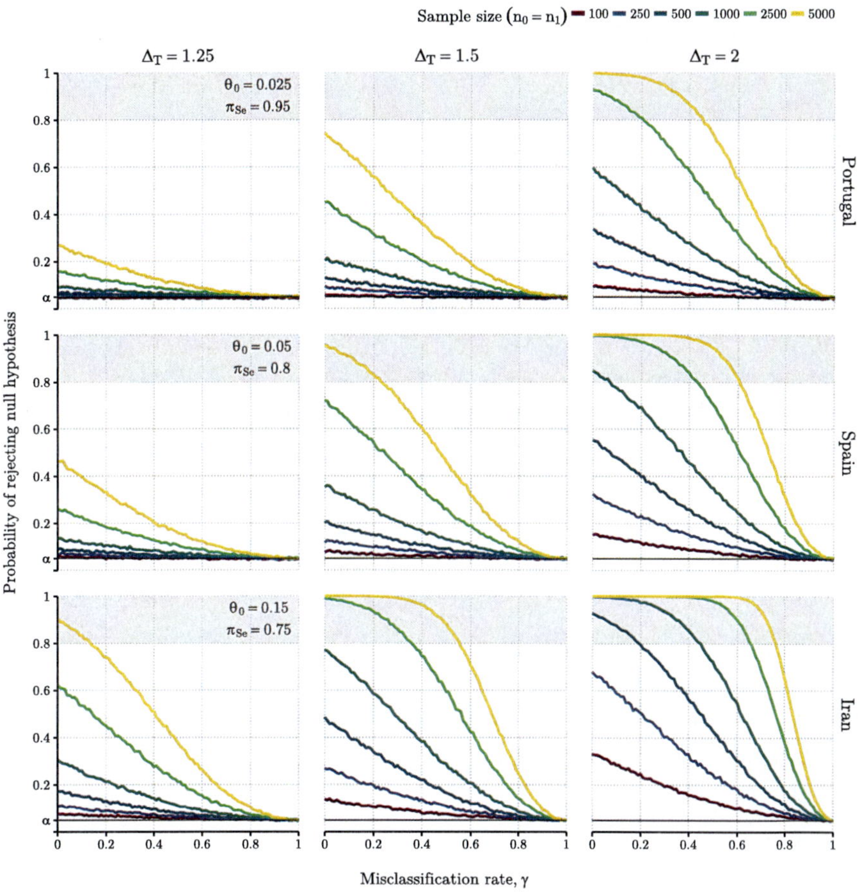

Fig. 1 Probabilities of rejecting the null hypothesis, i.e. absence of association between the two populations as function of the misclassification rate. Each column represents the values attributed to the true odds ratio for COVID-19 exposure and true ME/CFS, assessed between true positive cases and healthy controls. Each row indicates a country serologic survey, with distinct values of θ_0 and π_{se} identified in the first column of each survey, and fixed $\pi_{sp} = 0.98$ across all simulations. Power analysis was estimated for different cohort sample sizes of 100, 250, 500, 1000, 2500, and 5000 individuals ($n_0 = n_1$), represented by the lines of different colours in each scenario. Grey filled area indicates scenarios where the probability of rejecting the null hypothesis is above 80%. Dark horizontal line indicates the level of significance used, $\alpha = 0.05$

Table 3 Maximum values of misclassification rate, γ, that maintain power if at least 80% to reject the null hypothesis of lack of association, for different values of true odds ratio, Δ_T, country of serological survey, and sample sizes, n_i, $i = (0, 1)$. Cells with no value indicate the inability to reach the power threshold between cohort, even at $\gamma = 0$

Country	Δ_T			
	1.25	1.50	2.00	n_i
Portugal	–	–	–	100
Spain	–	–	–	
Iran	–	–	–	
Portugal	–	–	–	250
Spain	–	–	–	
Iran	–	–	–	
Portugal	–	–	–	500
Spain	–	–	–	
Iran	–	–	0.19	
Portugal	–	–	–	1000
Spain	–	–	0.07	
Iran	–	–	0.45	
Portugal	–	–	0.20	2000
Spain	–	–	0.43	
Iran	–	0.35	0.65	
Portugal	–	–	0.20	2500
Spain	–	–	0.43	
Iran	–	0.35	0.65	
Portugal	–	–	0.45	5000
Spain	–	0.22	0.60	
Iran	0.13	0.55	0.76	

4 Discussion

Focusing on ME/CFS, our simulation results showed how misclassification of patients poses an impact on the ability to consistently recognise true associations to a triggering viral exposure, prior to the disease onset. While still researching for biomarkers able to discriminate the disease, the power is very likely to suffer from limited statistical power due to possible misclassification of the suspected ME/CFS cases. The proposed solution to this problem is to take into account for misclassification in the respective statistical analysis.

The results evidenced how increasing a study's sample size can increase its power. Until now, misclassification studies mostly focused on identifying the extent of misdiagnosed of patients when using distinct diagnosis criteria, not particularly looking at sample sizes [12]. With MEC/FS research being usually underfunded [27, 28], case-control studies are frequently performed on sample sizes below 250 patients.

This allows for potential sporadic associations that ultimately cannot be replicated in follow-up studies. Throughout efforts to raise awareness and laboratory collaborations, studies have been increasing their sampled populations. After all, our study showed that under the parameterised conditions, only cohorts with samples above 500 individuals were able to consistently reject the null hypothesis under some levels of misclassification (Table 3).

A more in depth study would be required to pose a more general conclusion on the influence of power caused by the prevalence of exposure and the sensitivity and specificity of the serology test. One can argue that increasing the prevalence will make for better comparisons between cohorts through Pearson's χ^2 test for independence, as it might improve the frequency distributions across the 2×2 contingency table cells. Whereas sensitivity and specificity will produce a lessened effect, as serology tests keep improving—but still impactful, if not from the estimated π_{se} and π_{sp}, then because the majority of serological cutoff values for seropositivity used arise from inherently arbitrary choices if the researchers and manufacturers of the serology tests [20, 29]. Nevertheless, diagnostic accuracy is still of extremely importance in the evaluation of medical diagnostic tests and should be taken into account when replication of a study—in this case, a scenario of a serology study—is necessary.

This hypothetical study was done in the context of the recent COVID-19 pandemic and the association of the long-term symptoms caused by the SARS-CoV-2 virus and ME/CFS diagnosis. With the lack of extensive information on this COVID-19 exposure—ME/CFS diagnosis relation premise, the parameter Δ_T was defined within low-to-mild values so as to not profoundly influence the simulation results. As more studies and serological surveys are published on the matter, focusing on different populations or even focusing on serology tests for different specific antibodies against COVID-19, one could better parameterise the simulation study.

ME/CFS is a complex disease and there is still a lack of understanding to the extension of the disease's aetiology and pathophysiology. Even under these uncertainties, accepting and accounting for a level of patient misclassification—however small—in association studies might help to improve the study designs and increase scientific reproducibility. Ultimately, the ability to replicate and reproduce the results proposed by a study is one of the most important aspects in research, and consistent results are what allow ideas to become postulates, continuously driving science forwards.

Acknowledgements JM and NS acknowledge funding by the Fundação para a Ciência e Tecnologia, Portugal (ref. SFRH/BD/149758/2019 and UIDB/00006/2020, respectively). NS also acknowledges funding by the Polish National Agency for Academic Exchange (ref. PPN/ULM/2020/1/00069/U/00001).

References

1. Nacul, L., Lacerda, E.M., Kingdon, C.C., Curran, H., Bowman, E.W.: How have selection bias and disease misclassification undermined the validity of Myalgic encephalomyelitis/chronic fatigue syndrome studies? J. Health Psychol. **24**(12), 1765–1769 (2017)
2. Fukuda, K.: The chronic fatigue syndrome: a comprehensive approach to its definition and study. Ann. Intern. Med. **121**(12), 953 (1994)
3. Carruthers, B.M., Jain, A.K., Meirleir, K.L.D., Peterson, D.L., Klimas, N.G., et al.: Myalgic encephalomyelitis/chronic fatigue syndrome. J. Chronic Fatigue Syndr. **11**(1), 7–115 (2003)
4. Lim, E.-J., Ahn, Y.-C., Jang, E.-S., Lee, S.-W., Lee, S.-H., et al.: Systematic review and meta-analysis of the prevalence of chronic fatigue syndrome/myalgic encephalomyelitis (CFS/ME). J. Transl. Med. **18**(1) (2020)
5. Morris, G., Maes, M.: Myalgic encephalomyelitis/chronic fatigue syndrome and encephalomyelitis disseminata/multiple sclerosis show remarkable levels of similarity in phenomenology and neuroimmune characteristics. BMC Med. **11**(1) (2013)
6. Lacerda, E.M., Geraghty, K., Kingdon, C.C., Palla, L., Nacul, L.: A logistic regression analysis of risk factors in ME/CFS pathogenesis. BMC Neurol. **19**(1) (2019)
7. Chu, L., Valencia, I.J., Garvert, D.W., Montoya, J.G.: Onset patterns and course of myalgic encephalomyelitis/chronic fatigue syndrome. Front. Pediatr. **7** (2019)
8. Smith, M.E.B., Nelson, H.D., Haney, E., Pappas, M., Daeges, M., et al.: Diagnosis and treatment of myalgic encephalomyelitis/chronic fatigue syndrome. Technical report (2014)
9. Brurberg, K.G., Fønhus, M.S., Larun, L., Flottorp, S., Malterud, K.: Case definitions for chronic fatigue syndrome/myalgic encephalomyelitis (CFS/ME): a systematic review. BMJ Open **4**(2), e003973 (2014)
10. Pheby, D.F., Araja, D., Berkis, U., Brenna, E., Cullinan, J., et al.: The development of a consistent Europe-wide approach to investigating the economic impact of myalgic encephalomyelitis (ME/CFS): A report from the european network on ME/CFS (EUROMENE). Healthcare **8**(2), 88 (2020)
11. Brown, D., Birch, C., Younger, J., Worthey, E.: ME/CFS: whole genome sequencing uncovers a misclassified case of glycogen storage disease type 13 previously diagnosed as ME/CFS. Mol. Genet. Metabolism **132**, S194–S195 (2021). https://doi.org/10.1016/S1096-7192(21)00388-7
12. Malato, J., Graça, L., Nacul, L., Lacerda, E., Sepúlveda, N.: Statistical challenges of investigating a disease with a complex diagnosis. In: de Estatística, S.P. (ed.), Estatística: Desafios Transversais ás Ciências com Dados, pp. 153–167 (2021)
13. Lorusso, L., Mikhaylova, S.V., Capelli, E., Ferrari, D., Ngonga, G.K., Ricevuti, G.: Immunological aspects of chronic fatigue syndrome. Autoimmun. Rev. **8**(4), 287–291 (2009). https://doi.org/10.1016/j.autrev.2008.08.003
14. Sotzny, F., Blanco, J., Capelli, E., Castro-Marrero, J., Steiner, S., et al.: Myalgic encephalomyelitis/chronic fatigue syndrome–evidence for an autoimmune disease. Autoimmun. Rev. **17**(6), 601–609 (2018)
15. Rasa, S., Nora-Krukle, Z., Henning, N., Eliassen, E., Shikova, E., et al.: Chronic viral infections in myalgic encephalomyelitis/chronic fatigue syndrome (ME/CFS). J. Transl. Med. **16**(1) (2018)
16. Blomberg, J., Gottfries, C.-G., Elfaitouri, A., Rizwan, M., Rosén, A.: Infection elicited autoimmunity and myalgic encephalomyelitis/chronic fatigue syndrome: an explanatory model. Front. Immunol. **9** (2018)

17. Bansal, A., Bradley, A., Bishop, K., Kiani-Alikhan, S., Ford, B.: Chronic fatigue syndrome, the immune system and viral infection. Brain Behav. Immun. **26**(1), 24–31 (2012)
18. Scheibenbogen, C., Freitag, H., Blanco, J., Capelli, E., Lacerda, E., et al.: The european ME/CFS biomarker landscape project: an initiative of the European network EUROMENE. J. Transl. Med. **15**(1) (2017)
19. Jason, L.A., Corradi, K., Torres-Harding, S., Taylor, R.R., King, C.: Chronic fatigue syndrome: the need for subtypes. Neuropsychol. Rev. **15**(1), 29–58 (2005)
20. Domingues, T.D., Grabowska, A.D., Lee, J.-S., Ameijeiras-Alonso, J., Westermeier, F., et al.: Herpesviruses serology distinguishes different subgroups of patients from the united kingdom myalgic encephalomyelitis/chronic fatigue syndrome biobank. J. Transl. Med. **8** (2021)
21. Komaroff, A.L., Bateman, L.: Will COVID-19 lead to myalgic encephalomyelitis/chronic fatigue syndrome? Front. Med. **7** (2021)
22. Kedor, C., Freitag, H., Meyer-Arndt, L., Wittke, K., Zoller, T., et al.: Chronic COVID-19 syndrome and chronic fatigue syndrome (ME/CFS) following the first pandemic wave in Germany—a first analysis of a prospective observational study (2021)
23. Kislaya, I., Gonçalves, P., Barreto, M., Sousa, R.D., Garcia, A.C., et al.: Seroprevalence of SARS-CoV-2 infection in Portugal in May-July 2020: results of the first national serological survey (ISNCOVID-19). Acta Med. Port. **34**(2), 87 (2021)
24. Pollán, M., Pérez-Gómez, B., Pastor-Barriuso, R., Oteo, J., Hernán, M.A., et al.: Prevalence of SARS-CoV-2 in spain (ENE-COVID): a nationwide, population-based seroepidemiological study. Lancet **396**(10250), 535–544 (2020)
25. Khalagi, K., Gharibzadeh, S., Khalili, D., Mansournia, M.A., Samiee, S.M., et al.: Prevalence of COVID-19 in Iran: results of the first survey of the Iranian COVID-19 serological surveillance programme. Clin. Microbiol. Infect. **27**(11), 1666–1671 (2021)
26. Core Team, R.: A Language and Environment for Statistical Computing. R Foundation for Statistical Computing, Vienna, Austria (2020)
27. Dimmock, M.E., Mirin, A.A., Jason, L.A.: Estimating the disease burden of ME/CFS in the United States and its relation to research funding. J. Med. Ther. **1**(1) (2016)
28. Mirin, A.A., Dimmock, M.E., Jason, L.A.: Research update: the relation between ME/CFS disease burden and research funding in the USA. Work **66**(2), 277–282 (2020)
29. Domingues, T.D., Mouriño, H., Sepúlveda, N.: Analysis of antibody data using finite mixture models based on scale mixtures of skew-normal distributions (2021)

Identification of Antibody Responses Predictive of Protection Against Clinical Malaria

André Fonseca, Clara Cordeiro, and Nuno Sepúlveda

Abstract Statistical pipelines have been proposed to discover antibody responses associated with protection against clinical malaria. However, these often produce inconsistent results due to the failure of the statistical assumptions, such as normality. In the present work, we have developed a new statistical pipeline to analyse data from IgG antibodies against 36 *Plasmodium falciparum* antigens from 121 Kenyan children. This pipeline was based on the identification of cut-off values in the antibody distributions that maximised the distinction between susceptible and protected individuals. Our pipeline enabled us to construct a classifier based on few antibodies, whose performance outperformed the previous ones based on a Random forest approach. The good performance of the pipeline suggests its applicability in antibody data analysis with the aim of identifying antimalarial vaccine candidates.

Keywords Random forest · Regression · Malaria · Regularisation strategies

1 Introduction

Malaria is caused by infections of *Plasmodium* parasites with the *Plasmodium falciparum* species (*P.falciparum*) being the most lethal one. It remains a global health problem that threatens millions of people worldwide [1, 2]. Malaria is endemic to tropical and subtropical regions where children under 5 years old are the most affected by severe symptoms [1, 3]. The vulnerability of these children has been mainly attributed to the slow process in acquiring natural immunity against malaria

A. Fonseca (✉) · C. Cordeiro
Faculty of Sciences and Technology, University of Algarve, Faro, Portugal
e-mail: a49406@ualg.pt

N. Sepúlveda
Faculty of Mathematics and Information Science, Warsaw University of Technology, Warsaw, Portugal

C. Cordeiro · N. Sepúlveda
Faculty of Sciences, University of Lisbon, Lisbon, Portugal

R. Bispo et al. (eds.), *Recent Developments in Statistics and Data Science*, Springer Proceedings in Mathematics & Statistics 398,
https://doi.org/10.1007/978-3-031-12766-3_16

parasites via specialised antibody responses upon repeated exposure to the infection [4–6]. Antibodies, also known as immunoglobulins, are proteins produced by B cells of the adaptive immune system upon antigen recognition [7]. In turn, antigens are small protein fragments ingested and presented to B cells by other immune cells. When bound to their antigen, antibodies are typically used as molecular signals delivered to specialised immune cells (i.e. phagocytes) with the ability to remove the culprit infectious agent by a process called opsonization [7].

Given their putative protective effect, antibodies have been extensively investigated in the context of natural immunity against malaria parasites [8, 9]. However, which set of antibodies confer individual-level protection to clinical malaria is still elusive [8, 10]. A possible reason for the limited knowledge on this research topic is the lack of reproducible results across different studies, as demonstrated by different studies [8, 10, 11]. This lack of reproducibility might be attributed to the failure of the underlying statistical assumptions invoked in the data. To aggravate, there are no standard statistical pipelines to analyse immunological data consistently and reliably in order to make different studies directly comparable.

In this scenario, we propose a new methodology to analyse malaria antibody data. Our working hypothesis is that a pipeline based on strong statistical principles may increase reproducibility across studies, thus, contributing to a reliable discovery of antibodies that promote natural protection to clinical malaria.

The paper is organised as follows: the following section presents a brief description of the data, the methodologies used and the pipeline. The following section shows the results, ending with the discussion, concluding remarks and future work.

2 Materials and Methods

2.1 KEN Dataset

We have analysed a prospective cohort study of 286 children conducted in Kenya (KEN) that arbours immune profiles of ELISA-based antibody titers against 36 *P.falciparum*-specific antigens. Children were monitored for clinical episodes of malaria and classified as **Susceptible** (Sus) ($n_s = 40$) if they had at least one recorded episode of symptomatic malaria (clinical disease[1]). Children with no clinical episode were classified as **Protected** (Prt) ($n_p = 81$). Based on the article by Osier et al. [12], the analysis was performed solely on 121 children ($N = n_s + n_p$) who were infected at screening; these children had $1, 2, \ldots, 10$ years of age. In this way, the bias that can arise from ascertaining exposure to infectious mosquitoes was minimised.

[1] Clinical disease was defined as an auxiliary temperature >37.5 °C, plus any parasitemia for children less than 1 year, and an auxiliary temperature of > 37.5 °C, plus parasitemia > 2500/μl for individuals older than 1 year, during the 6-month follow-up.

2.2 *Measuring Association*

The Chi-squared (χ^2) test of independence identified antibodies associated with clinical protection to malaria [13]. The latter was used to determine if individuals' seropositivity was related to clinical protection against clinical malaria.

2.3 *Predictive Methodologies*

2.3.1 Multiple Logistic and Probit Regression

Logistic/probit regressions were followed by stepwise selection (forward and backward) to select the subset of immune responses most associated with the clinical malaria status response variable. The Hosmer–Lemeshow (HL) test was used to evaluate the goodness-of-fit of the estimated regressions [14]. When performing the HL test, the number of bins to calculate quantiles was set to 10. Finally, the Akaike's information criterion (AIC) was used to select the best model.

2.3.2 Regularisation Strategies

Ridge, Least Absolute Shrinkage and Selection Operator (LASSO) and Elastic-Net regressions were concomitantly used to predict immune signatures underlying clinical protection to malaria [15–17] using the `glmnet` package [18] for the R software. These regression models apply a penalty function λ to the regression model, which reduces or shrinks coefficient estimates towards 0, thus allowing the less-contributing covariates to have a coefficient close to or equal to zero [19]. To obtain the λ that provided the highest accuracy for each model, we incremented λ from 0.001 to 1 with a lag of 0.001. Then, a 10-fold cross-validation was used to compute the model accuracy for each λ [19, 20], and the process was repeated one hundred times. Usually, two distinct λ values are chosen when performing the Ridge and LASSO regressions. However, when using the `glmnet` package, a single λ value can be selected and a second tunning parameter called α that ranges from 0 to 1 can be set to adjust the tunning parameter. To perform the Ridge regression, α is set to 0 while performing the LASSO regression an α equal to 1 is established. To perform the Elastic-Net regression, we increased α from 0 and to 1 with a lag of 0.1.

2.3.3 Random Forest

A machine learning technique known to provide good results in classification problems is Random forest. It works by constructing multiple decision trees trained on different parts of the same training set by a process called bagging or bootstrap aggregation [21]. The number of trees to grow and the number of predictors randomly sampled as candidates in each split was set to default. To obtain more robust results we performed one hundred iterations of 10-fold cross-validations.

2.4 Predictive Accuracy

Two measures were used to assess the accuracy of the predictive approaches: Receiving Operating Characteristic (ROC) curves and confusion matrices. The area under the ROC curves (AUC) were utilised as a measure of the predictive model accuracy (or discrimination performance) [22]. In this case, ROC curves were used to assess the antibodies' inherent ability to predict individuals' protection to clinical malaria. Confusion matrices are tables used to describe the performance of a classification model on a set of data for which the true values are known. The confusion matrix is a 2×2 table in which each cell shows the frequency of a different combination of predicted and observed values [23].

2.5 Pipeline

Identification of antibody signatures associated with protection to clinical malaria was achieved by developing, establishing and integrating a pipeline to the KEN dataset (Fig. 1). This pipeline starts by ordering the individuals according to their antibody quantity values and specifying each value as a possible cut-off to characterise patients as either seropositive or seronegative. Individuals' classified as seropositive had expression values above the cut-off point, while seronegative individuals had expression values below. Contingency tables of seropositivity against clinical malaria status were then constructed. Chi-squared tests of independence were used to determine if antibody seropositivity was associated with clinical protection to clinical malaria. Finally, the cut-off that provided the strongest association to protection (the cut-off with the smallest p-value) for each antibody was selected to characterise patients into seropositive and seronegative populations. This process was repeated for each of all the 36 antibodies initially present in our data set. The methodologies Logistic/Probit, Ridge, LASSO, Elastic-Net regressions, and the Random forest were then used to construct different classifiers for clinical malaria. Finally, the performance of each classifier was assessed by ROC curves.

All the analyses were performed using R version 4.0.4 [24] and their packages: `AID` [25], `caret` [26], `dplyr` [27], `ggplot2` [28], `glmnet` [18], `MASS` [29], `pROC` [30], `randomForest` [31], `stats` [24], `tidyr` [32]. A significance level of 0.05 was used.

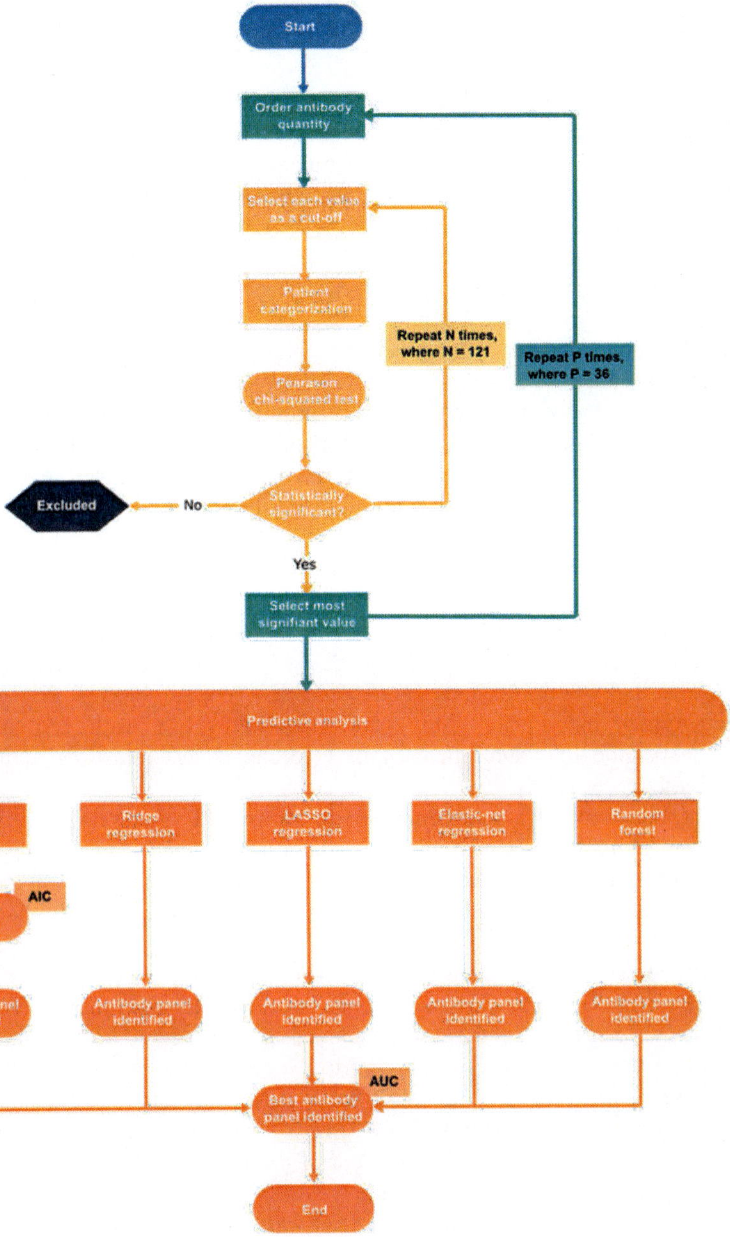

Fig. 1 **Pipeline**. The different steps of the analysis are displayed on the workflow using distinct coloured shapes. Blue colour identifies the beginning of the pipeline. Green indicate computational steps prior and after the loop for obtaining the χ^2 test p-value for each potential cut-off (light orange). Dark orange refers to the predictive performance step and dark grey indicates antibodies removed from the analysis. Additional information is provided by the faded light orange and dark orange coloured shapes

3 Results

The analysis was performed on the 121 children who were parasite-positive at screening, in line with both the original published article [12] and by Valletta and Recker [8]. Of the 121 children, 40 were considered susceptible, and 81 were protected against clinical malaria. The immune profiles for these individuals consisted of 36 *P.falciparum*-specific antigens taken at the start of the transmission season. Selection of immune profiles against the *P. falciparum* derives from the fact that this species is the most prevalent malaria one in the African continent, home to Kenya [33].

We started by ordering the individuals according to their antibody quantity levels and obtaining the antibody level that provided the best separation ability between the susceptible and protected group of individuals. Antibodies that were not statistically significant in the χ^2 test were removed from the analysis. The antibody data were replaced by a dichotomized seropositive/seronegative variable for the remaining antibodies, which was used later in the predictive performance analysis. According to our results, 28 out of 36 antibodies were able to differentiate susceptible from protected individuals with a 95% confidence, as seen in Table 1.

Considering the 28 antibodies, we proceeded to identify a panel of antibody signatures that could predict individuals' immune status to malaria. Therefore, five distinct methodologies: Logistic/probit, Ridge, LASSO, and Elastic-Net regressions and the Random forest were applied. The objective was to assure that the identification of the best classifier was not hindered by the predictive method selected. Regardless of the method used, individuals' status against malaria was used as the response variable. In contrast, the individuals dichotomized (seronegative/seropositive) data were used as predictive variables.

Logistic and probit regressions were performed. The subsets of antibodies with the highest association with clinical malaria were obtained by stepwise selection. Due to the similarity of the results, we present only the Logistic regression information. Our results showed that the best model was composed of antibodies against the *msp2*, *msp4*, *msp7 msp10*, *pf11_0373* and *pf113* antigens, with an accuracy of approximately 86% (as seen in Fig. 2a). Following this analysis, we included the variable "Age" into this classifier and it was statistically significant p-value <0.001; Mann–Whitney). Therefore, it was included in the model in order to understand its effect on the performance. According to the results, the accuracy of the classifier increased from 86 to 90%, reflecting the contributing effect of other antibodies that were not captured by the model (Fig. 2a). Overall, our method correctly classified a total of 102 (75 + 27) individuals out of the total 121 (Fig. 2b). In addition, for both the logistic models with (p-value = 0.450) and without Age (p-value = 0.9275) the p-value for the HL goodness of fit test was above 0.05, indicating that at a 95% confidence there was not enough evidence to say that our models were a poor fit.

Notwithstanding the predictive capability of the logistic/probit regression models, we also decided to perform the predictive analysis using regularisation strategies. Ridge regression ($\alpha = 0$) was the best performing model between the three regularisation methods utilised, reaching a predictive accuracy close to 80% when λ

Table 1 Patient Seroprevalence. The statistically significant results of the χ^2 test for the 28 antibodies. The antibody levels that provided the best separation ability between the susceptible and protected group of individuals (Cut-off), and the proportion of seropositive individuals for all (Total), Protected (Prt) and susceptible (Sus) children, respectively

Antibody	p-value	Cut-off	Total	Prt	Sus
msp1	0.013	0.15	0.85	0.91	0.73
msp2	<0.001	0.07	0.45	0.57	0.20
msp4	<0.001	0.13	0.86	0.96	0.65
msp5	0.020	0.09	0.56	0.64	0.40
msp10	<0.001	0.25	0.79	0.90	0.58
pf12	0.002	0.10	0.65	0.75	0.45
pf92	0.001	0.11	0.83	0.91	0.65
pf31	0.002	0.07	0.61	0.72	0.40
pf113	0.020	0.05	0.74	0.81	0.60
gama	0.002	0.05	0.61	0.72	0.40
ama1	0.001	0.16	0.74	0.84	0.53
eba175	<0.001	0.14	0.71	0.84	0.45
eba140	0.006	0.11	0.96	1.00	0.88
eba181	0.003	0.11	0.90	0.96	0.78
mtrap	0.013	0.05	0.85	0.91	0.73
asp	0.005	0.08	0.70	0.79	0.53
msp3	0.010	0.08	0.48	0.57	0.30
msp6	0.002	0.12	0.78	0.86	0.60
msp7	<0.001	0.24	0.71	0.86	0.40
msrp1	0.003	0.05	0.79	0.88	0.63
msrp3	0.006	0.04	0.96	1.00	0.88
h101	0.031	0.05	0.74	0.80	0.60
h103	0.001	0.07	0.50	0.60	0.28
pf41	0.002	0.12	0.38	0.48	0.18
pff0335c	0.003	0.05	0.88	0.95	0.75
rh5	0.046	0.16	0.39	0.46	0.25
ron6	0.016	0.04	0.81	0.88	0.68
pf11_0373	0.006	0.08	0.21	0.28	0.05

ranged from 0.526 to 0.839 (Fig. 3a). According to the Ridge regression model, the immune responses most associated with the clinical malaria status were similar to the ones obtained with logistic regression, with the antibody against the *msp7* antigen appearing as the most important variable (importance = 100), followed by the antibody against *msp4* (importance = 85) (Fig. 3a). The antibody against the *msp10* antigen appeared on the fourth position (importance = 78), followed by the antibody against *pf11_0373* in the fifth position (importance = 70) and the antibody against

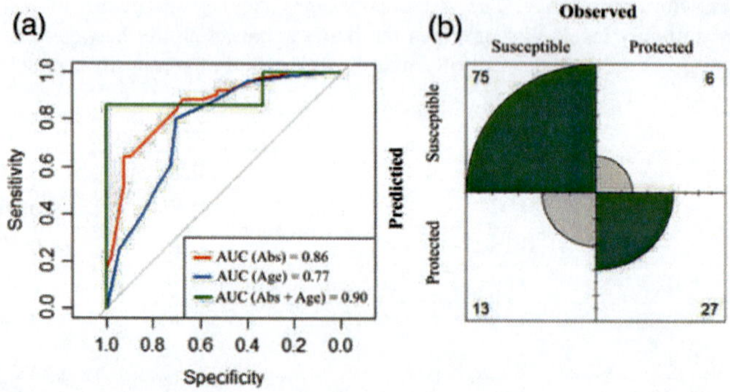

Fig. 2 **Predictive performance of the best antibody signature.** **a** ROC curve for the best antibodies signature comprising only the antibodies against *msp2*, *msp4*, *msp7*, *msp10*, *pf11_0373* and *pf113* antigens (red), only Age (blue) and the best antibodies signatures together with Age (green). **b** Confusion matrices derived from the model built with the best antibodies signature together with Age (Abs and Age)

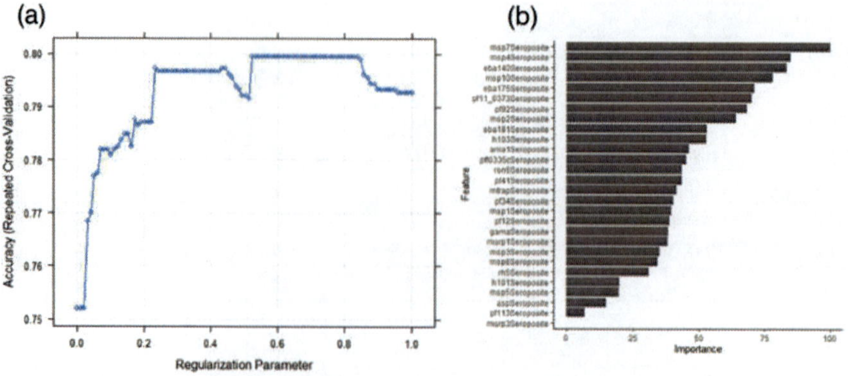

Fig. 3 **Ridge regression regularisation strategy results.** **a** The mean accuracy for each regularisation parameter (λ) after one hundred runs of 10-fold cross-validation are given by a blue circle. **b** Importance of each antibody in the model

msp2 on the eight position (importance = 64). The antibody against *Pf113* appeared well below the importance scale in the twenty-seventh position, with an importance of just 6.64 (see Fig. 3b). However, Ridge regression kept all antibodies in the final classifier with an exception for *asp*.

The results for both the LASSO and Elastic-Net regression will not be discussed here since the main objective was to identify the method that provides the highest accuracy. To further compare the results of the traditional regression techniques with more complex technologies such as machine learning model, the Random forest was used. This approach was able to provide an accuracy of 81% (Fig. 4a). Like the Ridge regression, the Random forest approach kept all antibodies in the final classi-

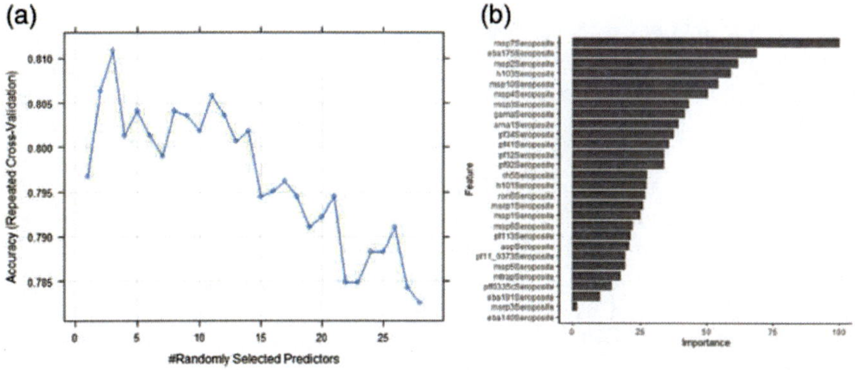

Fig. 4 **Random forest results. a** The mean accuracy for each value of randomly selected predictors when performing each tree after one hundred runs of 10-fold cross-validation are given by a blue circle. **b** Importance of each antibody in the model

fier except the antibody against *eba140* (Fig. 4b). Even more, the immune responses most associated with the clinical malaria status resembled the ones obtained by the Ridge regression, with the antibody against *msp7* once again appearing as the most important variable (importance = 100), the antibody against *msp2* on the third position (importance = 61), the antibody against *msp10* on the fifth position (importance = 54), followed by the antibody against *msp4* on the sixth (importance = 50). Interestingly the antibody against *pf113*, however, had more weight in the Random forest (importance = 21) than in the Ridge regression. Oppositely, however, the antibody against *pf11_0373* had significantly lower importance on the Random forest (importance = 19).

4 Discussion

Despite tremendous efforts in the malaria field, it is still unclear which antibodies are essential for developing immune responses that lead to clinical malaria protection [8, 12]. The inconsistent results amongst studies regarding which set of antibodies are responsible for individual-level protection to clinical malaria highlight the need for novel approaches to analysing immunological data. Here we set to establish and implement a pipeline to analyse immunological data in a consistent and replicable manner, thus obtaining reproducible results. We hypothesise that pipelines such as the one proposed may finally help identify clear relationships between the measured immune responses and the level of protection against malaria. Our pipeline was able to identify an immunological classifier against clinical malaria using 86% using antibody information solely against 6 antigens (*msp2*, *msp4*, *msp7*, *msp10*, *pf11_0373*, *pf113*). Adding "Age" to our classifier increased its accuracy to 90%. This reveals that there were antibody responses associated with clinical protection to malaria that our model could not identify. While age itself does not confer protection against malaria, older individuals are more to have been exposed to the malaria parasite, therefore developing different antibody responses [5]. In this sense, age is a proxy of additional antibodies that the model did not capture. Nevertheless, this effect could also come from the fact that the antibodies responsible for adding this additional explainability to the model were not found in the dataset (due to the small number of features). Comparing our results with the ones obtained by Valletta and Recker [8], our pipeline systematically outperformed their approach independently of the predictive technique used. This increase in accuracy provides clear evidence that an alternative approach to just blindly applying a Random forest approach without any selection criterion may not be best suitable. The benefit of doing a more thorough data analysis before applying a predictive model becomes even more evident when we consider the performance of the Random forest technique in our analysis, which was also used by Valletta and Recker [8]. While they obtained only a predictive performance of 68%, we, on the other hand, obtained a predictive performance of 81%. Concerning the antibody panel associated with protection to clinical malaria here identified, *msp2*, *msp4*, *msp7*, and *msp10* belong to the group of Merozoite Surface Proteins (MSPs) [34]. The MSPs are expressed on the surface of the merozoite, providing great therapeutic targets for malaria mainly because they are repeatedly and directly exposed to the host humoral immune system [34, 35]. In fact, *msp2* has been extensively associated with protection from clinical malaria in a vast number of independent studies. As an example, *msp2* has been demonstrated to be strongly associated with protection against clinical malaria in two independent cohorts of Kenyan children [10]. *Msp4* has too been already identified as a potential candidate component of the malaria vaccine. In a Senegalese community living in an area of moderate, seasonal malaria transmission, high antibody levels against msp4 constructs were associated with reduced morbidity [36]. Moreover, the protective effect of*msp4* against symptomatic malaria has been already reported in Kenyan children on two occasions [12, 37]. On the other hand, the association between *msp7* and protection against clinical malaria in the literature is less extensive, however *msp7* protection against malaria have already been identified in the Kenyan population [37]. For the *pf113* antigen, however, the literature is more prominent. Using sera from a longitudinal study in a cohort of Kenyan children, Osier et al. have identified 10 antigens amongst which *pf113* were associated with protection against clinical episodes of malaria [12].Furthermore, several other studies refer *pf113* as a promising malaria vaccine candidate [38, 39]. These findings further corroborate our results, as commonly malaria vaccine candidates identified in other studies were also identified here. Interestingly, *msp10* and *pf11_0373* have not been associated with clinical malaria protection so far, as we were unable to identify a single study with such information. This evidence may suggest that there may be antibodies associated with protection against clinical malaria that has not yet been identified. Nevertheless, further studies are necessary to validate our analysis. Immune responses commonly associated with malaria protection and often referred to as potential vaccine candidates such as the merozoite surface protein-1 (*msp1*) and the apical membrane antigen-1 (*ama1*) were not amongst the best predictors of clinical protection malaria in children, none being incorporated in any of our panel of antibodies [34, 40]. These findings have already been reported in other studies, where antibodies against *msp1* and *ama1* have been described to show low or no associations with protection to clinical malaria [8]. These inconsistent findings further suggest the need for sturdier pipelines that may help to increase reproducibility amongst studies.

5 Concluding Remarks and Future Work

Although we have provided a suggestive approach here, it should be noted that this pipeline is simplistic and will not provide the most sturdy results in every scenario. A situation where this pipeline may not perform well is if there are numerous antibodies related to the outcome under analysis, as a large number of antibodies will be available for the predictive analysis phase. This may reduce the strength of the analysis and consequently lead to less powerful results. One solution to overcome this problem might be to implement correction techniques (such as Bonferroni) for multiple testing. Nevertheless, the implementation of these correction techniques remains to be done. Note that, the question of multiple testing can also be raised for each 121 chi-squared tests when analysing a given antibody. However, this question can be reframed as an estimation problem where the cut-off value that best discriminates patients from healthy control is an unknown parameter that requires to be estimated. This idea is conceptually similar to the application of the profile likelihood method with cut-off as an unknown parameter.

Work to improve our pipeline to be more suitable for a broader range of datasets is already ongoing. Implementation of other approaches has been considered, where we are trying to make our pipeline more robust. We have also developed another pipeline that relies on traditional statistical techniques after appropriate data transformation and flexible finite mixture models for determining antibody positivity. The former has also shown promising results. Additionally, it is worth mentioning that by proposing a methodology to analyse antibody data instead of just identifying the exact antibody threshold, any differences in the results may arise due to different sample handling, different sequencing instruments, or other factors that may alter the results. As experimentally conditions are complex to recreate, providing a value that would differentiate patients is a less sensible strategy than providing a methodology that can systematically reproduce the findings of the antibodies associated with antibodies in various studies.

To conclude, although promising, we propose that this pipeline should be tested in other data sets to assess its robustness in different settings. Moreover, we believe that pipelines such as the one presented here may allow the identification of the antibodies that confer protection against clinical malaria in a reproducible manner. Finally, since antibody data are an essential research component of any infectious disease, it is expected that the impact of this work transverses the field of malaria.

Acknowledgements André Fonseca has a Ph.D. fellowship by FCT—Fundação para a Ciência e a Tecnologia (ref. SFRH/BD/147629/2019).

Clara Cordeiro and Nuno Sepúlveda are partially financed by national funds through FCT under the project UIDB/00006/2020.

Nuno Sepúlveda is funded by Polish National Agency for Academic Exchange (ref. grant: PPN/ULM/2020/1/00069/U/00001).

References

1. Talapko, J., Škrlec, I., Alebić, T., Jukić, M., Včev, A.: Malaria: the past and the present. Microorganisms **7**(6), 179 (2019)
2. Ashley, E.A., Phyo, A.P., Woodrow, C.J.: Malaria. The Lancet **391**(10130), 1608–1621 (2018)
3. Greenwood, B.M., Fidock, D.A., Kyle, D.E., Kappe, S.H., Alonso, P.L., et al.: Malaria: progress, perils, and prospects for eradication. J. Clin. Investig. **118**(4), 1266–1276 (2008)
4. Moormann, A.M.: How might infant and paediatric immune responses influence malaria vaccine efficacy? Parasite Immunol. **31**(9), 547–559 (2009)
5. Doolan, D.L., No, C.D., Baird, J.K.: Acquired immunity to malaria. Clin. Microbiol. Rev. **22**(1), 13–36 (2009)
6. Barry, A., Hansen, D.: Naturally acquired immunity to malaria. Parasitology **143**(2), 125–128 (2016)
7. Schroeder, H.W., Cavacini, L.: Structure and function of immunoglobulins. J. All. Clin. Immunol. **125**(2), S41–S52 (2010)
8. Valletta, J.J., Recker, M.: Identification of immune signatures predictive of clinical protection from malaria. PLoS Comput. Biol. **13**(10), e1005812 (2017)
9. Hviid, L.: Naturally acquired immunity to plasmodium falciparum malaria in Africa. Acta Trop. **95**, 270–275 (2005)
10. Osier, F.H.A., Fegan, G., Polley, S.D., Murungi, L., Verra, F., et al.: Breadth and magnitude of antibody responses to multiple plasmodium falciparum merozoite antigens are associated with protection from clinical malaria. Infect. Immun. **76**(5), 2240–2248 (2008)
11. Proietti, C., Krause, L., Trieu, A., Dodoo, D., Gyan, B., et al.: Immune signature against plasmodium falciparum antigens predicts clinical immunity in distinct malaria endemic communities. Mol. & Cell. Proteomics **19**(1), 101–113 (2020)
12. Osier, F.H., Mackinnon, M.J., Crosnier, C., Fegan, G., Kamuyu, G., et al.: New antigens for a multicomponent blood-stage malaria vaccine. Sci. Trans. Med. **6**(247) (2014)
13. McHugh, M.L.: The chi-square test of independence. Biochem. Med. 143–149 (2013)
14. Nattino, G., Pennell, M.L., Lemeshow, S.: Assessing the goodness of fit of logistic regression models in large samples: a modification of the hosmer-lemeshow test. Biometrics **76**(2), 549–560 (2020)
15. Hoerl, A.E., Kennard, R.W.: Ridge regression: biased estimation for nonorthogonal problems. Technometrics **42**(1), 80–86 (2000)
16. Tibshirani, R.: Regression shrinkage and selection via the lasso. J. R. Stat. Soc.: Ser. B **58**(1), 267–288 (1996)
17. Zou, H., Hastie, T.: Regularization and variable selection via the elastic net. J. R. Stat. Soc.: Ser. B **67**(2), 301–320 (2005)
18. Friedman, J., Hastie, T., Tibshirani, R.: Regularization paths for generalized linear models via coordinate descent. J. Stat. Softw. **33**(1) (2010)
19. McNeish, D.M.: Using lasso for predictor selection and to assuage overfitting: a method long overlooked in behavioral sciences. Multivar. Behav. Res. **50**(5), 471–484 (2015)
20. Melkumova, L., Shatskikh, S.: Comparing ridge and LASSO estimators for data analysis. Proc. Eng. **201**, 746–755 (2017)

21. Sarica, A., Cerasa, A., Quattrone, A.: Random forest algorithm for the classification of neuroimaging data in alzheimer's disease: a systematic review. Front. Aging Neurosci. **9** (2017)
22. Tripepi, G., Jager, K.J., Dekker, F.W., Zoccali, C.: Diagnostic methods 2: receiver operating characteristic (ROC) curves. Kidney Int. **76**(3), 252–256 (2009)
23. Düntsch, I., Gediga, G.: Confusion matrices and rough set data analysis. J. Phys: Conf. Ser. **1229**(1), 012055 (2019)
24. R Core Team: R: A Language and Environment for Statistical Computing. R Foundation for Statistical Computing, Vienna, Austria (2021)
25. Özgür Asar, O.I., Dag, O.: Estimating Box–Cox power transformation parameter via goodness-of-fit tests. Commun. Stat. - Simul. Comput. **46**(1), 91–105 (2014)
26. Kuhn, M.: `caret`: Classification and Regression Training (2021). R package version 6.0-86
27. Wickham, H., François, R., Henry, L., Müller, K.: `dplyr`: A Grammar of Data Manipulation (2021). R package version 1.0.2
28. Wickham, H.: `ggplot2`: Elegant Graphics for Data Analysis. Springer, New York (2016)
29. Venables, W.N., Ripley, B.D.: Modern Applied Statistics with S, 4th edn. Springer, New York (2002). ISBN 0-387-95457-0
30. Robin, X., Turck, N., Hainard, A., Tiberti, N., Lisacek, F., et al.: `pROC`: an open-source package for R and S+ to analyze and compare ROC curves. BMC Bioinf. **12**, 77 (2011)
31. Liaw, A., Wiener, M.: Classification and regression by `randomForest`. R News **2**(3), 18–22 (2002)
32. Wickham, H.: `tidyr`: Tidy Messy Data (2020). R package version 1.1.2
33. Snow, R.W., Sartorius, B., Kyalo, D., Maina, J., Amratia, P., et al.: The prevalence of plasmodium falciparum in sub-Saharan Africa since 1900. Nature **550**(7677), 515–518 (2017)
34. Jäschke, A., Coulibaly, B., Remarque, E.J., Bujard, H., Epp, C.: Merozoite surface protein 1 from plasmodium falciparum is a major target of opsonizing antibodies in individuals with acquired immunity against malaria. Clin. Vaccine Immunol. **24**(11) (2017)
35. Lin, C.S., Uboldi, A.D., Epp, C., Bujard, H., Tsuboi, T., et al.: Multiple plasmodium falciparum merozoite surface protein 1 complexes mediate merozoite binding to human erythrocytes. J. Biol. Chem. **291**(14), 7703–7715 (2016)
36. Perraut, R., Varela, M.-L., Joos, C., Diouf, B., Sokhna, C., et al.: Association of antibodies to plasmodium falciparum merozoite surface protein-4 with protection against clinical malaria. Vaccine **35**(48), 6720–6726 (2017)
37. Dent, A.E., Nakajima, R., Liang, L., Baum, E., Moormann, A.M., et al.: Plasmodium falciparumProtein microarray antibody profiles correlate with protection from symptomatic malaria in Kenya. J. Infect. Dis. **212**(9), 1429–1438 (2015)
38. Chia, W.N., Goh, Y.S., Rénia, L.: Novel approaches to identify protective malaria vaccine candidates. Front. Microbiol. **5** (2014)
39. Imboumy-Limoukou, R.-K., Oyegue-Liabagui, S.L., Ndidi, S., Pegha-Moukandja, I., Kouna, C.L., et al.: Comparative antibody responses against three antimalarial vaccine candidate antigens from urban and rural exposed individuals in Gabon. Eur. J. Microbiol. Immunol. **6**(4), 287–297 (2016)
40. Miura, K., Zhou, H., Muratova, O.V., Orcutt, A.C., Giersing, B., et al.: Immunization with plasmodium falciparum apical membrane antigen 1, the specificity of antibodies depends on the species immunized. Infect. Immun. **75**(12), 5827–5836 (2007)

Statistical Challenges in Mutational Signature Analyses of Cancer Sequencing Data

Víctor Velasco-Pardo, Michail Papathomas, and Andy G. Lynch

Abstract Cancer is a disease driven and characterised by mutations in the DNA. Different categorisations of DNA mutations have allowed the identification of patterns that can act as signatures for the processes that have governed the life of the cancer. Over the last decade, research groups have identified more than 100 such signatures. Mutational signature analyses are improving our understanding of cancer aetiology and have the potential to play a role in diagnosis, prognosis, and treatment choice. Consisting of the estimation of probability mass functions or weights determining non-negative weighted combinations, they are perhaps unique among comparable analyses in the medical literature, in that no confidence intervals or other representations of uncertainty are demanded when reporting the results. Here, we review the key statistical challenges for the field, assess the potential of existing approaches to adapt to those challenges, and comment on what we think are promising directions. As we deal with data that are noisy and heterogeneous, we evaluate how to present them so that models use all the information available. Often posed as a matrix factorisation problem, we argue that a fully probabilistic approach is required to quantify uncertainty around model parameters and to underpin principled study design. Lastly, we argue that novel methodology is required to evaluate uncertainties in analyses where prior information is available.

Keywords Biostatistics · Bioinformatics · Cancer · Genomics · Next-generation sequencing · Whole genome sequencing

---

V. Velasco-Pardo (✉) · M. Papathomas · A. G. Lynch
School of Mathematics and Statistics, University of St Andrews, St Andrews, U.K.
e-mail: vvp1@st-andrews.ac.uk

M. Papathomas
e-mail: m.papathomas@st-andrews.ac.uk

A. G. Lynch
e-mail: andy.lynch@st-andrews.ac.uk

A. G. Lynch
School of Medicine, University of St Andrews, St Andrews, U.K.

R. Bispo et al. (eds.), *Recent Developments in Statistics and Data Science*,
Springer Proceedings in Mathematics & Statistics 398,
https://doi.org/10.1007/978-3-031-12766-3_17

1 Introduction

Cancers can result from relatively few changes to a cell's DNA, but typically carry many additional somatic (i.e. occurring within the life of the patient) mutations. We can identify these mutations by sequencing and then comparing DNA from the cancer and DNA from healthy tissue from the same individual [1, 2]. "Mutation", here, refers to a wide range of events ranging from single base substitutions to larger structural variants (e.g. genomic rearrangements where large segments of a chromosome might be deleted, duplicated, or have their orientation inverted [3]). See, e.g. [4] for a review of mutation classes.

Somatic mutations are the result of biological mechanisms, termed mutational processes, associated with characteristic patterns of mutations or mutational signatures, described by means of probability mass functions over mutational categories [5]. Therefore, the catalogue of somatic mutations observed in an individual cancer genome can be thought of as a mixture of the mutational signatures that have acted on the tumour over time.

Some mutational processes act continuously throughout life [6], while others arise as a result of exposures to carcinogens [7, 8]. They might be ongoing, intermittent, or might have stopped [4]. Some processes are associated with germline mutations in tumour suppressor genes, such as BRCA1/2 [5, 9]. Cancer genomes contain the imprint of many such processes to differing degrees. Consequently, the goals of mutational signature analyses are to infer from the somatic mutations in tumours (1) the signatures of mutational processes, (2) the contribution of each process to individual cancer genomes, and (3) when those processes contributed.

To achieve those goals, a range of mathematical methods have been, and are being, developed [10–21] (for a review, see, e.g. [22, 23]). Their application to data sets of ever-increasing size and complexity has resulted in a remarkable improvement of our understanding of cancer and its causes [24]. More than a hundred inferred mutational signatures are available to the wider research community [24, 25]. In the context of personalised medicine, these have a remarkable potential to stratify cancer patients [26, 27] and to predict response to treatment [28].

1.1 Modelling Framework

Data Gathering. In the context of mutational signature analyses, we investigate data sets generated using next-generation sequencing and analysis pipelines (involving (a) sequencing, (b) alignment to a reference genome, (c) often-probabilistic mutation calling, and (d) post-processing). The output is a list of "mutations" observed in the tumour. Often, data are not solely collected for the purpose of signature analysis.

In the sequencing step, short segments of DNA from both tumour and matched healthy tissue are read as base sequences. Each of those "reads" covers 100–250 base pairs and may contain errors. We define the *coverage* of an individual base to be the number of times it has been sequenced. Additionally, we define the *sequencing depth* of an experiment to be the average number of times a base is sequenced. While sequencing depth is typically set by the investigator, coverage is not uniform across genomic regions. In particular, regions with a high prevalence of Cs and Gs are susceptible to low coverage [29].

Sequence reads are then aligned to a *reference genome*, and aligned reads from both tissues are presented to a "mutation caller" that determines whether a mutation is present at a given locus by means of a statistical test. Thus, there must be a balance between sensitivity and specificity that will differ between cancer types. Additionally, that balance is unlikely to be uniform across mutation types. Thus, the systematic bias introduced in this step will be propagated to mutational signature analyses, affecting inferences. This problem can be exacerbated by the application of post-calling filters [30, 31].

Mutational Signatures and Mutational Catalogues. For the mutational class being considered, biologically meaningful categorisations must be defined (see, e.g. [4] for a review) and we denote the resulting categories by $k = 1, \ldots, K$. We define a mutational signature, $\boldsymbol{s}_n = (s_{1n}, \ldots, s_{Kn})^T$, to be a probability mass function over the K categories, with s_{kn} denoting the probability that a mutation generated by signature n is of type k.

We now consider the mutational catalogues of G cancer patients and assume that they have been exposed to N mutational processes. The observed number of mutations of category k in patient g, m_{kg}, is approximately

$$m_{kg} \approx \sum_{n=1}^{N} s_{kn} e_{ng} \tag{1}$$

where e_{ng} denotes the exposure of patient g to signature n, that is, the number of mutations attributed to that signature. In matrix form,

$$\boldsymbol{M} \approx \boldsymbol{S} \times \boldsymbol{E} \tag{2}$$

where $\boldsymbol{M} = [\boldsymbol{m}_1 \cdots \boldsymbol{m}_G]$, $\boldsymbol{S} = [\boldsymbol{s}_1 \cdots \boldsymbol{s}_N]$, and $\boldsymbol{E} = [\boldsymbol{e}_1 \cdots \boldsymbol{e}_G]$.

1.2 Mathematical Approaches to Mutational Signatures

We will consider two problems. The first, termed de novo signature extraction, consists in estimating $\boldsymbol{S}$ and $\boldsymbol{E}$ for known $\boldsymbol{M}$. The second, termed refitting, consists in estimating $\boldsymbol{E}$ for known $\boldsymbol{M}$ and $\boldsymbol{S}$.

De Novo Signature Extraction. This problem, consisting of estimating $\boldsymbol{S}$ and $\boldsymbol{E}$ given $\boldsymbol{M}$ in (2), was originally posed as the following non-convex optimisation problem:

$$\arg \min_{\boldsymbol{S} \geq 0, \boldsymbol{E} \geq 0} ||\boldsymbol{M} - \boldsymbol{S}\boldsymbol{E}|| \tag{3}$$

where $||\cdot||$ denotes an appropriate norm. This approach, termed Non-Negative Matrix Factorisation (NMF) [32], is taken by the original and arguably most popular method, `SigProfiler` [10, 24]. Several other software packages are available implementing similar solutions based on NMF [11, 25, 33–36]. An alternative method is `EMu` [14], which considers the exposures to be nuisance parameters and uses the EM algorithm to estimate the matrix $\boldsymbol{S}$.

A slightly different approach is to place (2) in a Bayesian setting, as done by `SignatureAnalyzer` [12, 13], `signeR` [15], and `sigfit` [16]. Briefly, prior distributions are placed on the elements of $\boldsymbol{S}$ and $\boldsymbol{E}$, and a likelihood function is assumed for the elements of $\boldsymbol{M}$. `SignatureAnalyzer` performs Maximum A Posteriori estimation of $\boldsymbol{S}$ and $\boldsymbol{E}$ using the methodology developed by Tan and Févotte [37]. Alternatively, the other two methods use different MCMC algorithms [38–40] to draw from the posterior distributions of $\boldsymbol{S}$ and $\boldsymbol{E}$.

Those methods also differ in their model selection criterion (Table 1). For brevity, we refer the reader to [22] for a thorough albeit somewhat dated summary.

Table 1 Overview of methods for de novo mutational signature analysis. The third column indicates, if relevant, a point estimation criterion, a posterior sampling method, and a model selection criterion. NMF, PCA, MLE, MAP, EM, BIC, and HMC stand for Non-negative Matrix Factorisation, Principal Component Analysis, Maximum Likelihood Estimation, Maximum A Posteriori, Expectation Maximisation, Bayesian Information Criterion, and Hamiltonian Monte Carlo

Software	Method	Estimation methods
`SigProfiler` [24]	NMF [32]	MLE – Ad hoc
`SomaticSignatures` [11]	NMF/PCA [32]	Optimisation – –
`SignatureAnalyzer` [12, 13]	Bayesian NMF [37]	MAP – Not needed
`EMu` [14]	Poisson model	MLE (EM) – BIC
`signeR` [15]	Bayesian NMF [38, 39]	– Gibbs BIC
`sigfit` [16]	Bayesian NMF	– HMC (`stan` [40]) Ad hoc
`SparseSignatures` [17]	Sparse NMF	– – Cross validation

The Bayesian Nonparametric Alternative. An alternative approach to the methods described above is the one by Roberts [18], implemented in the `R` package `hdp`, using the methodology of Teh et al. [41]. Here, we are not presented with vectors of counts but with lists of mutations.

Specifically, we are presented with a data set $X = (\boldsymbol{x}_1, \dots, \boldsymbol{x}_J)$ where $\boldsymbol{x}_j = (x_{j1}, \dots, x_{jn_j})^T$ is the list of mutations observed in the jth patient. Within this framework, patients are assumed to be exchangeable, i.e. the joint probability distribution $p(X)$ does not depend on the ordering of patients. Similarly, mutations are assumed to be partially exchangeable, meaning that $p(X)$ is independent of the ordering of mutations within a specific patient. Observations are assumed to be drawn from a categorical distribution:

$$x_{ji}|\boldsymbol{\theta}_{ji} \sim \text{Categorical}(\boldsymbol{\theta}_{ji}) \tag{4}$$

The parameters $\boldsymbol{\theta}_{ji}$ of the discrete distributions are drawn from G_j, a realisation of the Dirichlet Process associated with the jth patient, whose base measure G_0 is distributed according to a "global" DP with base measure H and concentration parameter γ. Formally,

$$\boldsymbol{\theta}_{ji}|G_j \sim G_j \tag{5}$$

$$G_j|\alpha, G_0 \sim \text{DP}(\alpha, G_0) \tag{6}$$

$$G_0|\gamma, H \sim \text{DP}(\gamma, H) \tag{7}$$

where DP$(\cdot, \cdot)$ denotes a Dirichlet Process [41]. That is a nonparametric hierarchical prior that does not assume a fixed number of components and has three hyperparameters: H is the mean of the prior distribution over the signatures, and γ and α control the variability around that mean at the global and patient level, respectively. Often, H is conveniently set to Dirichlet$(1, \dots, 1)$, a flat prior over the $(K-1)$-simplex, and non-informative Gamma hyper-priors are placed on γ and α. As with any Bayesian analysis, a sensitivity analysis is required to assess the prior choice for H. The model of Eqs. (4)–(7) is referred to as the Hierarchical Dirichlet Process Mixture Model (HDPMM).

This method has several advantages over the ones reviewed above: First, the number of components (signatures) is inferred from the data, rather than fixed. Second, it naturally models the hierarchical nature of patient data. Further, it assumes naturally that the number of components grows with the number of observations, explicitly modelling the rate of growth. However, the assumption that the number of clusters grows logarithmically with the number of patients and doubly-logarithmically with the number of mutations is unchecked [42]. The main disadvantage is that, even if MCMC samplers are available, inference from the raw MCMC output is non-trivial as it requires a post-processing procedure that is currently not available.

Additionally, it should be noted that the HDPMM allows for the assumption of exchangeability at the patient level to be relaxed by extending the hierarchy of Dirichlet Processes. Patients can then be considered partially exchangeable and grouped,

Table 2 Overview of challenges, grouped by proposed statistical solution

Proposed statistical approach	Challenge
Constructing the matrix M	1. Accounting for bias and variance in M
	2. Recognising intra-tumour heterogeneity
	3. Accounting for opportunities
	4. Going beyond the 96 categories
Bayesian nonparametrics	5. Uncertainty in the number of signatures
	6. Uncertainty around the signatures
	7. Sample size calculations
Novel statistical methodology	8. Uncertainty around the exposures
	9. Obtaining separated signatures
	10. Partial information about the signatures

e.g. according to the tissue where the tumour arose [18]. However, to relax the assumption of exchangeability at the mutation level would be more challenging.

Refitting of Mutational Signatures. This is a simpler problem which consists of solving for $\boldsymbol{e}_g$ for a single patient g in (2), assuming $\boldsymbol{m}_g$ and $\boldsymbol{S}$ are known. The most popular approach is perhaps `deconstructSigs` [19]. Alternatively, one can solve (2) using, e.g. non-negative least squares [20, 43]. An attempt to quantify uncertainty by using the Bootstrap within the context of refitting has been provided by `SignatureEstimation` [20]. A Bayesian alternative that also enforces sparsity in the solution is `sigLASSO` [21]. For brevity, we do not detail these approaches here.

Statistical Challenges. Despite the advances in this area over the last decade, it is a concern that within this field, uncertainty quantification is not receiving enough attention. Even if the effort to develop new methods has been substantial, recognition of uncertainty within the discipline is surprisingly limited. While previous reviews have focused on a mathematical description of the methods [22] and their performance [23], here we focus on the key statistical challenges for the field, enumerated in Table 2. In the forthcoming sections, we describe these challenges, highlighting the potential of different methods to address these challenges.

The first group of challenges (Sect. 2) concerns the uncertainties arising from data collection. The second group (Sect. 3) concerns uncertainties in de novo analyses and how accounting for them could inform data collection. We will argue that the Bayesian Nonparametric approach is suitable to address those challenges. The third group (Sect. 4) concerns uncertainty in analyses where partial information is available. While we will highlight that progress has been made, the need to address these challenges demands the development of new methodology.

2 Challenges in Constructing *M*

2.1 Challenge 1: Accounting for Bias and Variance in M

Sequencing experiments are stochastic events, and the identification of mutations, necessary for constructing $\boldsymbol{M}$, is often based on probabilistic models [31]. $\boldsymbol{M}$ is itself therefore also an observation of a random variable. While uncertainty around the mutation calls is unavoidable, it can be reduced by increasing sequencing depth [29]. High sequencing depth increases the chance of calling subclonal mutations (see also Sect. 2.2) and reduces disagreements between mutation callers [31]. Typically, it is beneficial to increase the depth of sequencing as it results in the identification of mutations that are present in a fraction of cells. However, the benefits of doing so are marginal after a certain depth threshold, which differs across individual tumours [30]. Therefore, allocating extra resources to recruit more patients might be more cost-efficient.

As well as exhibiting variation, $\boldsymbol{M}$ will be a biased estimate of the true value. Different callers [31] and sequencing pipelines [30] can return systematically different results. Genomic context affects the power to detect mutations (via variation of sequencing coverage [44]) and the false discovery rate [31], meaning that some classes of mutation are less likely to be called correctly than others. There is potential for novel statistical developments to estimate more accurate catalogues.

Going back to the identification of mutations present in a small fraction of cells, these are more likely to have occurred more recently—and thus they are more likely to be overlooked due to insufficient coverage. If there is a change in mutational patterns over time [45], then this will cause a bias in $\boldsymbol{M}$. On the other hand, if the tumour has recently diverged into subclones, then recent mutational processes might have their impact measured on each subclone, and these processes will be over-represented relative to the truth for any cell present.

2.2 Challenge 2: Recognising Intra-Tumour Heterogeneity

Intra-tumour heterogeneity (ITH) poses a difficulty with mutational signature analyses that is not always acknowledged. Briefly, tumours are heterogeneous mixtures of cells, and we are often able to identify mutations only at the patient level (i.e. not with single cell resolution). We can sometimes infer whether a mutation is *clonal* (meaning it is present in every sampled cancer cell) or *subclonal*. Every subclonal mutation belongs to one or more *subclones*, subpopulations of cells that carry the same variants. Subclones can be inferred by clustering on the space of the *cancer cell fraction* (CCF), the unobserved proportion of tumour cells in which a mutation is present [46].

ITH in De Novo Signature Extraction. All de novo methods ignore ITH. They consider, explicitly or implicitly, mutations to be exchangeable at the patient level, ignoring their clonal status. Ideally, we would relax the assumption of exchangeability by incorporating available information regarding ITH. An interesting approach has been taken in recent studies of normal and non-neoplastic colon biopsies [47, 48] and consists of extending the tree-like hierarchical structure of the HDPMM to a further level. Then, mutations are grouped according to their subclone, which is in turn grouped according to patients. However, it remains to be shown whether this approach is applicable to cancer data.

ITH in Signature Refitting. By combining the estimation of subclones with refitting methods we can learn about the evolution of cancers [45]. One approach is to infer the subclones and then apply a refitting algorithm to each of them [49]. An alternative is implemented by `TrackSig` [50], and consists of sorting mutations by CCF (a surrogate for "age"). Refitting is then applied to "time points" of 100 mutations each. Lastly, subclones are inferred at boundaries between time points.

The first approach fails to propagate the uncertainty around subclones to the second step of the analysis. Performing inference on the subclones and the subclone-specific exposures jointly, as done by `TrackSig`, seems sensible but the current approach ignores uncertainty in the estimation of the CCF.

2.3 Challenge 3: Accounting for Opportunities

A mutation category implies a "reference state" and a "variant state". For example, consider the category "A[C>T]G" in the standard categorisation of SBSs. That category implies a reference state "ACG" and a variant state "ATG". Reference states are not uniformly distributed across the human genome and their distribution varies across cancer patients (due to copy number variation and loss of heterozygosity events).

Fischer et al. [14] have proposed to adjust the observed number of mutations of category k by the relative prevalence of that category's reference state. That relative prevalence is termed "opportunity" and, for patient g, is denoted o_{kg}. Adjusting for opportunities, (1) becomes

$$m_{kg} \approx o_{kg} \sum_{n=1}^{N} s_{kn} e_{ng} \tag{8}$$

While this approach is available in several de novo methods [14–16], it does not seem to be widely used in practice.

Opportunities, when measured, are informative about the distribution of mutations that might occur contemporaneously, but are used to analyse mutations that have occurred in the past. Copy-Number gains change the opportunities for late mutations, while loss of heterozygosity events and copy number losses effectively change the opportunities for early events. By contrast, other processes can gradually shift the balance of opportunities. An SBS event can change three local contexts, so a hypermutation event with 1,000,000+ similar mutations would noticeably change the opportunities.

2.4 Challenge 4: Going Beyond the 96 Categories

As mentioned in Sect. 1.1, signature analyses are applicable to a range of mutational classes. Most, though, have been performed on single base substitutions (SBS) for which a canonical categorisation with 96 categories is available. Six basic categories result from considering the pyrimidine in the mutated base pair and the base to which it mutates (C>A, C>G, C>T, T>A, T>C, T>G). Considering this and the four possible nucleotides before and after the mutated base, we obtain the most common categorisation, with $4 \times 6 \times 4 = 96$ mutation types.

Further Categorisations of SBS. We could consider four flanking bases instead of two. The number of categories in this taxonomy is then $6 \times 4^4 = 1536$. While it has been shown that the two bases immediately flanking the mutated base carry a stronger signal, in some cases using this extended taxonomy has led to further resolution [24]. This taxonomy comes with its own challenges. First, we would not expect MCMC-based methods to scale to this level of resolution. Second, we would expect matrix $\boldsymbol{M}$ to contain many zeroes, requiring methods that can account for such sparsity.

A related problem is that there is currently no distance structure between mutation categories. A mutation A[C>T]G is as different from C[C >T]G as it is from T[T>A]T. While the NMF approach offers no obvious way of creating such distance structure, the one-dimensional categorical observations $x_{ji} \in \{1, \ldots, 96\}$ in the HDPMM could be replaced with three-dimensional observations $\boldsymbol{x}_{ji} = (x_{ji1}, x_{ji2}, x_{ji3})$ with $x_{ji2} \in \{1, \ldots, 6\}$ and $x_{ji1}, x_{ji3} \in \{1, \ldots, 4\}$.

Integrating Mutation Classes. Whether it would be informative for signatures to integrate all the mutation classes is a matter of debate [4, 24]. A cross-class categorisation, such as the one with 1,697 categories proposed by Alexandrov et al. [24], ignores the difference in noise and degree of sparsity between mutational classes. Performing separate analyses for each class followed by post-hoc association analysis of exposures has the drawback of ignoring uncertainty in signature attribution. Instead, we would suggest a strategy of information sharing, using class-specific categorisations and catalogues to extract signatures, but incorporating an association parameter that would quantify which signatures of diverse classes tend to occur together.

Accounting for Genomic Properties. So far, we have considered mutations from a given patient to be exchangeable. That is reasonable if we lack information to distinguish them, other than the category we are measuring. However, that is not entirely true, as each mutation has *genomic properties* (e.g. chromosome, chromatin state, proximity to a particular binding site, etc.) that we might be able to measure. Those properties can help elucidate the aetiology of a signature, as well as help determine whether a signature is an artefact of the extraction algorithm.

Categorisations can be augmented to account for these genomic properties, but increasing the number of categories comes at a price. With that strategy, we are likely to be able to consider one genomic property at a time. Vöhringer et al. have suggested an alternative based on *non-negative tensor factorisation*, `TensorSignatures` [51]. This method scales to a large number of genomic properties. However, it has the disadvantage of not being a probabilistic method. Further methods may arise, in the spirit of `TensorSignatures`, perhaps modelling mutation categories and genomic properties with a joint probability distribution and thus relaxing the assumption of exchangeability.

3 Challenges Addressed with Bayesian Nonparametrics

3.1 Challenge 5: Uncertainty in the Number of Signatures

Parametric methods such as those based on NMF, reviewed in Sect. 1.2, assume a fixed number of signatures. Therefore, uncertainty around the number of signatures is not modelled or evaluated. Moreover, it has been argued that uncertainty around the model dimension should be disregarded as its influence in the estimation of the main signatures is marginal [4].

We argue that as the number of signatures is unknown, there is uncertainty about the true model dimension. This uncertainty can be modelled and evaluated after collecting data. A Bayesian clustering approach relaxes the assumption of a fixed number of signatures and lets this number be a parameter whose value is to be learned. This is achieved by placing a prior on the number of signatures. A nonparametric prior implies that the model dimension increases with the number of observations [52]. The assumed rate of growth depends on the chosen nonparametric prior, as briefly discussed for the HDPMM in Sect. 1.2.

The latter approach has, in our opinion, several advantages. First, avoiding an upper bound on the number of signatures is intuitively appealing, as we expect to see more signatures as more observations arrive. However, the assumption about the rate of growth is rather strong and must be checked. Second, it allows for inference to be performed on model parameters and model dimension jointly. Hence, uncertainty intervals around model parameters will reflect the uncertainty around the number of signatures (see also Sect. 3.2).

Provided with a data set, a sampler for the HDPMM will produce draws from a posterior distribution, each of them with a different number of signatures. From those draws, it is straightforward to produce a (marginal) posterior distribution over the number of signatures. As that posterior will help quantify the strength of the signal in the data set, it must be reported along with the "most representative set of signatures". Relatedly, the required evaluation of uncertainty around signatures in that representative set is not trivial (see Sect. 3.2).

3.2 Challenge 6: Uncertainty Around the Signatures

Contrary to the usual practice in the biomedical literature, estimates of mutational signatures have typically been reported without intervals of uncertainty [5, 9, 24]. This is undesirable, as we are often interested in the possible range of values that might have generated the data. First, even if we were only interested in the "centre" of the signatures, uncertainty in estimating that centre is unavoidable. Second, if there is any randomness in the biological mechanism under which mutational processes generate mutations, we would expect them to leave slightly different "fingerprints" in each patient. Uncertainty intervals around signature probabilities should reflect that variability.

The Bayesian paradigm provides a natural setting to quantify that uncertainty. While this has been proposed in two contexts, Bayesian NMF [15, 16] and Bayesian clustering [18], we believe that the latter is more promising. This is because the Bayesian clustering approach accounts for the uncertainty in the model dimension when reporting uncertainty around the signatures (see Sect. 3.1). This can be useful considering study design (see Sect. 3.3).

The Bayesian clustering framework provides a posterior over the space of possible *partitions*. At every iteration of the MCMC sampler, every mutation is allocated to a cluster which is, in turn, characterised by $\boldsymbol{\theta}_{ji}$ in (5)–(7). The random vector $\boldsymbol{\theta}_{ji}$ represents the signature attributed to mutation x_{ji}. For ease of interpretation, a representative clustering must be determined from the MCMC output. An objective criterion must be defined to determine that "most representative set of signatures".

Once a representative set has been derived, the MCMC output can be used to determine the strength of the signal. If a signature is needed to explain the data, it will appear consistently across iterations of the sampler, and hence credible intervals around it will be narrow. Conversely, if a signature appears in the best set but does not appear throughout the MCMC output (e.g. because it might emerge admixed with similar signatures), it will be reported with wide credible intervals.

Such an approach, while needing development, would differ from the post-processing method of Roberts [18] that disregards uncertainty in clustering by assuming that every reported signature *is present across iterations of the sampler*. Rather, one of the strengths of the Bayesian clustering approach is that it allows one to assess *whether a given signature is present across iterations*.

3.3 Challenge 7: Sample Size Calculations

Since the first collection of 5 mutational signatures was found on a data set of 21 breast cancer whole genomes [9], the number of known mutational signatures has grown with the number of cancer genomes available for analysis. The first pan-cancer mutational signature study reported 21 SBS signatures in 507 genomes and 6535 exomes [5, 10], while the most recent large-scale study has reported 49 SBS signatures in 4645 genomes and 19184 exomes [24], suggesting that the rate at which new mutational signatures can be found shrinks as the number of patients and observed mutations grows. Heterogeneity within the cohort is also known to influence the power to extract signatures.

While we would expect the inventory of mutational signatures to keep increasing as new tumour samples are observed, it is good practice to make sample size calculations before collecting new samples. When making sample size calculations, it is advisable to consider (1) the number of new individuals recruited, (2) the number of mutations observed in each patient, and (3) heterogeneity within the cohort.

Whereas methods based on Non-negative matrix factorisation do not provide an obvious way of informing study design, the fully probabilistic approach of the HDPMM could be used to inform future sample collection. In particular, we would be interested in assessing the posterior probability of discovering a new signature, conditional on the data already observed and L future observations $\boldsymbol{x}_{J+1}, \boldsymbol{x}_{J+2}, \ldots, \boldsymbol{x}_{J+L}$.

The scaling properties of the HDPMM [42, 52], explained in Sects. 1.2 and 3.1, can be applied to assess that probability. Related probabilistic questions on future data collection could be answered, for example regarding heterogeneity within the cohort. This approach has been successful in other problems, such as single-cell sequencing experiments with competing budget constraints [53]. However, to avoid making false inferences, we must check that the newly discovered signatures are likely to be genuine, considering the level of support for them by the observed data.

4 Challenges Requiring a New Modelling Approach

4.1 Challenge 8: Uncertainty Quantification Around Exposures

Remember that the goal of a refitting analysis is to solve for $\boldsymbol{e}_g$ in (2) for a single patient g. In Sect. 1.2, we have briefly reviewed the mathematical methods available for performing this task. To date, it remains the case that most point estimates in refitting analyses are reported without an uncertainty interval (see, e.g. [54]).

So far, there has been one attempt to provide confidence intervals around the estimates of a refitting analysis, provided by `SignatureEstimation` [20], which uses the bootstrap to produce confidence intervals around the exposure estimates.

There is a concern though that this approach accounts at best for a fraction of the uncertainty.

Avoiding False Exposures and Obtaining a Sparse Solution. Because signatures overlap, different weighted combinations of signatures can explain a mutational catalogue equally well. Thus, it has been argued that $\boldsymbol{S}$ should include only the signatures that one could reasonably expect to see in the tissue where the tumour arose [4]. Moreover, any extra signature added to the $\boldsymbol{S}$ matrix will result in a fitted vector that better resembles the observed vector.

Those two difficulties are acknowledged and addressed by Alexandrov et al. [24]. Their solution consists in (a) including in $\boldsymbol{S}$ all the signatures that have been previously found in the relevant tissue, (b) removing signatures from $\boldsymbol{S}$ sequentially, until the removal of a single signature results in a reduction in the cosine similarity ≥ 0.01, and (c) adding to $\boldsymbol{S}$ the signatures that result in an increase in cosine similarity of ≥ 0.05, even if they have not been previously associated with the relevant tissue.

However, that approach is not without problems. First, the inference is based on ad-hoc rules and relies on cut-offs that appear arbitrary. The first suggestion from a statistical point of view would be to elucidate an informative prior distribution over the exposures. If prior information is limited to the tissue in which the tumour was observed, it might be possible to adopt a hierarchical modelling approach, with the ambition to borrow information across patients. Further, a penalty parameter could be included, ensuring that over-fitting is avoided.

Assessing All Sources of Uncertainty. In principle, to avoid underestimating uncertainty, all its sources should be modelled explicitly. Degasperi et al. [25] have argued that, even if most signatures occur in more than one tissue, the profile of each signature is tissue-specific. Therefore, the matrix $\boldsymbol{S}$ should contain signatures as extracted from tumours of the relevant tissue only. While this seems sensible, we would go further and argue that, if there is any randomness in the mechanism under which a given mutational process generates mutations, then the fingerprint of that process must differ at least slightly between patients. This must be accounted for when allocating mutations to signatures.

Another source of uncertainty that is often ignored has been termed "sampling uncertainty" by Li and colleagues [21]. It formalises the idea that uncertainty in the estimated exposures will decrease as more mutations are observed. A response to that is their method, `sigLASSO`. However, even if this method accounts for such "sampling uncertainty" in its modelling, it reports point estimates only. This is an appealing idea that could be incorporated into the other methods.

4.2 *Challenge 9: Obtaining Separated Signatures*

If we are looking to extract a representation of the true exposures and signatures, then it should be noted that two true but distinct signatures can be similar. This has been highlighted as problematic, as the presence of similar signatures in the matrix $\boldsymbol{S}$ prevents unambiguous attribution of mutations to signatures [24]. We should also note that the interpretation of similarity is very much dependent on the vector space in which we are representing signatures, which is a restrictive space due to the non-negativity constraint.

To avoid such ambiguity in post-hoc refitting analysis, we can impose a sparsity constraint on de novo methods by adding a penalty term to the optimisation problem (3), as suggested by Lal et al. [17]:

$$\lambda \sum_{n=1}^{N} ||\boldsymbol{s}_n||_1 \tag{9}$$

where $||\cdot||_1$ is the L1 norm and λ can be interpreted as the data set's *degree of sparsity*. This approach results in extracting signatures that are sparse, thus making pairs of signatures more likely to be *separated*. It should be noted however that, by imposing a sparsity constraint, a restriction that may not be supported by evidence is introduced for computational and interpretational convenience.

By shrinking the signature parameters towards zero, the aforementioned sparsity constraint results in a rather strong restriction over a space that is already restrictive. This has implications for the stability of present and future signatures: presented with additional data carrying novel signatures, a de novo method may fail to find space to accommodate those novel signatures, potentially distorting old ones.

4.3 Challenge 10: Partial Information About the Signatures

With the methodology available to date, a researcher has two options when attempting to analyse data—to rely on an external collection of signatures to perform a refitting analysis or to perform a de novo analysis. However, there are situations where it would be more natural to assume an intermediate setting, where the signatures are neither known nor unknown.

In this context, it might make sense to consider an intermediate approach where partial information about the signatures is available, but they are not known precisely. This is not the same as the approach termed *fit-ext* in [16] and also implemented in [18]. That approach, consisting in setting part of the signatures matrix to point estimates derived from previous studies, ignores the uncertainty associated with those point estimates. Moreover, it does not allow for those estimates to be updated.

Rather than considering previously discovered signatures to be fixed, it seems more appropriate to incorporate knowledge obtained from previous studies through means of an informative prior distribution. This setting has, to some extent, been explored also in [16], allowing informative Dirichlet priors over both signatures and the exposures. However, there is little guidance on how to take advantage of this method. We note however two possible lines of future research within this approach. First, the Dirichlet distribution might not be flexible enough to model prior knowledge about the signatures. Second, a hierarchical prior over the exposures might be worth considering, to borrow statistical strength between patients.

5 Conclusions

This review has set out what we perceive to be the main statistical challenges in the field of mutational signatures. While highlighting the achievements of the mutational signatures community in improving our understanding of cancer, we have drawn attention to the lack of estimates of uncertainty in such analyses. Motivated by this, and by related statistical challenges, we have highlighted the strengths of certain methods to address those challenges while also emphasising the need for future developments.

First, we have outlined four challenges involving potential errors or loss of information when constructing $\boldsymbol{M}$. We have highlighted that the problem of estimating the "true" $\boldsymbol{M}$ has been largely ignored (Sect. 2). As an alternative, we could have argued for a single Bayesian pipeline integrating mutation calling and signature analysis. However, that would set back the adoption of new methods, since mutation calling pipelines are established. Relatedly, we have underlined the promise of `TrackSig` in the study of tumour evolution, but further developments are required to account for all the uncertainties (Sect. 2.2). Similarly, we drew attention to the concept of mutational opportunities while calling for new developments to account for the opportunities' temporal evolution (Sect. 2.3).

Second, we have outlined three challenges related to uncertainty quantification in de novo applications. While NMF approaches have been augmented with probabilistic models, their lack of flexibility regarding model dimension is a drawback. We have argued that the Bayesian Nonparametrics approach, first suggested by Roberts, offers a more natural framework for assessing sources of uncertainty. However, we have argued that further study is needed to take advantage of the vast MCMC output resulting from this approach (Sects. 3.1 and 3.2). We have also discussed the potential of this fully probabilistic modelling to underpin study design, allowing practitioners to address trade-offs and optimise limited resources (Sect. 3.3).

Lastly, we have outlined three challenges for which no obvious statistical solution is available. We have highlighted the need for quantifying uncertainty in the context of refitting. We have also highlighted the recent application of statistical methods such as the Bootstrap to assess a fraction of such uncertainty, while identifying additional sources of uncertainty that are being ignored (Sect. 4.1). Finally, we have underlined the fit-ext approach as an attempt to pose an intermediate problem between de novo and refitting. However, that approach needs enhancement to account for the uncertainty around estimates obtained in previous studies (Sect. 4.3).

Acknowledgements We thank The Melville Trust for the Care and Cure of Cancer for providing financial support. We are grateful to the Editors and to an anonymous reviewer for valuable comments that helped to improve the manuscript.

References

1. Greenman, C., Stephens, P., Smith, R., et al.: Patterns of somatic mutation in human cancer genomes. Nature **446**, 153–158 (2007)
2. Stratton, M., Campbell, P., Futreal, P.: The cancer genome. Nature **458**(7239), 719–724 (2009)
3. Li, Y., Roberts, N., Wala, J., Shapira, O., Schumacher, S., et al.: Patterns of somatic structural variation in human cancer genomes. Nature **578**(7793), 112–121 (2020)
4. Koh, G., Degasperi, A., Zou, X., Momen, S., Nik-Zainal, S.: Mutational signatures: emerging concepts, caveats and clinical applications. Nat. Rev. Cancer **21**(10), 619–637 (2021)
5. Alexandrov, L.B., Nik-Zainal, S., Wedge, D.C., Aparicio, S.A.J.R., et al.: Signatures of mutational processes in human cancer. Nature **500**(7463), 415–421 (2013)
6. Alexandrov, L.B., Jones, P.H., Wedge, D.C., Sale, J.E., Campbell, P.J., Nik-Zainal, S., Stratton, M.R.: Clock-like mutational processes in human somatic cells. Nat. Genet. **47**(12), 1402–1407 (2015)
7. Brash, D.E., Rudolph, J.A., Simon, J.A., Lin, A., McKenna, G.J., et al.: A role for sunlight in skin cancer: UV-induced p53 mutations in squamous cell carcinoma. Proc. Natl. Acad. Sci. **88**(22), 10124–10128 (1991)
8. Denissenko, M.F., Pao, A., Tang, M., Pfeifer, G.P.: Preferential formation of benzo[a]pyrene adducts at lung cancer mutational hotspots in p53. Science **274**, 430–432 (1996)
9. Nik-Zainal, S., Alexandrov, L.B., Wedge, D.C., Van Loo, P., Greenman, C.D., et al.: Mutational processes molding the genomes of 21 breast cancers. Cell **149**, 979–993 (2012)
10. Alexandrov, L.B., Nik-Zainal, S., Wedge, D.C., Campbell, P.J., Stratton, M.R.: Deciphering signatures of mutational processes operative in human cancer. Cell Rep. **3**, 246–259 (2013)
11. Gehring, J.S., Fischer, B., Lawrence, M., Huber, W.: SomaticSignatures: inferring mutational signatures from single-nucleotide variants. Bioinformatics **31**, 3673–3675 (2015)
12. Kasar, S., Kim, J., Improgo, R., Tiao, G., Polak, P., et al.: Whole-genome sequencing reveals activation-induced cytidine deaminase signatures during indolent chronic lymphocytic leukaemia evolution. Nat. Commun. **6**(1), 8866 (2015)
13. Kim, J., Mouw, K.W., Polak, P., Braunstein, L.Z., Kamburov, A., et al.: Somatic ERCC2 mutations are associated with a distinct genomic signature in urothelial tumors. Nat. Genet. **48**, 600–606 (2016)
14. Fischer, A., Illingworth, C.J.R., Campbell, P.J., Mustonen, V.: EMu: probabilistic inference of mutational processes and their localization in the cancer genome. Genome Biol. **14**(4), R39 (2013)
15. Rosales, R.A., Drummond, R.D., Valieris, R., Dias-Neto, E., Da Silva, I.T.: signeR: an empirical Bayesian approach to mutational signature discovery. Bioinformatics **33**(1), 8–16 (2017)
16. Gori, K., Baez-Ortega, A.: sigfit: flexible Bayesian inference of mutational signatures. bioRxiv 372896 (2020)
17. Lal, A., Liu, K., Tibshirani, R., Sidow, A., Ramazzotti, D.: De novo mutational signature discovery in tumor genomes using SparseSignatures. PLoS Comput. Biol. **17**(6), e1009119 (2021)
18. Roberts, N.: Patterns of somatic genome rearrangement in human cancer. Ph.D. Thesis, University of Cambridge (2018)
19. Rosenthal, R., McGranahan, N., Herrero, J., Taylor, B.S., Swanton, C.: DeconstructSigs: delineating mutational processes in single tumors distinguishes DNA repair deficiencies and patterns of carcinoma evolution. Genome Biol. **17**, 31 (2016)
20. Huang, X., Wojtowicz, D., Przytycka, T.M.: Detecting presence of mutational signatures in cancer with confidence. Bioinformatics **34**, 330–337 (2018)
21. Li, S., Crawford, F.W., Gerstein, M.B.: Using sigLASSO to optimize cancer mutation signatures jointly with sampling likelihood. Nat. Commun. **11**(1), 3575 (2020)
22. Baez-Ortega, A., Gori, K.: Computational approaches for discovery of mutational signatures in cancer. Brief. Bioinform. **20**, 77–88 (2019)

23. Omichessan, H., Severi, G., Perduca, V.: Computational tools to detect signatures of mutational processes in DNA from tumours: a review and empirical comparison of performance. PLoS ONE **14**(9), e0221235 (2019)
24. Alexandrov, L.B., Kim, J., Haradhvala, N.J., Huang, M.N., Tian Ng, A.W., et al.: The repertoire of mutational signatures in human cancer. Nature **578**(7793), 94–101 (2020)
25. Degasperi, A., Amarante, T.D., Czarnecki, J., Shooter, S., Zou, X., et al.: A practical framework and online tool for mutational signature analyses show inter-tissue variation and driver dependencies. Nat. Cancer **1**, 249–263 (2020)
26. Davies, H., Glodzik, D., Morganella, S., Yates, L.R., Staaf, J., et al.: HRDetect is a predictor of BRCA1 and BRCA2 deficiency based on mutational signatures. Nat. Med. **23**, 517–525 (2017)
27. Zou, X., Koh, G.C.C., Nanda, A.S., Degasperi, A., Urgo, K., Roumeliotis, T.I., Agu, C.A., Badja, C., Momen, S., Young, J., Amarante, T.D., Side, L., Brice, G., Perez-Alonso, V., Rueda, D., Gomez, C., Bushell, W., Harris, R., Choudhary, J.S., Consortium, G.E.R., Jiricny, J., Skarne, W.C., Nik-Zainal, S.: A systematic CRISPR screen defines mutational mechanisms underpinning signatures caused by replication errors and endogenous DNA damage. Nat. Cancer **2**, 643–657 (2021)
28. Zhao, E.Y., Shen, Y., Pleasance, E., Kasaian, K., Leelakumari, S., et al.: Homologous recombination deficiency and platinum-based therapy outcomes in advanced breast cancer. Clin. Cancer Res. **23**, 7521–7530 (2017)
29. Sims, D., Sudbery, I., Ilott, N.E., Heger, A., Ponting, C.P.: Sequencing depth and coverage: key considerations in genomic analyses. Nat. Rev. Genet. **15**(2), 121–132 (2014)
30. Alioto, T.S., Buchhalter, I., Derdak, S., Hutter, B., Eldridge, M.D., et al.: A comprehensive assessment of somatic mutation detection in cancer using whole-genome sequencing. Nat. Commun. **6**(1), 10001 (2015)
31. Krøigård, A.B., Thomassen, M., Lænkholm, A.-V., Kruse, T.A., Larsen, M.J.: Evaluation of nine somatic variant callers for detection of somatic mutations in exome and targeted deep sequencing data. PLoS ONE **11**, e0151664 (2016)
32. Lee, D.D., Seung, H.S.: Learning the parts of objects by non-negative matrix factorization. Nature **401**(6755), 788–791 (1999)
33. Ardin, M., Cahais, V., Castells, X., Bouaoun, L., Byrnes, G., et al.: MutSpec: a Galaxy toolbox for streamlined analyses of somatic mutation spectra in human and mouse cancer genomes. BMC Bioinform. **17**(1), 170 (2016)
34. Mayakonda, A., Lin, D.-C., Assenov, Y., Plass, C., Koeffler, H.P.: Maftools: efficient and comprehensive analysis of somatic variants in cancer. Genome Res. **28**, 1747–1756 (2018)
35. Blokzijl, F., Janssen, R., van Boxtel, R., Cuppen, E.: MutationalPatterns: comprehensive genome-wide analysis of mutational processes. Genome Med. **10**(1) (2018)
36. Wang, S., Tao, Z., Wu, T., Liu, X.-S.: Sigflow: an automated and comprehensive pipeline for cancer genome mutational signature analysis. Bioinformatics **37**, 1590–1592 (2021)
37. Tan, V.Y., Févotte, C.: Automatic relevance determination in nonnegative matrix factorization with the /spl beta/-divergence. IEEE Trans. Pattern Anal. Mach. Intell. **35**(7), 1592–1605 (2013)
38. Cemgil, A.T.: Bayesian inference for nonnegative matrix factorisation models. Comput. Intell. Neurosci. 785152 (2009)
39. Schmidt, M.N., Winther, O., Hansen, L.K.: Bayesian non-negative matrix factorization. In: International Conference on Independent Component Analysis and Signal Separation, pp. 540–547. Springer (2009)
40. Gelman, A., Lee, D., Guo, J.: Stan: a probabilistic programming language for Bayesian inference and optimization. J. Educ. Behav. Stat. **40**(5), 530–543 (2015)
41. Teh, Y.W., Jordan, M.I., Beal, M.J., Blei, D.M.: Hierarchical Dirichlet Processes. J. Amer. Stat. Assoc. **101**(476), 1566–1581 (2006)
42. Antoniak, C.E.: Mixtures of Dirichlet processes with applications to Bayesian nonparametric problems. Ann. Stat. 1152–1174 (1974)
43. Krüger, S., Piro, R.M.: decompTumor2Sig: identification of mutational signatures active in individual tumors. BMC Bioinform. **20**(4), 1–15 (2019)

44. Barbitoff, Y.A., Polev, D.E., Glotov, A.S., Serebryakova, E.A., Shcherbakova, I.V., et al.: Systematic dissection of biases in whole-exome and whole-genome sequencing reveals major determinants of coding sequence coverage. Sci. Rep. **10**(1), 1–13 (2020)
45. Gerstung, M., Jolly, C., Leshchiner, I., Dentro, S.C., Gonzalez, S., et al.: The evolutionary history of 2,658 cancers. Nature **578**(7793), 122–128 (2020)
46. Dentro, S.C., Wedge, D.C., Van Loo, P.: Principles of reconstructing the subclonal architecture of cancers. Cold Spring Harb. Perspect. Med. **7**(8), a026625 (2017)
47. Lee-Six, H., Olafsson, S., Ellis, P., Osborne, R.J., Sanders, M.A., et al.: The landscape of somatic mutation in normal colorectal epithelial cells. Nature **574**(7779), 532–537 (2019)
48. Olafsson, S., McIntyre, R.E., Coorens, T., Butler, T., Jung, H., et al.: Somatic evolution in non-neoplastic IBD-affected colon. Cell **182**(3), 672–684 (2020)
49. Yates, L.R., Knappskog, S., Wedge, D., Farmery, J.H., Gonzalez, S., et al.: Genomic evolution of breast cancer metastasis and relapse. Cancer Cell **32**(2), 169–184 (2017)
50. Rubanova, Y., Shi, R., Harrigan, C.F., Li, R., Wintersinger, J., et al.: Reconstructing evolutionary trajectories of mutation signature activities in cancer using TrackSig. Nat. Commun. **11**(1), 1–12 (2020)
51. Vöhringer, H., Hoeck, A.V., Cuppen, E., Gerstung, M.: Learning mutational signatures and their multidimensional genomic properties with TensorSignatures. Nat. Commun. **12**(1), 1–16 (2021)
52. Teh, Y.W., Jordan, M.I.: Hierarchical Bayesian nonparametric models with applications. In: Bayesian Nonparametrics, vol. 1, pp. 158–207. Cambridge University Press, Cambridge (2010)
53. Camerlenghi, F., Dumitrascu, B., Ferrari, F., Engelhardt, B.E., Favaro, S.: Nonparametric Bayesian multiarmed bandits for single-cell experiment design. Ann. Appl. Stat. **14**(4), 2003–2019 (2020)
54. Riaz, N., Havel, J.J., Makarov, V., Desrichard, A., Urba, W.J., et al.: Tumor and microenvironment evolution during immunotherapy with nivolumab. Cell **171**(4), 934–949 (2017)

PCR Duplicate Proportion Estimation and Consequences for DNA Copy Number Calculations

Andy G. Lynch, Mike L. Smith, Matthew D. Eldridge, and Simon Tavaré

Abstract The volume of DNA in a sequencing experiment is often amplified by PCR, leading to the possibility that the same original DNA fragment will be sequenced twice—a "PCR duplicate". Sometimes indistinguishable from these are multiple sequences arising from identical but independent molecules, which can lead to an over-estimation of the PCR duplicate proportion. The PCR duplicate proportion, and other measures derived from it, are important statistics for quality assurance, experimental design, and interpretation of sequencing experiments. Here, we provide a full likelihood basis for a combinatorial approach using heterozygous SNPs as implemented in our R package and demonstrate the efficacy of the approach. We also discuss the association with DNA copy number and demonstrate the impact on a question of inferring mitochondrial DNA copy number that has recently been a feature of several high-profile cancer studies. This is explored through a simulation study.

Keywords Cancer · DNA copy number · Likelihood · Mitochondria · Quality control · Whole-genome sequencing

A. G. Lynch (✉)
School of Mathematics and Statistics, University of St Andrews, St Andrews KY16 9SS, UK

School of Medicine, University of St Andrews, St Andrews KY16 9TF, UK
e-mail: andy.lynch@st-andrews.ac.uk

M. L. Smith
Genome Biology Unit, EMBL, 69117 Heidelberg, Germany
e-mail: mike.smith@embl.de

M. D. Eldridge
CRUK Cambridge Institute, University of Cambridge, Li Ka Shing Centre, Robinson Way, Cambridge CB2 0RE, England
e-mail: matthew.eldridge@cruk.cam.ac.uk

S. Tavaré
Irving Institute for Cancer Dynamics, Columbia University, New York, NY 10027, USA
e-mail: st3193@columbia.edu

R. Bispo et al. (eds.), *Recent Developments in Statistics and Data Science*, Springer Proceedings in Mathematics & Statistics 398,
https://doi.org/10.1007/978-3-031-12766-3_18

1 Duplicate Sequencing Reads

A simple DNA whole-genome sequencing (WGS) experiment might consist of sampling DNA from several cells, breaking the DNA up into fragments, increasing the number of fragments by creating copies, using a sequencer to identify the sequences of a random sample of those fragments, and mapping them to a reference genome. Once this is done, we can assume that the number of reads mapping to a genomic region is proportional to the average DNA copy number for that region and that the degree of evidence for a particular feature of the genome is measured in the number of sequenced fragments (reads) that support the feature.

It is desirable for the accuracy of these quantitative methods that no original small molecule ends up being counted more than once in the analysis, for which reason "duplicate reads" are typically removed from analyses.

Typically, duplicate reads are defined by the locations to which they map in the genome. Broadly, there are three ways in which such reads can arise. The first is an error in the imaging or image processing (hereafter referred to as "optical duplicates", although our definition may be broader than that usually associated with this term). The second is that the same original DNA fragment can give rise to multiple clusters on the sequencing flow cell—most likely because the fragment was duplicated in a Polymerase Chain Reaction (PCR) amplification step—and so we refer to these as PCR duplicates. The third is that two independent DNA molecules happen to fragment in the same positions and both give rise to clusters on the flow cell (hereafter referred to as "fragmentation duplicates").

Since fragmentation duplicates represent independent molecules, we wish to retain them in analyses. By contrast, ideally, we would wish to retain only one of a set of PCR duplicates, and so all others are typically removed. As fragmentation duplicates are generally indistinguishable from PCR duplicates but fewer in number, fragmentation duplicates are typically removed along with PCR duplicates. Optical duplicates by their nature are typically identifiable and can be removed as a separate process, but could also reasonably be combined with the PCR duplicates in an "undesirable" duplicate category. We will ignore optical duplicates for the rest of the manuscript.

1.1 An Example Data Set

We illustrate this article with WGS data sets previously published by the Oesophageal Cancer Clinical and Molecular Stratification (OCCAMS) consortium [1]. In particular, we focus on 22 "control" WGS data sets that we can assume to be broadly diploid (i.e. they have two copies of each of the autosomal chromosomes). These were generated from blood ($n = 12$) and non-cancerous oesophageal tissue ($n = 10$) from 22 Oesophageal Adenocarcinoma (OAC) patients. DNA from oesophageal tissue was extracted using the DNeasy kit (Qiagen) and from blood using the NucleonTM

Genomic Extraction kit (Gen-Probe) (according to the manufacturers' instructions). A single library was created for each sample and was sequenced to a nominal depth of 50x, using paired-end reads of length 100. Read-pairs were aligned to the human reference genome GRCh37 using the Burrows-Wheeler Aligner (BWA) [2].

The median duplicate percentage (counting both PCR and Fragmentation) across these samples, as derived using Picard [3], is 6.5% (ranging from 3.73 to 14.49%). As might be anticipated, these values are skewed by areas of the genome that are not diploid (e.g. mitochondria), or which (due to problems with aligning reads and discrepancies between the reference genome and the true genome) do not behave as diploid (e.g. telomeres). Such regions need to be removed before calculating and correcting the values.

2 Approaches to Separating Out the Duplicate Types

When classifying specific duplicate reads as being fragmentation duplicates is not possible, i.e. when random tags have not been appended to the original molecules in the mix, it is sufficient for some analyses merely that we can estimate the numbers in each class.

A probabilistic approach for estimating the numbers of fragmentation duplicates, through considering the distribution of insert sizes, read lengths, and coverage, has been presented in the context of high-coverage targeted sequencing experiments [4]. This makes such reasonable assumptions about the independence of reads, the independence of insert size and depth of coverage, and the lack of external limiting factors (e.g. constraints imposed by starting with few molecules). While it is possible to apply an approach comparable to Zhou et al.'s [4] to WGS data, the nature of these data allows for an empirical estimate of the proportion of fragmentation duplicates.

Specifically, we take advantage of knowing that many loci in a WGS experiment will be heterozygous, with a known allele fraction (often 0.5), and that the definition of duplicate reads makes use of their genomic locations rather than their sequences. PCR duplicates covering a heterozygous site should show the same allele, while fragmentation duplicates are neither constrained to show the same allele nor compelled not so to do. This was a characteristic that we exploited in our 2016 software and the update accompanying this manuscript [5], and which has been similarly exploited by others [6]. This latter application is notable for suggestions of application also to RNA-seq data.

3 A Likelihood Approach Based on Allele Patterns at Heterozygous Loci

Here, we set out a likelihood methodology for estimating the proportion of duplicate reads that are PCR duplicates (or equivalently the proportions that are fragmentation duplicates). This is the same approach as implemented in our software [5].

3.1 A Simple Approach Using Only Pairs of Duplicates

We first simplify the problem by imagining that where duplicate reads exist, there are precisely two reads mapping to the locus and no more.

We will consider such pairs of reads that overlay the sites of heterozygous Single Nucleotide Polymorphisms (SNPs). In each case, one of the pair will have been marked as a duplicate. In practice, we will consider only a predefined set of potential sites of heterozygous SNPs in order to simplify computations. Our aim is to identify the proportion, P_D, of duplicate reads that do not represent an observation arising from a novel molecule and to separate this from the proportion that do.

If we assume that we are dealing only with a pair of fragments, then with probability P_D (the quantity we wish to estimate) they are observations of the same original molecule, while with probability $F_D = 1 - P_D$ they are observations representing different starting molecules. We exploit the fact that at these locations, if we are restricting ourselves to parts of the genome that are in allelic balance (i.e. the same number of copies of paternal and maternal sequence), then we can make the following statements:

If the two reads are observations of the same original molecule, then they should report the same nucleotide at the locus of the heterozygous SNP (excepting for sequencing errors, the inclusion of which we assume we can control by filtering on the base-calling quality score). This scenario we denote AA regardless of the allele being reported.

If the reads arise from different starting molecules, then they will report the same nucleotide (AA) half of the time and different nucleotides (denoted AB) half of the time (assuming that the number of cells contributing to the sequencing library is such that removing one molecule from one cell does not noticeably affect the balance of available alleles).

If we observe counts of N_{AA} pairs of reads where the duplicate is reporting the same nucleotide, and N_{AB} where it is reporting different nucleotides, giving a total number $N = N_{AA} + N_{AB}$, then equating the observed and expected proportions of AA and AB patterns gives

$$N_{AA}/N = P_D \times 1 + F_D \times 0.5$$
$$N_{AB}/N = F_D \times 0.5$$

which we can rearrange to gain an estimate of P_D:

$$P_D = 1 - 2 \times N_{AB}/N. \tag{1}$$

3.2 A Likelihood Approach for Pairs of Duplicates

We can explicitly frame this in terms of a likelihood model. There are $Q = 2$ distinct observable allele patterns ($AP_1 = AA$ and $AP_2 = AB$). We wish to calculate the probabilities of observing each of the Q allele patterns given a value of P_D, denoted $\Pr(AP_k|P_D)$ for allele pattern k of Q. Coupled with the observed counts of each allele pattern, $N(AP_k)$, these allow us to define the log-likelihood of P_D to within an additive constant:

$$l(P_D) = \sum_{k=1}^{Q} N(AP_k) \log \Pr(AP_k \mid P_D). \tag{2}$$

We can write down $\Pr(AP_k \mid P_D)$ in a straightforward manner. When $Q = 2$,

$$\Pr(AA \mid P_D) = \frac{1}{2}(1 + P_D)$$
$$\Pr(AB \mid P_D) = \frac{1}{2}(1 - P_D).$$

The log-likelihood is then

$$l(P_D) = N_{AA} \log((1 + P_D)/2) + N_{AB} \log((1 - P_D)/2),$$

and if we seek the maximum likelihood estimate by equating the first derivative to zero, we obtain $0 = N_{AA}(1 - \hat{P}_D) + N_{AB}(1 + \hat{P}_D)$, whence

$$\hat{P}_D = (N_{AA} + N_{AB})/N = 1 - 2 \times N_{AB}/N$$

as required to match the estimate in Eq. (1).

3.3 The Full Model

If we have more than two fragments in our duplicate set, then we can extend the log-likelihood approach in a natural manner. For each size M of duplicate set, we still sum over all $Q = Q_M$ potential allele patterns the number of times that allele pattern was seen multiplied by the log of the probability of seeing that allele pattern.

We simply have to extend this by summing also over all values of M. The challenge is to calculate the probabilities of the allele patterns, $\Pr(AP_k \mid P_D)$.

This calculation can be facilitated by conditioning on the underlying partition of the M reads into the, at most M, original molecules contributing to the set. We consider every possible partitioning of M fragments into m non-identifiable bins representing m original molecules, to obtain

$$\Pr(AP_k \mid P_D) = \sum_i \Pr(AP_k \mid \text{PART}_i) \Pr(\text{PART}_i \mid P_D), \tag{3}$$

allowing us to calculate the log-likelihood and to find the maximum likelihood estimate of P_D.

Determining the Number of Partitions Details of the sequence of partition numbers can be found at http://oeis.org/A000041/. Since the task needs only to be performed once, and the largest value of M observed will typically not be very large, the numbers can be determined by recursively deriving all possible partitions.

Determining the Probability of an Allele Pattern Given a Partition Given a partition, we know the number of molecules present, and the number of read-pairs each molecule contributes (this is in essence our definition of a partition). Every pattern of assignment of alleles ("A" or "B") to the molecules is given an equal probability. Without loss of generality, we can initially assign "A" to the first molecule, so the number of allele assignments to be considered is only 2^{m-1} where m is the number of molecules in the partition. Similarly, for reasons of identifiability, if necessary we relabel the alleles within a pattern so that the number of "A" alleles is at least as great as the number of "B" alleles. See Fig. 1 and supplementary materials for example calculations. The probability of an allele pattern is the sum of probabilities of assignments that give rise to that pattern.

When M read-pairs are partitioned among m molecules, it is straightforward to see that the form of $\Pr(\text{PART}_i \mid P_D)$ must be

$$\Pr(\text{PART}_i \mid P_D) = K F_D^{(m-1)} P_D^{(M-m)} \tag{4}$$

since m molecules imply that we have $(m-1)$ fragmentation duplicates (the "-1" since one read-pair is regarded as an original and not a duplicate of anything) and the remaining $(M-m)$ read-pairs in the set must be PCR duplicates.

The value of K is

$$K = \left(\sum_j \nu_j\right)! \Big/ \prod_j \nu_j! \tag{5}$$

where ν_j is the number of molecules from which exactly j read-pairs have originated. This may be intuited via combinatorial arguments, or a proof is given in the appendix.

As a concrete example, consider the case when there are four fragments ($M = 4$) partitioned among three molecules ($m = 3$) such that two read-pairs arise from one

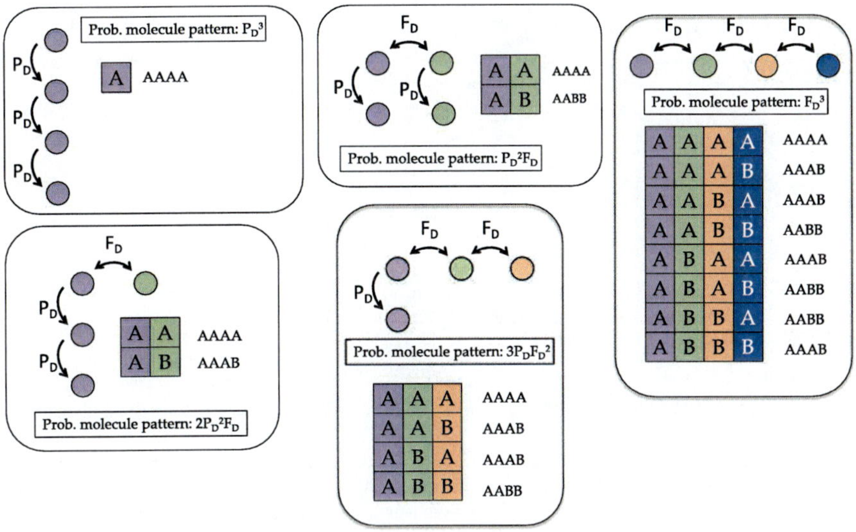

Fig. 1 Details for the case when $M = 4$. For example, if the 4 read-pairs arose from two original molecules, then they must partition into a 3 and 1, or into 2 lots of 2. In the latter case, the only two patterns that can be seen are "AAAA" and "AABB" depending on whether the two original molecules exhibited the same or different alleles, respectively. Each has equal probability when arising from this partitioning, but the same observed patterns can also result from other partitionings

molecule and one read-pair arises from each of the other two (as in the lower-middle case of Fig. 1). Then $\nu_1 = 2$ and $\nu_2 = 1$ ($\nu_j = 0 \; \forall j > 2$). The value of K is then $3!/(2!1!)$
$= 3$.

3.4 Application to Our Example Data

Our method relies on identifying heterozygous SNPs in regions of constant copy number. In this case, we seek regions that are well-behaved and diploid. We also require an observation of the proportion of duplicates that we can correct. The basic observation of the percentage of duplicates for the samples (the total number of duplicates seen, minus optical duplicates, divided by the total number of read-pairs examined) varies from 3.7 to 14.5% with a median of 6.5%. However, as highlighted above, the proportion of duplicates seen is affected by the inclusion of regions that are not representative of the regions in which our SNPs are located, and we may then choose to replace our basic observation with a "masked" observation.

With the removal of masked regions, the median duplicate percentage seen in our 22 samples is 5.0% (ranging from 2.3 to 13.2%). The reduction in the percentage is quite uniform across samples (Fig. 2) but, additionally, we have a third observation.

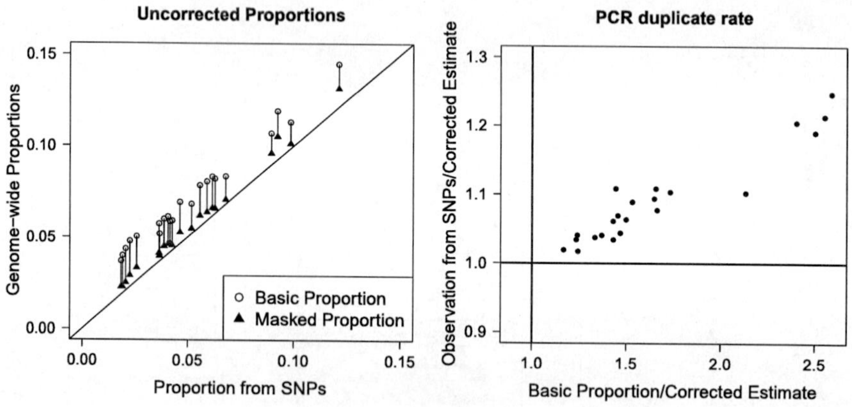

Fig. 2 **Left**: Showing the basic and masked observations of duplicate proportions to be unsatisfactory estimates of the proportions at our SNP loci. **Right**: Showing the degree to which the basic observation and observation from our SNP loci over-estimate our best, corrected, estimate

To apply the methods described above, we investigate 2,500 common SNPs in anticipation of identifying 1,000 heterozygous sites for each sample: In fact, the numbers seen per sample vary from 942 to 1,093. From these approximately 1,000 heterozygous SNPS, we can calculate an observed proportion of duplicates that directly relates to the correction we will make. On average there are 70,000 read-pairs considered per sample, which is sufficient to estimate the duplicate proportion well.

As seen in Fig. 2, masking the genome brings the observed proportion much more in line with that observed from the SNP loci (median 4.5%, range 1.9 to 12.1%), but the observations remain over-estimates of the duplicate proportions at the SNPs. Therefore, our calculations that follow will take the direct observation at the SNP loci as the combined PCR and fragmentation duplicate rate.

In total, 78,173 sets of duplicates are observed across our 22 samples, with the largest set containing six duplicate read-pairs. The percentage of observed duplicates attributed to fragmentation varied from 1.7 to 19.8% and was higher in blood samples (which have a lower observed duplicate proportion than the tissue samples). As seen in Fig. 2, the "corrected" estimate for PCR duplicate proportion is overestimated by more than a tenth in several samples if the fragmentation contribution is not removed, but more noticeably it is overestimated by a factor of up to 2.5 if, additionally, over-influential regions of the genome are not masked, or some other approach to establishing a representative observation of duplicate proportion is not used.

Single versus Paired-End Sequencing. We have, to this point, been considering read-pairs, those reads arising from DNA fragments where both ends of the fragment are sequenced. It is possible also to conduct sequencing such that only one end of the fragment is read ("Single-end sequencing"). In the case of single-end sequencing, the definition of a duplicate is based on only the coordinate of one end of the fragment,

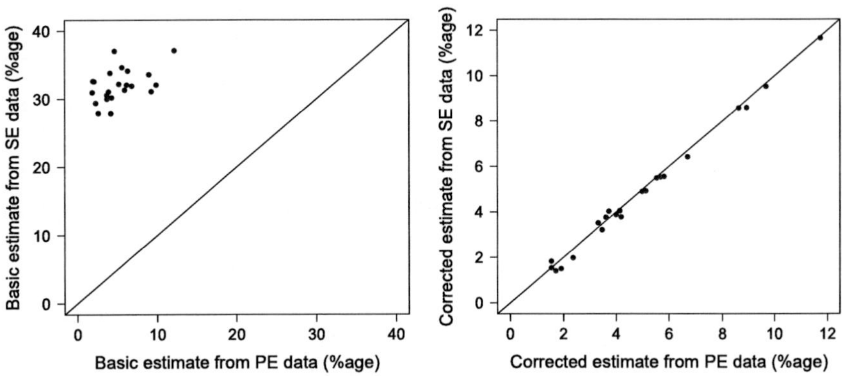

Fig. 3 **Left**: Comparing the basic observations of duplicate proportions from our paired-end example data and simulated single-end sequencing data. **Right**: Showing the agreement between corrected estimates of PCR duplicate proportion from the two data sets

and not the length of the fragment. With this laxer criterion reads will be classed as fragmentation duplicates more readily.

We can simulate a single-end read data set by discarding the second end from each read in our example data. Crucially, in doing this, we are simulating a single-end data set with the same PCR duplicate proportion as the paired-end data set, because these are the same DNA fragments represented in both. One property of our correction method then is that it should return the same value when applied to each data set in turn.

In Fig. 3, we see that the observed duplicate proportion is indeed substantially higher in the single-end data, and not even highly correlated with the observation in the paired-end data. After applying the correction methods presented here, the estimates show remarkable agreement (also Fig. 3).

A Cancer Sample We have until now been considering "normal" diploid samples, but much interest lies in the study of cancer samples that are not diploid. We will illustrate now the application of this methodology to an OAC sample. Specifically, we consider sequencing library SS6003314 from the same study [1] as the blood and benign tissue samples that have been the examples so far.

SS6003314 appears to be generated from a broadly tetraploid tumour with approximately 74% tumour purity (i.e. 26% of cells in the sample are contaminating normal tissue). While a copy number stage of "AABB" (i.e. two copies of both the paternal and maternal genome) is most frequently observed (Fig. 4, there are noticeable regions with copy numbers ranging from one to six and ranging from balanced to exhibiting loss of heterozygosity (i.e. for a given region, only one of the maternal or paternal genome is present). Importantly for this analysis, there are regions present with inferred copy number state "AB".

So long as the SNP loci selected are from regions with the same copy number, and are balanced, then we can apply the methods outlined in this paper. For this

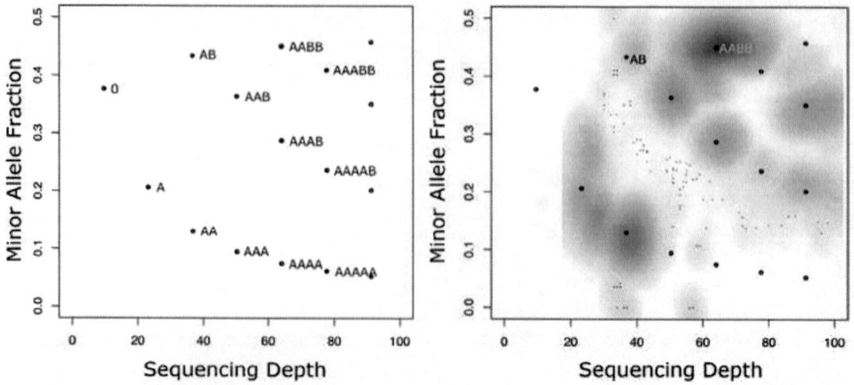

Fig. 4 **Left**: Illustrating the expected patterns to be seen when plotting minor allele frequency against sequencing depth for a sample that is 74% tumour. Genomic regions that, in the tumour, share the same copy number state in all cells are expected to appear at the points indicated, and the copy number state associated with each point is annotated. For example, "AAABB" indicates a region of copy number five with three paternal and two maternal copies or vice versa, while "0" indicates regions that are entirely missing in the tumour genome. Note that since the minor allele fraction is bounded at 0.5, the expected value for balanced regions has to be less than this, and the bias is more extreme, the lower the copy number count. **Right**: A scatter plot illustrating the observed relationship between smoothed minor allele fraction and smoothed sequencing depth for sequencing library SS6003314; an oesophageal adenocarcinoma sample with inferred tumour purity of 74%. Darker regions indicate that more of the genome lies at this position. The grid from the left-hand plot is superimposed. Clouds of points lying off the grid may indicate regions of the genome that do not have a common copy number state in all cancer cells, artefacts from the smoothing, or that the tumour purity has been misidentified

Table 1 Reporting the percentage of observed duplicates and the estimated PCR and fragmentation duplicate percentages both for regions of the genome that have copy number pattern "AABB" and those with copy number pattern "AB"

	Observed duplicates (%)	Proportion due to fragmentation	PCR duplicates (%)	Fragmentation duplicates (%)
AABB	3.76	0.047	3.58	0.18
AB	3.68	0.017	3.62	0.06

example, we can apply them independently to the "AB" and "AABB" copy number states. For the "AABB" regions, we have identified 8,396 heterozygous SNPs to use in the analysis, while for the "AB" regions, we have identified 759.

The results from the analysis in Table 1 show that the inferred proportion of duplicates due to fragmentation is still, for this data set, low at a copy number of four. Therefore, the duplicate proportions are similar before and after correction and also when comparing "AABB" and "AB" regions. While still small, the proportion of duplicates due to fragmentation did increase going from "AB" to "AABB".

Note that the likelihood models presented here could be extended to any copy number state where both alleles are present, but (a) this is more complicated and (b) most cases have a region that can be identified as balanced. Note also that even if the assignment of copy number states was wrong (perhaps we have actually been considering regions that were "AABB" and "AAABBB"), we are not affected, because all we have made use of is the knowledge that the regions were balanced.

4 Effects on the Estimation of DNA Copy Number

While the effects of copy number may sometimes be minimal when comparing diploid and tetraploid genomes, there are circumstances in considering duplicate proportions when it is important to distinguish DNA copy number and depth of sequencing coverage despite the linear relationship we anticipate (as in Fig. 4).

Local to a region of constant copy number, the PCR duplicate proportion will be trivially linked to the depth of coverage since duplicate sequences count towards that coverage, and if fewer than two reads are present, then there cannot be a duplicate. There may also be factors such as GC content that have the potential to influence both properties locally within a genome. Beyond this, there is no reason to expect the PCR duplicate proportion to vary with copy number. The variation of our observed duplicate proportion with copy number we then attribute to the fragmentation duplicates.

At high values, it is clear that the depth of sequencing will drive the proportion of fragmentation duplicates we see. There are only a finite number of positions in which sequencing read-pairs can be positioned and that there must be a depth of coverage, beyond which all additional reads will be classed as duplicates. That is, we achieve saturation, and there is a depth beyond which our sequencing will reveal only additional duplicates. Consequently, if we remove duplicates from an analysis, we place an artificial threshold on the copy number we can call. Moreover, as one approaches that threshold, reads will be classed as duplicates more frequently. Depth of sequencing for a region of the genome will depend on the DNA copy number locally (as shown in Fig. 4) and the overall number of sequences generated for the sample.

For a given DNA copy number, there are three key aspects of the sequencing that determine the numbers of reads that are lost after being classed as fragmentation duplicates. These are as follows: (a) The depth of sequencing associated with a region of copy number one: More depth is generally a good thing in sequencing experiments, but leads us to problems with fragmentation duplicates sooner. (b) The standard deviation (or more generally the distribution) of the fragment sizes: Less variable fragment lengths are conceptually useful for identifying some types of structural variant, but increase the numbers of fragment duplicates. (c) The lengths of the sequencing reads: For most purposes, it is beneficial that these are long, and minimizing fragmentation duplicates is no exception.

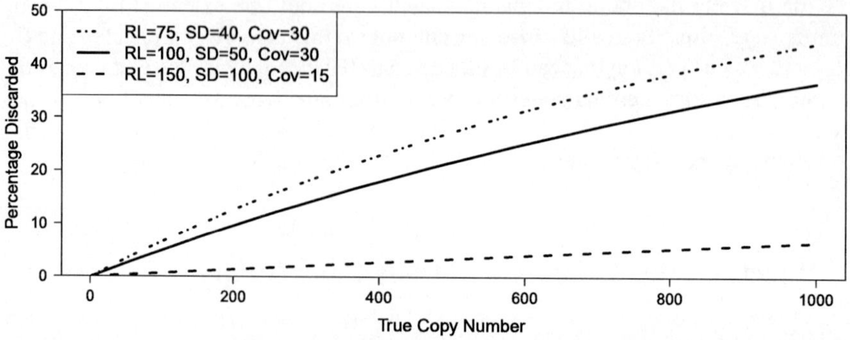

Fig. 5 Showing the percentages of reads incorrectly discarded due to being identified as fragmentation duplicates under three simulation schemes. The parameters varied are read length (RL), standard deviation of the fragment lengths (SD), and depth of coverage for a region of copy number one (Cov)

If we simulate some not-unrealistic data, where the sequencing coverage associated with one copy of DNA is 30 reads (achieved using paired-end 100 base pair (bp) reads and a DNA fragment length standard deviation of 50, and with no PCR duplicates), then we see that the removal of duplicates (all due to fragmentation) has an increasingly large effect as the copy number increases. At moderate copy numbers, taking a copy number of 2 as the baseline, there is little effect—regions of copy number 8 for example will be estimated to have a copy number of 7.98 in these conditions. A true copy number of 50 would be estimated to be 49, 100 would be estimated to be 96, 500 would be estimated to be 410, and a copy number of 1000 would be estimated to be 686. This "compression" of observed copy numbers in high-copy-number-states will naturally result in increased uncertainty in the inference of true copy number, even before saturation is reached.

In Fig. 5, we show the percentages of reads that are lost through being fragmentation duplicates for three simulated examples. One example matches the scenario given above where the parameters provide an approximation to our real data. The second example is a more extreme case with shorter reads and a tighter distribution of insert sizes, while the third shows the effect for a case with longer reads, more variable fragment length, but lower coverage per DNA copy (perhaps because the sample being studied is tetraploid not diploid). From this figure, we can see that the effects can vary from extreme to possibly ignorable.

Although most of the genome is of a copy number where these effects are small, it is worth noting that (a) the PCR duplicate proportion is also small, and the effect on this (and downstream characteristics such as inferred sequencing library size) can be considerable, (b) that only a small region of the genome at very high copy number can greatly increase the number of fragmentation duplicates present in samples, and (c) the inference of copy number states can sometimes be finely balanced between multiple credible solutions, and any discrepancy between the assumptions of the model and the true nature of the data could affect the proffered solution.

5 The Estimation of Mitochondrial DNA Copy Number

Mitochondria are organelles within a cell that contain their own small (∼17 kB) genome (mtDNA). There will be many mitochondria within a cell and each can have several copies of the mtDNA. Thus, the mtDNA is expected to be present in a cell at a high copy number.

That different cell types have different mtDNA copy numbers has been known for nearly half a century [7] and "next-generation" sequencing data have been used to investigate this since the early days of the technology using targeted sequencing [8] or WGS [9]. A review of the changes in mtDNA copy number in cancers of various tissues highlights the potential importance of this quantity and also highlights the range of copy numbers that are possible (0–100,000) [10]. A recent pan-cancer analysis of over 2000 tumour samples estimated values from 8 in a pancreatic cancer to > 1750 in a cancer originating in the central nervous system [11].

Clearly then, we can be of an order of copy number where the saturation effects described above could have an effect, in underestimating the mtDNA copy number.

5.1 *PCAWG Copy Number*

Assuming that appropriate measures of coverage for the nuclear genome and mitochondrial genome can be identified, the recent Pan Cancer Analysis of Whole Genomes (PCAWG) survey of mitochondrial changes in cancer [11] used the following approach for the estimation of mtDNA copy number (mtDNA-CN):

$$\text{mtDNA-CN}_{\text{tumour}} = \frac{\text{mtDNA coverage}}{\text{nuclear coverage}} \times \text{mean nuclear copy number} \tag{6}$$

where the mean nuclear copy number is defined as

$$f \times \text{`Tumour mean nuclear copy number'} + (1 - f) \times 2,$$

f being the proportion of tumour within the sample.

Tumour Purity We note that the term

$$\frac{\text{nuclear coverage}}{\text{mean nuclear copy number}}$$

is simply a measure of the coverage per copy number, and while it has been calculated taking into account the tumour purity, when we rearrange Eq. 6, it becomes clear that there is no further correction for tumour purity in the mitochondrial copy number:

$$\text{mtDNA-CN}_{\text{tumour}} = \frac{\text{mtDNA coverage}}{\text{coverage per copy number}}. \tag{7}$$

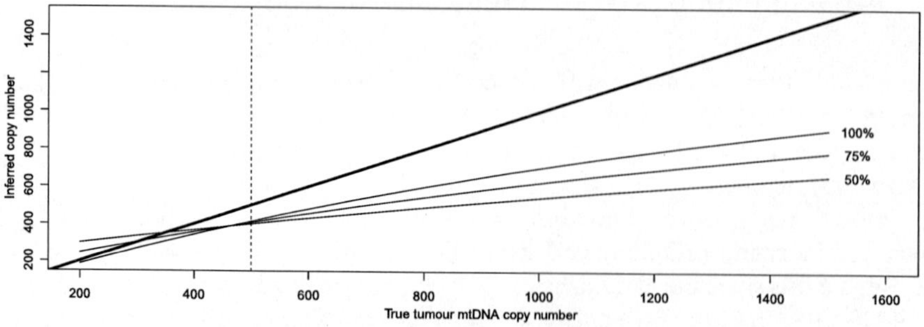

Fig. 6 Showing how the effect of removing duplicates can quickly outstrip the effect of impurity in the sample. For a range of true tumour mtDNA-CN values and a fixed mtDNA-CN of 500 for contaminating benign tissue (indicated with a vertical dotted line), three curves are depicted for the copy number inferred from simulation with three different levels of tumour purity. A line of agreement is shown in bold for contrast

Thus, the estimated mtDNA copy number is that averaged over the tumour and contaminating benign tissue. This is natural if, as is often the case, the mtDNA copy number for benign tissue is not known (unlike for the nuclear genome where the copy number for benign tissue can be assumed to be 2), but since it has long been known that mtDNA copy number can differ between malignant and benign tissue [12], trends between estimated mtDNA copy number and tumour purity would seem inevitable.

In particular, the tumour mtDNA-CN will be shrunk towards the benign value. A process that accentuates any bias due to duplicate removal if the mtDNA-CN is higher in the tumour than surrounding benign tissue, but may apparently compensate for it if the mtDNA-CN is lower. Nevertheless, in that scenario, the two competing biases cannot be relied upon to "cancel out" (Fig. 6). These two effects clearly have the potential to mask or reduce the differences in mtDNA-CN observed between groups.

Consideration of Duplicates It seems clear that in calculating the ratio of coverages in Eq. 6, duplicates should either be retained in both numerator and denominator, or duplicates should be removed from both numerator and denominator. Early examples of research into mitochondria using sequencing technologies retained the duplicates [8, 13, 14], but many more recent investigations have been secondary analyses. It is almost certainly the case that reported values pertaining to the nuclear genome will have been calculated after removing duplicates and revisiting an entire WGS data set to recalculate values for the nuclear genome will be costly. Therefore, it may be more convenient to remove duplicates from both numerator and denominator, as indeed appears to have been done in the recent pan-cancer characterization [11] and in other studies.

5.2 *An Approach to Correct the Estimate of mtDNA Copy Number*

The problem with removing duplicates in both denominator and numerator is that it is only the PCR duplicates that we would wish to remove, and we have seen that while the contribution of fragmentation duplicates will have minimal effect on the nuclear genome calculations, it will have a potentially great effect on the mitochondrial calculations (Fig. 6).

Assuming that we do not wish to pay the cost of reanalysing the complete data set, then we are typically in the position of having the nuclear coverage with PCR and fragmentation duplicates removed, and mitochondrial coverage with PCR and fragmentation duplicates removed. For little cost, it is possible to extract and reprocess the mitochondrial-mapping sequences, while applying the methods of this paper to the nuclear genome.

We are then left with observations of the nuclear coverage with PCR and fragmentation duplicates removed, an estimate of the corresponding fragmentation duplicate proportion, an estimate of the PCR duplicate proportion, and the observed mitochondrial coverage with no duplicates removed. From these, it is clearly possible to obtain an estimate either of the ratio of coverages with no duplicates removed, or the ratio of coverages with PCR duplicates removed.

Note that the fragmentation duplicate proportion in the mitochondrial genome cannot be estimated directly using our methods due to the lack of heterozygous SNPs in the mtDNA. Note also that in many cases, the correction of the nuclear genome with the nuclear fragmentation duplicate proportion will have minimal effect and might be dropped for even greater computational simplicity.

5.3 *Example*

We contrast the mtDNA-CN calculated with duplicates removed with a corrected estimate for our example data in Fig. 7. In this figure, we can see that not only are the absolute values of mtDNA-CN poorly estimated if all duplicates are removed, but the general reduction in copy number will shrink differences between groups, making comparisons less powerful (although a contrast as striking as blood versus tissue still shows a clear difference).

In calculating the coverages, we have assumed that the alignment process was well-behaved and that there are minimal biases—enabling a natural measure of coverage to be used. Note also that since these are benign samples, we do not need to worry about tumour purity or ploidy in the calculations.

Applying the method to cancer samples is only marginally trickier, but as previously mentioned, the inference of nuclear copy number can often present multiple credible solutions. For example, distinguishing between a copy number of 2 and a high tumour purity and a copy number of 4 and lower tumour purity can sometimes

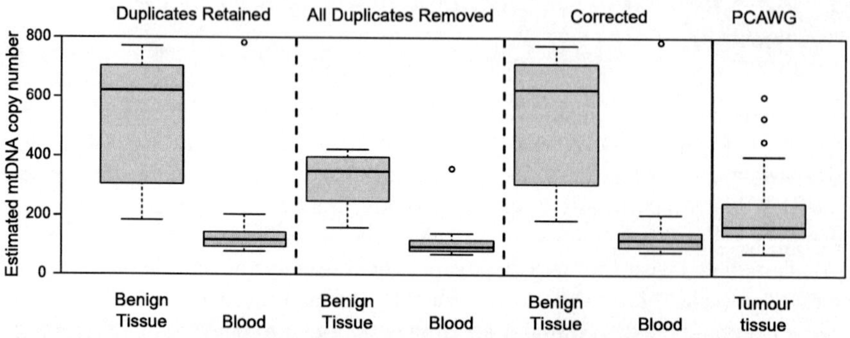

Fig. 7 Showing estimates of mtDNA-CN in the gold standard scenario that no duplicates (excepting optical duplicates) are removed from either coverage estimate, the scenario that all duplicates are removed, and then also estimates corrected using the approach described above. For comparison, the estimates for OAC tumour tissue recently reported [11] are also shown

be nearly impossible (consider sequencing a sample immediately following a nuclear genome doubling event). It should be noted that such uncertainty will naturally lead to a reciprocal change in the inferred mtDNA copy number, and so uncertainty in the nuclear copy number is something of which one should be aware. Although the ranges of mtDNA copy number for a cancer type typically range by more than a factor of two, the inferred mtDNA copy number may be a tool for distinguishing between competing nuclear copy number solutions.

6 Conclusions

We have set out a framework for estimating the PCR duplicate proportion in a WGS library. This we have argued from basic principles, but have also demonstrated to provide sensible and consistent results. We have updated our software [5], better to make these methods available. Our approach relies on being able to identify a subset of the genome where the PCR duplicate to fragmentation duplicate ratio is constant (i.e. regions of constant copy number state), and we require knowledge of the minor allele fraction (which should preferably be 0.5).

Should we not know the true minor allele fraction or should the number of cells being sequenced be such that removing one DNA fragment greatly changes the minor allele fraction, then these methods will be biased. For all reasonable experimental scenarios, their application would still be an improvement over attributing the basic observed duplicate proportion to be the PCR duplicate proportion.

There are implications too for quality control metrics that rely on the PCR duplicate proportion, e.g. sequencing library complexity. Complexity is an important metric, allowing comparison with previously sequenced libraries in order to detect out-of-control library preparation [15]. It also predicts the value of generating further sequencing from a sample, making it invaluable for experimental design (especially adaptive designs), and will be underestimated if fragmentation duplicates are not corrected for.

We have also shown that the estimation of DNA copy number is affected by the removal of fragmentation duplicates and that regions of high copy number can be severely affected. Additionally, we have demonstrated a computationally effective way to make corrections when the copy number estimation is a secondary analysis on WGS data for which duplicates have been removed.

Appendix 1: Proof That $K = (\sum_j \nu_j)!/\prod_j \nu_j!$

The proof of Eq. 5 is by induction.

1.1 The Base Case ($M = 2$)

If $M = 2$, we either have the case where two fragments have been observed from the same starting molecule (and so $\nu_2 = 1,\ \nu_j = 0$ for all $j > 2$), or we have the right-hand case where one fragment is observed from each of two original molecules (and so $\nu_1 = 2$, $\nu_j = 0$ for all $j > 1$). In the first case, $K = 1!/1! = 1$ and in the second $K = 2!/2! = 1$ as required.

1.2 The Assumption ($M = G - 1$, $G > 2$)

For typographical convenience, we write $\nu_+ = \sum_j \nu_j$ in what follows. We assume that, for all partitions where $M = G - 1$, the relationship

$$K = \nu_+! \,/ \prod_j \nu_j! \tag{8}$$

holds.

1.3 The Inductive Step ($M = G$)

We assume that our partition of G duplicates is represented by the vector (ν_1, ν_2, ν_3, ...). We view the set of G duplicates as having arisen from a set of $G - 1$ fragments and then sequencing one more. We must distinguish between the two cases: (1) where the new duplicate in the set is the first from a previously unseen molecule (only possible if $\nu_1 > 0$), and (2) where the new duplicate is a further PCR duplicate from a previously seen molecule.

Case 1: A New Molecule If we have observed a new molecule with our Gth fragment, then the previous set of $G - 1$ duplicates must have been represented by the vector $(\nu_1 - 1, \nu_2, \nu_3, ...)$. Clearly, this is only possible if $\nu_1 > 0$ and, since observing a new molecule in this situation will always result in our observed partition, the full coefficient is inherited from the previous set (there will of course be a factor of F_D as well).

Hence, the contribution to a from this case is

$$\frac{\mathbb{I}(\nu_1 > 0)\,(\nu_+ - 1)!}{(\nu_1 - 1)!\prod_{j>1} \nu_j!} \tag{9}$$

where $\mathbb{I}()$ is the indicator function.

Case 2: A PCR Duplicate from a Previously Observed Molecule In this case, the previous set of $G - 1$ duplicates must have been represented by the vector $(..., \nu_{k-1} + 1, \nu_k - 1, ...)$ for some k such that $\nu_k > 0$ and $k > 1$.

The coefficient, K', associated with that vector is

$$K' = \frac{\mathbb{I}(\nu_k > 0)\,\nu_+!}{(\nu_{k-1} + 1)!\,(\nu_k - 1)!\prod_{j \notin k,(k-1)} \nu_j!}$$

but a new PCR duplicate added to that set might create patterns other than the one in which we are interested, so only a portion of the coefficient makes a contribution to our estimate of K. It would only have led to our observed pattern if the PCR duplicate had been of a molecule of which there previously existed $k - 1$ copies. The fraction of the coefficient, K', that contributes to our value of K (not withstanding a factor P_D) is therefore the proportion of molecules of which there were previously $k - 1$ copies: $(\nu_{k-1} + 1)\,/\nu_+$.

The additive contribution to K for this value of k is therefore

$$\frac{(\nu_{k-1} + 1)}{\nu_+}\frac{\mathbb{I}\,(\nu_k > 0)\nu_+!}{(\nu_{k-1} + 1)!\,(\nu_k - 1)!\prod_{j \notin k,(k-1)} \nu_j!}$$

and in total the contributions from this second case are

$$\sum_{k>1}\left(\frac{(\nu_{k-1} + 1)}{\nu_+}\frac{\mathbb{I}(\nu_k > 0)\nu_+!}{(\nu_{k-1} + 1)!\,(\nu_k - 1)!\prod_{j \notin k,(k-1)} \nu_j!}\right). \tag{10}$$

Combining The Two Cases. If we combine the terms from the two cases as represented by expressions (9) and (10), then we get

$$K = \frac{\mathbb{I}(\nu_1 > 0)\,(\nu_+ - 1)!}{(\nu_1 - 1)!\prod_{j>1}\nu_j!} + \sum_{k>1}\left(\frac{(\nu_{k-1}+1)}{\nu_+}\frac{\mathbb{I}(\nu_k > 0)\,\nu_+!}{(\nu_{k-1}+1)!\,(\nu_k - 1)!\prod_{j\notin k,(k-1)}\nu_j!},\right)$$

which we can simplify by removing the terms in the first fraction on the right-hand side to get

$$K = \frac{\mathbb{I}(\nu_1 > 0)\,(\nu_+ - 1)!}{(\nu_1 - 1)!\prod_{j>1}\nu_j!} + \sum_{k>1}\left(\frac{\mathbb{I}(\nu_k > 0)\,(\nu_+ - 1)!}{(\nu_{k-1})!\,(\nu_k - 1)!\prod_{j\notin k,(k-1)}\nu_j!}\right)$$

and this can be tidied to

$$K = \frac{\mathbb{I}(\nu_1 > 0)\,(\nu_+ - 1)!}{(\nu_1 - 1)!\prod_{j>1}\nu_j!} + \sum_{k>1}\left(\frac{\mathbb{I}(\nu_k > 0)\,(\nu_+ - 1)!}{(\nu_k - 1)!\prod_{j\neq k}\nu_j!},\right).$$

Adjusting the products to be independent of 1 and k, we get

$$K = \frac{\mathbb{I}(\nu_1 > 0)\,(\nu_+ - 1)!\,\nu_1!}{(\nu_1 - 1)!\prod_{j}\nu_j!} + \sum_{k>1}\left(\frac{\mathbb{I}(\nu_k > 0)\,(\nu_+ - 1)!\,\nu_k!}{(\nu_k - 1)!\prod_{j}\nu_j!}\right).$$

Tidying up the other terms,

$$K = \frac{\mathbb{I}(\nu_1 > 0)\,(\nu_+ - 1)!\,\nu_1}{\prod_{j}\nu_j!} + \sum_{k>1}\left(\frac{\mathbb{I}(\nu_k > 0)\,(\nu_+ - 1)!\,\nu_k}{\prod_{j}\nu_j!}\right).$$

We can now combine everything into one sum over k:

$$K = \sum_{k}\left(\frac{\mathbb{I}(\nu_k > 0)\,(\nu_+ - 1)!\,\nu_k}{\prod_{j}\nu_j!}\right).$$

Moving the terms that are independent of k out of the sum,

$$K = \frac{(\nu_+ - 1)!}{\prod_{j}\nu_j!}\sum_{k}(\nu_k\mathbb{I}(\nu_k > 0)) = \frac{(\nu_+ - 1)!}{\prod_{j}\nu_j!}\,\nu_+,$$

whence

$$K = \frac{\nu_+!}{\prod_{j}\nu_j!}$$

as was to be shown.

Appendix 2: Data Availability

The raw data are archived in the European Genome-Phenome Archive [EGA: EGAD00001000704]. Processed data and code to generate these values, alongside code to reproduce the figures in this text, have been added to the GitHub repository containing the `fragmentationDuplicates` R Package [16].

Appendix 3: OCCAMS Consortium

For membership of the OCCAMS Consortium, see [17].

References

1. Weaver, J.M.J., Ross-Innes, C.S., Shannon, N., Lynch, A.G., Forshew, T., et al.: Ordering of mutations in preinvasive disease stages of esophageal carcinogenesis. Nat. Genet. **46**(8), 837–843 (2014)
2. Li, H., Durbin, R.: Fast and accurate short read alignment with burrows-wheeler transform. Bioinformatics **25**(14), 1754–1760 (2009)
3. Broad Institute.: Picard toolkit (2019). https://broadinstitute.github.io/picard/
4. Zhou, W., Chen, T., Zhao, H., Eterovic, A.K., Meric-Bernstam, F., et al.: Bias from removing read duplication in ultra-deep sequencing experiments. Bioinformatics **30**(8), 1073–1080 (2014)
5. Lynch, A., Smith, M., Eldridge, M., Tavaré, S.: Duplicates (2016). https://github.com/dralynch/duplicates
6. Bansal, V.: A computational method for estimating the PCR duplication rate in DNA and RNA-seq experiments. BMC Bioinform. **18**(S3) (2017)
7. Bogenhagen, D., Clayton, D.: The number of mitochondrial deoxyribonucleic acid genomes in mouse l and human hela cells. Quantitative isolation of mitochondrial deoxyribonucleic acid. J. Biol. Chem. **249**(24), 7991–7995 (1974)
8. Vasta, V., Ng, S.B., Turner, E.H., Shendure, J., Hahn, S.H.: Next generation sequence analysis for mitochondrial disorders. Genome Med. **1**(10), 1–10 (2009)
9. Castle, J.C., Biery, M., Bouzek, H., Xie, T., Chen, R., et al.: DNA copy number, including telomeres and mitochondria, assayed using next-generation sequencing. BMC Genomics **11**(1), 244 (2010)
10. S. Meng and J. Han, "Mitochondrial DNA copy number alteration in human cancers," *North American Journal of Medicine and Science*, vol. 6, no. 1, 2013
11. Yuan, Y., Ju, Y.S., Kim, Y., Li, J., Wang, Y., et al.: Comprehensive molecular characterization of mitochondrial genomes in human cancers. Nat. Genet. **52**(3), 342–352 (2020)
12. Heddi, A., Faure-Vigny, H., Wallace, D.C., Stepien, G.: Coordinate expression of nuclear and mitochondrial genes involved in energy production in carcinoma and oncocytoma. Biochimica et Biophysica Acta (BBA)—Molecular Basis of Disease **1316**(3), 203–209 (1996)
13. Calvo, S.E., Compton, A.G., Hershman, S.G., Lim, S.C., Lieber, D.S., et al.: Molecular diagnosis of infantile mitochondrial disease with targeted next-generation sequencing. Sci. Transl. Med. **4**(118) (2012)
14. Lindberg, J., Mills, I.G., Klevebring, D., Liu, W., Neiman, M., et al.: The mitochondrial and autosomal mutation landscapes of prostate cancer. Eur. Urol. **63**(4), 702–708 (2013)

15. Guo, Y., Ye, F., Sheng, Q., Clark, T., Samuels, D.C.: Three-stage quality control strategies for DNA re-sequencing data. Brief. Bioinform. **15**(6), 879–889 (2013)
16. Lynch, A., Smith, M., Eldridge, M., Tavaré, S.: FragmentationDuplicates: R package (2022). https://github.com/dralynch/duplicates
17. Frankell, A.M., Jammula, S., Li, X., Contino, G., Killcoyne, S., et al.: The landscape of selection in 551 esophageal adenocarcinomas defines genomic biomarkers for the clinic. Nat. Genet. **51**(3), 506–516 (2019)

A Retrospective Study on Obstructive Sleep Apnea

Ricardo São João, Andreia Cardoso, Tiago Dias Domingues, Marta Fradinho, Vânia Silva, and Amélia Feliciano

Abstract Obstructive sleep apnea (OSA) is a sleep-related breathing disorder with worldwide increasing prevalence. Polysomnography is the traditional gold standard for the diagnosis of OSA, but the fact that it is a complex, time-consuming, and expensive test contributes to the underdiagnosis of this pathology. For this reason, one usually opts for the simpler, less labor-intensive, and cheaper cardiorespiratory sleep test for the diagnosis of this syndrome. The manual analysis of these tests, which usually involves two or more qualified observers, is one of the aspects that most contributes to the amount of time spent in the analysis and, consequently, to diagnostic delay. Automatic analysis emerges as a faster alternative to the manual analysis. Based on a sample of 2559 patients monitored by the Pulmonology Department—Sleep Unit of the Hospital da Luz Setúbal during the period 2011–2019, this research concludes that there is no agreement between the manual and automatic readings of two popular OSA classification indexes.

Keywords Automatic reading · Association measures · Concordance measures · Manual reading · OSA

R. São João (✉) · T. D. Domingues
Polytechnic Institute of Santarém, Complexo Andaluz, Ap. 295, 2001-904 Santarém, Portugal
e-mail: ricardo.sjoao@esg.ipsantarem.pt

CEAUL, Faculdade de Ciências, Universidade de Lisboa, Lisbon, Portugal

A. Cardoso · M. Fradinho · V. Silva
Hospital da Luz Setúbal, Setúbal, Portugal

A. Feliciano
Lusíadas Cluster Clinics & Trofa Saúde Loures/Amadora, Loures, Portugal

R. Bispo et al. (eds.), *Recent Developments in Statistics and Data Science*,
Springer Proceedings in Mathematics & Statistics 398,
https://doi.org/10.1007/978-3-031-12766-3_19

1 Introduction

Sleep has multiple functions, from preventing multiple diseases (cardiovascular, metabolic, neurological, psychiatric), contributing to the body's immune response and weight regulation to the consolidation of memory and learning and physical recovery for daily life activities. Thus, when sleep is insufficient or of poor quality, there is an alteration in the entire homeostasis of the body with consequences on daily activities and quality of life, as well as at the systemic level, increasing the propensity for certain diseases and aggravating pre-existing ones [1]. Sometimes breathing pauses occur during sleep, reflecting a pathology called sleep apnea. According to the International Classification of Sleep Disorders (ICSD-3), sleep apnea can be classified into two main groups: obstructive sleep apnea and central sleep apnea [2]. OSA is a frequent sleep-related breathing disorder that can be present at any age. It is characterized by recurrent episodes of partial collapse (hypopnea) or complete collapse (apnea) of the upper airway during sleep and translates to changes in the quality of sleep and daily life [3]. OSA is a very heterogeneous disease, resulting from the interaction between different pathophysiological mechanisms, anatomical characteristics, genetic and environmental factors resulting in diverse clinical manifestations.

The prevalence of OSA is estimated to be 4–6% in men and 2–3% in women, values that may, however, be underestimated. There are data that indicate a significant increase in prevalence of OSA in the last 20 years, partly related to the increase in the prevalence of obesity [3]. In Portugal, the prevalence of OSA is not known. Considering the data from Spain, it is observed a high prevalence corresponding to moderate/severe disease (82.4%) [4]. As the Spanish population is demographically similar to the Portuguese, specialists believe that the prevalence of OSA may be identical. Currently, OSA is considered a public health problem, not only due to the associated comorbidities, but also due to the risk of traffic and work accidents resulting from poor and/or insufficient sleep quality.

The gold standard sleep exam for evaluating sleep apnea is polysomnography (PSG), which is a time-consuming exam. The cardiorespiratory studies (manual scoring) are simpler exams that are indicated in patients who have a higher suspicion and probability of having this disease. However, these exams are also time-consuming. The aim of this study is to evaluate if the manual scoring of cardiorespiratory exams could be replaced by automatic scoring. Previous studies have already confirmed that cardiorespiratory studies are inferior in terms of diagnosis comparing to PSG. PSG is a more complete test than the cardiorespiratory test, as it comprehends the analysis of a greater number of physiological variables. In this way, the time spent in the analysis of the PSG test is always higher than the one spent in the analysis of the cardiorespiratory test. In addition, because the PSG allows for a much more comprehensive diagnosis than the cardiorespiratory test it is substantially more costly. A patient with a negative cardiorespiratory study should perform a PSG. In this article, we can suggest to compare with the gold standard (PSG), but we already know that cardiorespiratory exams are inferior in terms of diagnosis comparing to PSG.

OSA diagnosis as well as its treatment depends on the Apnea Hypopnea Index (AHI) classification, i.e., the average number of apneas and hypopneas per hour of sleep [5, 6]. The AHI classification can be made by a manual analysis (performed by the physician) or in an automatic way using specific software [7–9]. The manual analysis, although more reliable, is a very time-consuming method that contributes to OSA being an underdiagnosed pathology worldwide. Several studies have been performed in order to verify the effectiveness of automatic analysis of sleep studies in OSA diagnosis with the performance of the two methods varying [7, 10, 11]. The severity of sleep apnea is based on AHI and also on the oxygen desaturation index (ODI). ODI is defined as the number of episodes of oxygen desaturation per hour of sleep, with oxygen desaturation defined as a decrease in blood oxygen saturation (SpO2) to lower than 3% or 4% below clinical baseline. As ODI is an important parameter in assessing the severity of OSA, its manual and automatic readings were also considered in this study. Another factor that contributes to the onset of OSA is obesity which is considered in this study [12].

This study is a retrospective observational study based on patient data from the Sleep Unit of Hospital da Luz Setúbal (Portugal). Here, we intend to compare: (i) the agreement between the AHI and ODI manual and automatic readings; and (ii) OSA diagnosis based on the automatic readings to OSA diagnosis based on the manual readings, which are taken in this study as gold standard.

2 Data

The data under analysis is based on a sample of 2979 patients monitored by the Sleep Unit of the Pulmonology Department of Hospital da Luz, Setúbal, during the period 2011–2019 and refers to: age (in years), sex, Body Mass Index (BMI), and manual and automatic readings of AHI and ODI. As eligibility criteria for statistical analysis, we consider only the records of users who had complete information in terms of the values of the manual and automatic readings of AHI and ODI, which resulted in a final sample with 2559 records, i.e., a reduction of 14.13%. These patients were submitted to type-III cardiorespiratory sleep tests with the manual readings of AHI and ODI being performed by two physicians and the automatic readings of these indexes obtained from the Embla RemLogic Software [13]. The study was authorized by the hospital's ethics committee.

3 Statistical Analysis

Considering the aim of the study, an association analysis between the two reading methods was performed using the χ^2 test of independence and Cramer's V coefficient. The Concordance Correlation Coefficient (CCC) and the Bland–Altman analysis were also used in the agreement analysis of the two reading methods.

3.1 Association Analysis

Automatic and manual reading performance was compared using the Mann-Whitney test for continuous variables. In the case of the apnea-hypopnea index (AHI), data were grouped into class intervals and an association analysis was performed using the χ^2 test for independence. When an association is verified, the Cramer's V coefficient is calculated.

3.2 Agreement Analysis

In addition to the association analysis, one of the objectives of this study is to understand whether manual reading can be replaced by automatic reading, taking into account the subdiagnoses of OSA. In particular, given the possibility of reading the AHI values can be performed by two different techniques (manual vs. automatic) and being the AHI values used in the classification of the diagnosis of OSA (AHI: [0;5[—no apnea; [5;15[—mild apnea; [15;30[—moderate apnea; ≥30—severe apnea) it is relevant to know if these techniques lead to similar results, i.e., if there is an agreement between the readings. Therefore the CCC proposed by Lin was calculated as well as the Bland–Altman plot reporting both the limits of agreement and the percentage error [14–16].

3.2.1 Concordance Correlation Coefficient of Agreement

The CCC is based on the distance in the plane of the pair of variables relative to the 45° line through the origin, which allows us to evaluate the degree of agreement between two techniques, with manual reading being considered the gold standard. Considering the bivariate Normal random sample $(X_{i1}, X_{i2}),\ i = 1, ..., n$ with means μ_1 and μ_2, respectively, and covariance matrix

$$\begin{pmatrix} \sigma_1^2 & \sigma_{12} \\ \sigma_{21} & \sigma_2^2 \end{pmatrix},$$

the CCC is given by

$$\rho_C = \frac{2\sigma_{12}}{\sigma_1^2 + \sigma_2^2 + (\mu_1 - \mu_2)^2}.$$

The value of ρ_C ranges between -1 and 1 where the value of 1 is interpreted as perfect positive agreement, 0 as no agreement, and -1 as perfect negative agreement. The method of moments is used to estimate the parameters [15, 16]. In addition to assessing the degree of agreement between two readings, the CCC also takes into account the assessment of precision, which is the deviation of observations from the fitted line, but also the measurements of accuracy, which is the deviation of the fitted line from the concordance line [15, 16]. Considering $\widehat{\rho}_C$ the estimator of ρ_C and using the Fisher's Z-transformation to approximate the distribution of $\widehat{\rho}_C$ to the normal distribution, we obtain

$$\widehat{\lambda} = \tanh^{-1}(\widehat{\rho}_C) = \frac{1}{2}\ln\left(\frac{1+\widehat{\rho}_C}{1-\widehat{\rho}_C}\right). \tag{1}$$

The variance of $\widehat{\rho}_C$ is estimated by

$$S^2_{\widehat{\lambda}} = \frac{1}{n-2}\left\{\frac{(1-r^2)\widehat{\rho}^2_C}{(1-\widehat{\rho}^2_C)r^2} + \frac{4\widehat{\rho}^3_C(1-\widehat{\rho}_C)u^2}{r(1-\widehat{\rho}^2_C)^2} - \frac{2\widehat{\rho}^4_C u^4}{r^2(1-\widehat{\rho}^2_C)^2}\right\}, \tag{2}$$

where $u = \frac{|\overline{X}_1 - \overline{X}_2|}{\sqrt{S_1 S_2}}$ and r is the Pearson correlation coefficient. Accordingly with (1) and (2), a $(1-\alpha)\times 100\%$ confidence interval is given by $(\widehat{\lambda} \pm z_{1-\alpha/2} S_{\widehat{\lambda}})$ [15].

3.2.2 Bland–Altman Analysis

The Bland–Altman analysis consists of determining the differences between measurements and the resulting averages of both measurements, information which will subsequently be represented in a two-dimensional graph where it will be possible to identify biases in relation to a pair of measurements used. Let X_{i1} and X_{i2}, $(i = 1, ..., n)$, the measures used in the measurement of a given variable referring to a random sample of n individuals, where X_{i1} represents the value of the gold standard measure in i-individual while X_{i2} represents the alternative measures. The Bland–Altman plot consists in considering the pair $((X_{i1} + X_{i2})/2, diff)$, where $diff = X_{i1} - X_{i2}$. The lower (LL) and upper (UL) limits of agreement are also considered and are calculated as

$$LL = \overline{diff} - z_{(1-\alpha/2)}\sigma_{\overline{diff}}; \quad UL = \overline{diff} + z_{(1-\alpha/2)}\sigma_{\overline{diff}},$$

where, $\overline{diff} = \sum_{i=1}^{n}(X_{i1} - X_{i2})/n$; $\sigma_{\overline{diff}} = \sqrt{\frac{\sum_{i=1}^{n}[(X_{i1}-X_{i2})-\overline{diff}]^2}{n}}$ and $z_{(1-\alpha/2)}$ denotes the $1-\alpha/2$ quantile of the standard normal distribution. A higher level of agreement between the measures used is visible by the distribution of most pairs of observations along the line $y = 0$ or by the overlapping of the lines $y = \overline{diff}$ and $y = 0$. On the other hand, if the observations are located between the two limits of agreement, which are clinically admissible limits, the variable may be measured with any of the measurements. The existence of observations that are outside the limits of agreement indicates deviations of the alternative measure from the gold standard measure, and this difference is more pronounced depending on the higher number of observations outside the recommended limits [17, 18].

A significance level of 0.05 was considered and the data analysis was performed using the R software version 4.0.2 [19].

4 Results

Two thousand, five hundred fifty-nine individuals were retrospectively included. Most patients are male ($n = 1433$; 56%). Table 1 shows some basic characteristics of the sample by sex, namely age (years) and BMI (kg/m^2). The comparisons between genders in relation to the variables age and BMI were made using Mann-Whitney test, where statistically significant differences were identified in age, observing that women presented a higher median value than men.

Since the AHI corresponds to the sum of the number of apneas (pauses in breathing) and hypopneas (periods of shallow breathing) that occur on average per hour, its value allows the severity of OSA to be measured. According to the International Classification of Sleep Disorders (ICSD-3) one of the criteria for the diagnosis of sleep apnea consists of AHI values $\geq$15. A first analysis shows that the automatic reading of the AHI underestimates the diagnosis of OSA. The AHI values more than triple from manual to automatic approach (17.8 *vs.* 5.3; $p < 0.001$). Also, we observe a possible relation between the values of AHI and the two readings (Fig. 1). Figure 1 shows the automatic readings (y-axis) of AHI plotted against the corresponding manual readings (x-axis). The dashed lines represent the threshold AHI values, where, according to the International Classification of Sleep Disorders (ICSD-3), values $\geq$ than 15 represent a diagnosis of OSA. Since we are trying to assess the agreement between the two readings, we would have perfect agreement only if the points in the plot would lie along the line of equality ($y = x$). This is clearly not the case here, with the manual readings showing higher values than the automatic ones, results that are inline with those from the literature [10, 20].

The average manual reading of AHI values was 23.59 ($\pm$19.38) per hour, with distinct values in both genders (male: 27.06 $\pm$ 19.73; female: 19.15 $\pm$ 17.99; $p < 0.001$). The literature corroborates differences in AHI values taking into account gender as well as in the prevalence of OSA itself [21]. OSA prevalence differs between male and female, even more if we consider values of AHI $\geq$ 5 events/hour verses AHI $\geq$ 15 events/hour. Thus, the more reliability of the results obtained through automatic analysis vs manual analysis, the closer to reality will be the difference in prevalence

Table 1 Sample characteristics

	Total ($n = 2559$)	Male ($n = 1433$)	Female ($n = 1126$)	p-value
Age (years)	57.57 $\pm$ 13.03	56.97 $\pm$ 13.26	58.33 $\pm$ 12.69	< 0.001
BMI (kg/m^2)	29.35 $\pm$ 5.32	29.07 $\pm$4.77	29.71$\pm$ 5.94	0.10

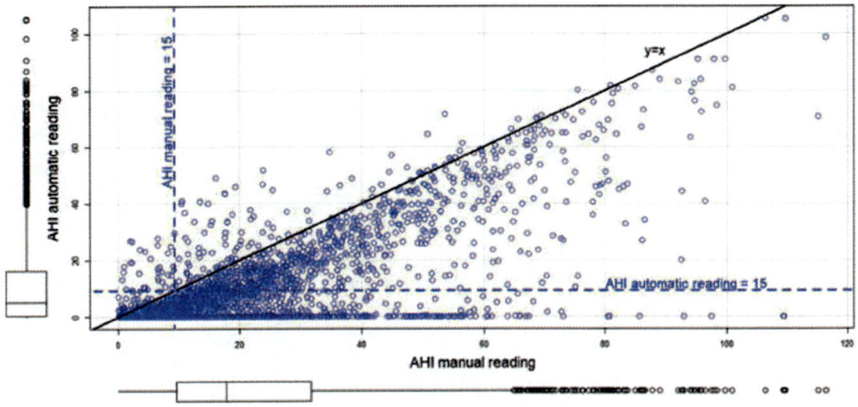

Fig. 1 AHI values for manual (x axis) and automatic (y axis) readings. The solid black line represents the line of equality ($y = x$) and the dashed lines the AHI threshold at which OSA is diagnosed

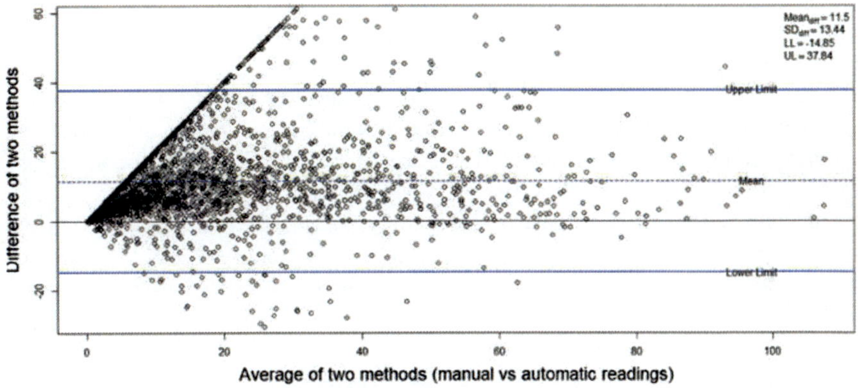

Fig. 2 Bland–Altman's plot depicts a bias in the AHI values comparing manual and automatic readings

between genders. Figure 2 displays the Bland–Altman's plot, which represents the differences between two paired manual and automatic readings against the average of the paired readings. We observe a positive bias ($\overline{diff} = 11.5$), which corroborates that manual AHI readings tend to be higher than the automatic, and that seems to be due to AHI readings above 20 units. Indeed, because the mean of the differences in the measurements is non-zero this indicates an absence of absolute agreement between the measurements, otherwise all pairs of observations would be arranged under the straight line $y = 0$. The existence of observations (163) outside the limits of agreement [−14.84; 37.85] corresponds to about 6.36% (163/2559) of pairs of measurements whose difference exceeds the expected tolerance limits.

Table 2 Number of individuals by OSA severity, type of reading and by AHI values

AHI automatic reading		AHI manual reading			
		[0–5[	[5–15[	[15–30[	≥30
No apnea	[0–5[	241	575	269	158
Mild apnea	[5–15[	17	203	340	53
Moderate apnea	[15–30[	9	28	162	174
Severe apnea	≥30	0	6	18	306

A pertinent issue in clinical practice is the identification of misdiagnoses of OSA based on reading the automatic AHI values. Our attention will focus on the number of patients counted in the AHI class [0-5[with automatic reading. This is justified because values in this class correspond to a diagnosis of absence of OSA. We, therefore, confronted these values with those obtained in the manual reading deserving another classification. 19.39% of the results in the automatic AHI are correct (80.61% of misdiagnosis); 33.12% keep mild sleep apnea; 43.43% keep moderate sleep apnea and 92.73% keep severe sleep apnea (Table 2).

Additionally, it can be seen that the higher the severity of OSA, the greater the agreement between readings. The percentage of concordant classifications in both readings is 35,52%. The chi-square test was used to assess the existence of an association between the two reading classes. We concluded that there was a statistically significant association between the two AHI readings (χ^2= 1427.1, df = 9, $p < 0.001$). Once the existence of a statistically significant association between readings was verified, the intensity of this relationship was measured using the Cramer's V coefficient, whose value was 0.431. The value of the Cramer's V coefficient reveals a very strong association between the readings [22].

Another parameter evaluated was the ODI measurement. In Fig. 3 it can be seen that there is no agreement in the manual and automatic readings of the ODI values, justifying the Bland–Altman and CCC analysis. We observe the existence of statistically significant differences between manual and automatic readings regarding the ODI values (median: 17.7 *vs.* 5.4; $p < 0.001$). Considering the analysis by sex we observe statistically significant differences in both genders (male: 21.1 *vs.* female: 14.1; $p < 0.001$). As with the AHI values in the automatic reading, we observe differences in the ODI values in both genders (male: 6.8 *vs.* female: 4.3; $p < 0.001$). The Bland–Altman's plot (Fig. 4) depicts a bias in the ODI values when comparing the two readings (manual vs. automatic), in line with the conclusions drawn from the analysis of the AHI values. It is verified that the mean of the differences in the measurements is non-zero ($diff = 11.41$) which means an absence of absolute agreement between the measurements indicating that ODI values in manual reading are systematically higher compared to automatic reading. The existence of observations (130) outside the limits of agreement [-10.84;33.66] corresponds to about 5% of pairs of measurements whose difference exceeds the expected tolerance limits.

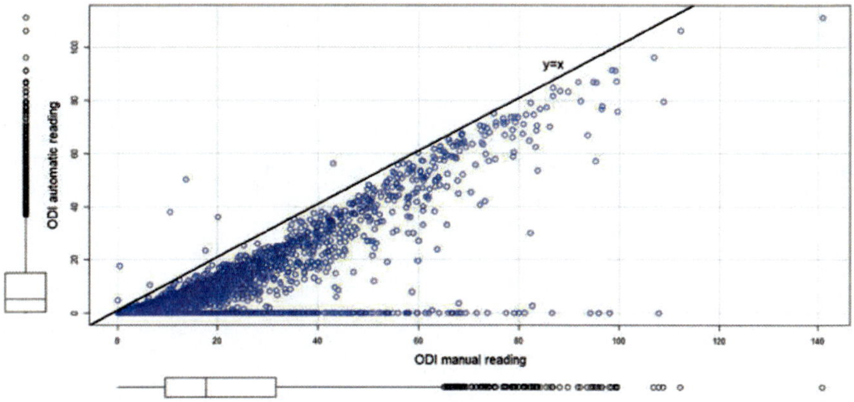

Fig. 3 ODI values for manual (x axis) and automatic (y axis) readings. The solid black line represents the line of equality ($y = x$). There is no fixed threshold for the diagnosis of OSA based on ODI values

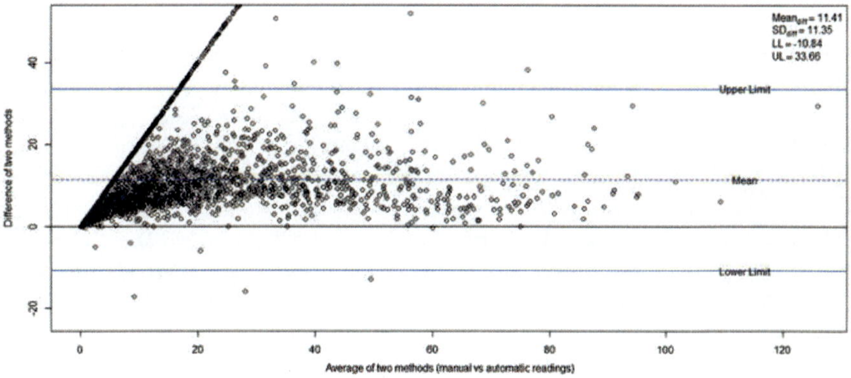

Fig. 4 Bland–Altman's plot depicts a bias in the ODI values comparing manual and automatic readings

In a properly administered exam, the literature points to the AHI and ODI values being positively correlated [23]. Our data further confirms this as one obtains Spearman correlation coefficients r_S of 0.76 and 0.99 for the automatic and manual readings of AHI and ODI, respectively (both association test p-values<0.001). In addition, we observe that the correlation between manual readings of both indexes is higher than the one obtained between automatic readings.

One question that arose naturally in the course of this investigation was whether the automatic reading of AHI and ODI values emerges as a credible alternative to the current gold standard represented by manual reading, which is performed by two clinicians independently. We obtained the Lin's Concordance Correlation Coefficient r_c for AHI reading: $r_c = 0.557$ ($CI_{95\%}^{\rho_c}$: [0.534; 0.578]) while for the ODI was $r_c =$

Table 3 Number of individuals by BMI classes and by AHI values considering the manual reading

BMI classes		AHI manual reading			
		[0–5[	[5–15[	[15-30[	≥30
Low	<18.5	5	5	9	5
Normal	[18.5–25.0[	114	190	81	28
Overweight	[25.0–30.0[	100	386	375	229
Grade I	[30.0–35.0[	36	180	230	264
Grade II	[35.0–40.0[	8	37	68	119
Morbid	≥40	4	14	26	46

0.626 ($CI_{95\%}^{\rho_c}$: [0.599; 0.651]). Given the absence of a high concordance between readings evidenced by both the Bland–Altman analysis and the CCC coefficient, there is a natural need for comparison with a third method, a method recognized as a gold standard. These results revealed that automatic reading alone is not yet an alternative solution to the manual reading [14].

Since obesity is a risk factor for OSA, the BMI was determined for each patient and the following classes and classifications were adopted: < 18.5 (low weight), [18.5–25.0[(normal weight), [25.0–30.0[(overweight), [30.0–35.0[(grade I obesity), [35.0–40.0[(grade II obesity) and ≥ 40 (morbid obesity). We note that the BMI thresholds and classifications considered, are in conformity with those defined by WHO [24] and in line with the guidelines of the National Institute of Health (NIH). Accordingly, we found that 82.3% of the patients ($n = 2122$) are obese or overweight. Further, we observed an association between the BMI and the AHI values obtained from manual reading (Table 3; χ^2= 418.43, df = 15, $p < 0.001$). This association translates into a strong relationship between the two variables by Cramer's V coefficient ($C = 0.233$).

5 Conclusions

OSA is still an underdiagnosed disease and is currently considered a public health problem, not only because of the associated comorbidities but also because of the risk of accidents that result from insufficient and/or poor sleep quality. In order to help prevent these and other possible consequences, it is thus essential to improve upon the accuracy of OSA diagnosis and consequently effectively decide on the adequate type of treatment.

In our study, the AHI values are greater than ODI values independently of the reading method. Also we observed a high correlation between AHI values and ODI values for each technique. Since the severity of OSA is evaluated by the AHI, we can conclude that the automatic analysis, using the Embla Remlogic software, undervalued the diagnosis of the disease. Although there is a significant agreement between automatic and manual analysis when OSA severity is higher (higher AHI), the same is not true for the remaining stages of severity, with a high percentage of patients with falsely normal AHI. So, the greater the severity of OSA the greater the agreement between the analyses (manual and automatic).

Automatic analysis with the Embla RemLogic Software is reliable for the diagnosis of OSA but should still be complemented with manual analysis by qualified professionals, in order to decrease the number of false negative results and thus mitigate the underdiagnosis of OSA via this automated method.

In addition, because manual analysis is time-consuming due to its complexity, any improvement in the algorithm of the software that enhances its accuracy, could help, not only to alleviate the amount of time that is currently spent on manual review, but also to speed up OSA diagnosis and subsequent treatment protocols.

Acknowledgements This study is partially financed by national funds through FCT Fundação para a Ciência e Tecnologia under the project UIDB/00006/2020. We thank the reviewer for all the comments and suggestions that enriched this study.

References

1. Bassetti, C.: Sleep Medicine Textbook. European Sleep Research Society (ESRS), Regensburg, Germany (2021)
2. Sateia, M.J.: International classification of sleep disorders. Chest **146**(5), 1387–1394 (2014)
3. Epstein, L.J., Kristo, D., Strollo, P.J.J., Friedman, N., Malhotra, A., et al.: Adult obstructive sleep apnea task force of the American academy of sleep medicine. Clinical guideline for the evaluation, management and long-term care of obstructive sleep apnea in adults. J. Clin. Sleep Med. **5**(3), 263–276 (2009)
4. Santos, A., Barreto, C., Barata, F., Froes, F., Carvalho, I. et al.: 13° relatório do observatório nacional das doenças respiratórias 2016/2017—panorama das doenças respiratórias em Portugal—retrato da saúde, pp. 84–88 (2018)
5. Shahar, E.: Apnea-hypopnea index: time to wake up. Nature and Science of Sleep, p. 51 (2014)
6. Secretariat, M.A.: Polysomnography in patients with obstructive sleep apnea: an evidence-based analysis. Ont. Health Technol. Assess. Ser. **6**, 1–38 (2006)
7. Valério, M.P., Pereira, S., Moita, J., Teixeira, F., Travassos, C., et al.: Is the nox-t3 device scoring algorithm accurate enough for the diagnosis of obstructive sleep apnea? Adv. Respir. Med. **89**, 262–267 (2021)
8. Kristiansen, S., Traaen, G.M., Øverland, B., Plagemann, T., Gullestad, L. et al.: Comparing manual and automatic scoring of sleep monitoring data from portable polygraphy. J. Sleep Res. 30(2) (2020)
9. Magalang, U.J., Johns, J.N., Wood, K.A., Mindel, J.W., Lim, D.C., et al.: Home sleep apnea testing: comparison of manual and automated scoring across international sleep centers. Sleep and Breathing **23**(1), 25–31 (2018)
10. Park, D.Y., Kim, H.J., Kim, C.-H., Kim, Y.S., Choi, J.H., et al.: Reliability and validity testing of automated scoring in obstructive sleep apnea diagnosis with the embletta x100. Laryngoscope **125**(2), 493–497 (2014)
11. Ernst, G., Bosio, M., Salvado, A., Nogueira, F., Nigro, C., et al.: Comparative study between sequential automatic and manual home respiratory polygraphy scoring using a three-channel device: Impact of the manual editing of events to identify severe obstructive sleep apnea. Sleep Disord. **2015**, 1–5 (2015)

12. Shah, N., Roux, F.: The relationship of obesity and obstructive sleep apnea. Clin. Chest Med. **30**(3), 455–465 (2009)
13. "Embla remlogic psg software."
14. Mahon, G.M.: A proposal for strength-of-agreement criteria for Lin's concordance correlation coefficient, (New Zealand), National Institute of Water & Atmospheric Research Hamilton (2005)
15. Lin, L.I.: A concordance correlation coefficient to evaluate reproducibility. Biometrics **45**, 255–268 (1989)
16. Nickerson, C.A.E.: A note on "a concordance correlation coefficient to evaluate reproducibility". Biometrics **53**(4), 1503 (1997)
17. Karun, K.M., Puranik, A.: `BA.plot`: an R function for Bland–Altman analysis. Clin. Epidemiol. Global Health **12**, 100831 (2021)
18. Bland, J.M., Altman, D.G.: Measuring agreement in method comparison studies. Stat. Methods Med. Res. **8**(2), 135–160 (1999)
19. R Core Team: R: A Language and Environment for Statistical Computing. R Foundation for Statistical Computing, Vienna, Austria (2020)
20. Barreiro, B., Badosa, G., Quintana, S., Esteban, L., Heredia, J.: Comparación entre el análisis automático y manual de la polisomnografía convencional en el diagnóstico del síndrome de apnea-hipopnea obstructiva del sueño. Arch. Bronconeumol. **39**(12), 544–548 (2003)
21. Bonsignore, M.R., Saaresranta, T., Riha, R.L.: Sex differences in obstructive sleep apnoea. Eur. Respir. Rev.: Offic. J. Eur. Respir. Soc. **28** (2019)
22. Akoglu, H.: User's guide to correlation coefficients. Turk. J. Emerg. Med. **18**, 91–93 (2018)
23. Zou, D., Grote, L., Peker, Y., Lindblad, U., Hedner, J.: Validation a portable monitoring device for sleep apnea diagnosis in a population based cohort using synchronized home polysomnography. Sleep **29**(3), 367–374 (2006)
24. Obesity: preventing and managing the global epidemic. report of a who consultation. World Health Organization Technical Report Series, vol. 894, pp. i–xii, 1–253 (2000)

Censored Multivariate Linear Regression Model

Rodney Sousa, Isabel Pereira, and Maria Eduarda Silva

Abstract Often, real-life problems require modelling several response variables together. This work analyses a multivariate linear regression model when the data are censored. Censoring distorts the correlation structure of the underlying variables and increases the bias of the usual estimators. Thus, we propose three methods to deal with multivariate data under left censoring, namely Expectation Maximization (EM), Data Augmentation (DA) and Gibbs Sampler with Data Augmentation (GDA). Results from a simulation study show that both DA and GDA estimates are consistent for low and moderate correlation. Under high correlation scenarios, EM estimates present a lower bias.

Keywords Censored data · Multivariate linear regression

1 Introduction

Linear regression (LR) is one of the most widely used models in Econometrics to analyse the relationship between two sets of variables. Often, real-life problems can be best described by considering several (say $m \geq 2$) correlated response variables, that is, experiments are performed to analyse the variation of m characteristics of the same phenomenon. In these cases, we should consider the multivariate LR model, which is a natural extension of the univariate regression model. An essential aspect of multivariate analysis is the dependence between the different variables, which may involve the covariance between them [1].

R. Sousa (✉) · I. Pereira
Center for Research and Development in Mathematics and Applications, University of Aveiro, Aveiro, Portugal
e-mail: rodney@ua.pt

M. E. Silva
Center for Research and Development in Mathematics and Applications, University of Porto, Porto, Portugal

R. Bispo et al. (eds.), *Recent Developments in Statistics and Data Science*, Springer Proceedings in Mathematics & Statistics 398,
https://doi.org/10.1007/978-3-031-12766-3_20

Additionally, some or all of the response variables can be censored, meaning that they are only accessible in a restricted interval. Censored data can arise for a variety of reasons, such as limitations of the measuring device or of the experimental design [2]. Examples occur in environmental studies where mineral concentration in air/water may be subjected to lower detection limits [3], in Medicine, where [4] studied the relationship between two cytokines (pro-inflammatory and anti-inflammatory) when both variables are censored or in Economics where hours worked is usually treated as censored variable [5]. We might note that in the literature, the terminology censored data is also used in the survival data analysis, in which the variable of interest is the time to an event. In these cases, unexpected interruptions of scheduled experiments create fully missing values or censored survival (or failure time) data. The structure of such data and the censored data described above are quite different and require different statistical techniques for their analysis [6, 7]. Our discussion will focus on the first type of censored data in which the outcome or variable of interest is below (or above) a limit of detection (LOD).

Censoring makes the observed dataset incomplete and therefore direct analysis using standard complete data methods inadequate, resulting in inconsistent estimates. To overcome these issues, a variety of methods have been proposed to handle censored univariate data (see [8–10]). Filling in censored data in order to apply standard complete data methods has a strong intuitive appeal, because this strategy greatly reduces the burden of developing specialized methods and computer code for analysing incomplete data [3].

Methods for creating complete data via filling in censored data can be single imputation (one value for each observation) or multiple imputations. In single imputation, it is common to fill in the censored observation by its expected value, predicted mean or the centre of the detection interval. More statistically sound approaches are based on the EM and DA algorithms [8, 11]. However, the extension of methods to handle censored data in multivariate settings confronts a significant practical barrier. Indeed, there are very few works is this subject [3, 7, 12]. In particular, to the best of our knowledge, there is no specific work in the literature about the censored multivariate linear regression model (CMLR).

Muthén [13] pointed out that, in addition to inconsistent estimates, censoring also distorts the correlation structure of the response variables. Aiming to develop more suitable methods to handle this problem, in this work we propose three methods to estimate CMLR, mainly Expectation Maximization (EM), Data Augmentation (DA) and Gibbs sampler with Data Augmentation (GDA). All of these methods are based on filling in censored data in order to create a complete dataset, which is the most widely used strategy when the data are missing or censored, both in Classical and Bayesian approaches.

The paper is organized as follows: Sect. 2 presents the CMLR model, Sect. 3 analyses three methods to estimate CMLR model, in Sect. 4 we present the simulation study, in which we analyse the accuracy of the proposed methods and, finally, we present some final remarks.

2 Censored Multivariate Linear Regression

In this section, we define the multivariate linear regression model in order to introduce censored multivariate linear regression.

2.1 *The Multivariate Linear Regression Model*

In matrix form, the Multivariate Linear Regression Model (MLR) can be written as follows:

$$\mathbf{W} = \mathbf{X}\beta + \varepsilon, \tag{1}$$

where $\mathbf{W} = [\mathbf{W}_{(1)} \ \dots \ \mathbf{W}_{(m)}]$ is a $n \times m$ matrix of m response variables, $\mathbf{X}$ is a $n \times (k+1)$ matrix of k predictors, whose rows are $\mathbf{x}_i = (1, x_{i1}, \dots, x_{ik})', \ i = 1, \dots, n$, β is a $(k+1) \times m$ coefficients matrix and $\varepsilon = [\varepsilon_{(1)} \ \dots \ \varepsilon_{(m)}]$ is a $n \times m$ matrix of the errors associated with each response variable, where each $\varepsilon_i = (\varepsilon_{i1}, \dots, \varepsilon_{im})', \ i = 1, \dots, n$ is assumed to be iid $m-$variate normal variable with mean $\mathbf{0}$ and $m \times m$ covariance matrix $\boldsymbol{\Sigma} = [\sigma_{ij}]$ [14]. Then, the model (1) may be written as

$$\begin{bmatrix} W_{11} & \dots & W_{1m} \\ \vdots & \ddots & \vdots \\ W_{n1} & \dots & W_{nm} \end{bmatrix} = \begin{bmatrix} 1 & x_{11} & \dots & x_{1k} \\ \vdots & \vdots & \ddots & \vdots \\ 1 & x_{n1} & \dots & x_{nk} \end{bmatrix} \cdot \begin{bmatrix} \beta_{01} & \dots & \beta_{0m} \\ \vdots & \ddots & \vdots \\ \beta_{k1} & \dots & \beta_{km} \end{bmatrix} + \begin{bmatrix} \varepsilon_{11} & \dots & \varepsilon_{1m} \\ \vdots & \ddots & \vdots \\ \varepsilon_{n1} & \dots & \varepsilon_{nm} \end{bmatrix} \tag{2}$$

where $E[\varepsilon_{(j)}] = 0$ and $Cov(\varepsilon_{(i)}, \varepsilon_{(j)}) = \sigma_{ij}\mathbf{I}_n, \sigma_{jj} = \sigma^2, \ i, j = 1, \dots, m$ and $\mathbf{I}_n$ is the $n \times n$ identity matrix. This is the generalization of multiple LR ($m = 1$), where each response variable $\mathbf{W}_{(j)}, \ j = 1, \dots, m$, follows a multiple LR model.

In the MLR model (2), observations from different individuals are uncorrelated, but the errors for different responses of the same individual can be correlated [14]. By using the multivariate model, the covariance of the response variables can be modelled, which is not possible in the case of separate univariate regression models.

2.2 *The Censored Multivariate Linear Regression Model*

Let's assume that the latent variable $\mathbf{W}_i = (W_{i1}, \dots, W_{im})'$ denotes the m multivariate measure on subject $i = 1, \dots, n$, and that each component vector $W_{(j)}$ of the hypothetical multivariate data $\mathbf{W}$ is subjected to left censoring at fixed limit of detection (LOD), $L_j \in \mathbf{R}, \ j = 1, \dots, m$. Rather than $\mathbf{W}_i$, we actually observe $\mathbf{Y}_i = (y_{i1}, \dots, y_{im})'$, where $y_{ij} = \max\{w_{ij}, L_j\}$ and corresponds to the $j-$th record on the subject i, for $i = 1, \dots, n$ [7, 12]. Here we are assuming that the censoring patterns vary across the component vectors, but are fixed within each $W_{(j)}$, for $j = 1, \ldots, m$.

Now, given a dataset $\mathbf{Y} = (\mathbf{y}_1', \ldots, \mathbf{y}_n')'$, each observation $\mathbf{y}_i = (y_{i1}, \ldots, y_{im})'$ of the CMLR model can be defined as follows:

$$\begin{aligned} \mathbf{Y} =&[y_{ij}] = [\max(w_{ij}, L_j)], \;\; i = 1, \ldots, n \text{ and } j = 1, \ldots, m, \\ \mathbf{W} =&\mathbf{X}\boldsymbol{\beta} + \varepsilon. \end{aligned} \tag{3}$$

For simplicity of notation, the remaining of the text focus on the bivariate case, $m = 2$, defined as follows:

Censored Bivariate Linear Regression. We assume that the errors term ε_i, $i = 1, \ldots, n$ has bivariate normal distribution $N_2(\mathbf{0}, \boldsymbol{\Sigma})$, the probability density function (pdf) of the latent variable $\mathbf{W}_i$ is $N_2(\boldsymbol{\beta}'\mathbf{x}_i, \boldsymbol{\Sigma})$ and has the form

$$\begin{aligned} f(W_{i1}, W_{i2}) =& \frac{1}{2\pi\sigma_1\sigma_2\sqrt{1-\rho^2}} \exp\Big\{ -\frac{1}{2(1-\rho^2)} \Big[\Big(\frac{W_{i1} - \mathbf{x}_i'\boldsymbol{\beta}_1}{\sigma_1}\Big)^2 \\ &+ \Big(\frac{W_{i2} - \mathbf{x}_i'\boldsymbol{\beta}_2}{\sigma_2}\Big)^2 - 2\rho \frac{(W_{i1} - \mathbf{x}_i'\boldsymbol{\beta}_1)(W_{i2} - \mathbf{x}_i'\boldsymbol{\beta}_2)}{\sigma_1\sigma_2} \Big] \Big\}, \end{aligned} \tag{4}$$

while the observed $\mathbf{Y}_i$ variable has a bivariate truncated normal distribution, with support $[L_1, \infty] \times [L_2, \infty]$ and pdf

$$f(Y_{i1}, Y_{i2} | W_{i1} \geq L_1, W_{i2} \geq L_2) = \frac{f(W_{i1}, W_{i2})}{P(W_{i1} \geq L_1, W_{i2} \geq L_2)} \times I_{(W_{i1} \geq L_1, W_{i2} \geq L_2)}. \tag{5}$$

Although there are several approaches and methods to estimate CLR in the univariate case, extensions to multivariate settings confront a significant practical barrier. Muthén [13] observed that censoring distorts the correlation structure of the underlying variable and presented results on a general formula for truncation in the standard bivariate normal distributions. Cohen [15] found a maximum likelihood solution for the truncated bivariate normal where the truncation is with respect to only one variable, while Tallis [16] gave general formulas for multivariate truncation from below in the multivariate normal distribution using the moment-generating function.

3 Estimation of CMLR Model

In this section, we propose three methods to estimate the CMLR model, focusing on left-censored bivariate data. All these methods are based on filling in the censored data in order to obtain complete data.

3.1 EM Algorithm for Multivariate Data

The EM (*Expectation Maximization*) algorithm is an iterative method to maximize the expected value of the likelihood function, given the observed data, $\mathbf{Y}$ [11]. In the case of censored bivariate data, the algorithm requires the computation of the expected value of the truncated bivariate variable, in order to fill up the data. If the latent variable $\mathbf{W}_i = (W_{i1}, W_{i2})'$ is left-censored, then the values below the LOD have right-truncated distribution, with expected value given by

$$E[(W_{i1}, W_{i2})'|W_{i1} \leq L_1, W_{i2} \leq L_2] = \\ (E[W_{i1}|W_{i1} \leq L_1, W_{i2} \leq L_2], E[W_{i2}|W_{i1} \leq L_1, W_{i2} \leq L_2])' \tag{6}$$

for $i = 1, \ldots, n$. Using the moment-generating function, Tallis [16] gave general formulas for truncated multivariate multivariate normal distribution. Let $\alpha = P(W_1 \leq L_1, W_2 \leq L_2) = F(L_1, L_2)$ represent the probability that the random variable $\mathbf{W} = (W_1, W_2)'$ takes on a value less than or equal to $\mathbf{L} = (L_1, L_2)'$. Taking $\mu_j = E[W_{(j)}]$, $\eta_j = (W_j - \mu_j)/\sigma_j$ and $\gamma_j = (L_j - \mu_j)/\sigma_j, \quad j = 1, 2$, the probability α can be written as

$$\alpha = P(\eta_1 \leq \gamma_1, \eta_2 \leq \gamma_2), \tag{7}$$

where $\eta_j, \quad j = 1, 2$, are standardized normal variables, truncated at $\gamma = (\gamma_1, \gamma_2)$. Thus, we can write

$$\alpha = \Phi(\gamma; \mathbf{R}), \tag{8}$$

where

$$\mathbf{R} = \begin{bmatrix} 1 & \rho \\ \rho & 1 \end{bmatrix} \tag{9}$$

is the correlation matrix with $\rho = corr(\eta_1, \eta_2)$ [16] and the expected value of the truncated standardized bivariate variable, $\boldsymbol{\eta} = (\eta_1, \eta_2)'$, is given by

$$E[\eta_i|\boldsymbol{\eta} \leq \gamma] = \frac{1}{\alpha} \times \left\{\rho_{i1}\phi(\gamma_1)\Phi(A_{12}; \mathbf{R}_1) + \rho_{i2}\phi(\gamma_2)\Phi(A_{21}; \mathbf{R}_2)\right\}, \quad i = 1, 2, \tag{10}$$

where $A_{ij} = (\gamma_j - \rho_{ji}\gamma_i)/\sqrt{1 - \rho_{ji}^2}$, for $i, j = 1, 2$ and $i \neq j$ [16].

From (10) results that

$$\begin{aligned} E[\eta_1|\eta \le \gamma] &= \frac{1}{\alpha}\{\rho_{11}\phi(\gamma_1)\Phi(A_{12}) + \rho_{12}\phi(\gamma_2)\Phi(A_{21})\} \\ E[\eta_2|\eta \le \gamma] &= \frac{1}{\alpha}\{\rho_{21}\phi(\gamma_1)\Phi(A_{12}) + \rho_{22}\phi(\gamma_2)\Phi(A_{21})\}, \end{aligned} \tag{11}$$

where $\phi(.)$ and $\Phi(.)$ are, respectively, the pdf and distribution function of a standard normal variable.

Using the result in Eq. (11), the expected value of each component W_{ij} of the truncated variable $\mathbf{W}_i = (W_{i1}, W_{i2})$ is given by

$$E[W_{ij}|\mathbf{W} \le \mathbf{L}] = \mathbf{x}_i'\boldsymbol{\beta}_{(j)} + \sigma_j \times E[\eta_j|\boldsymbol{\eta} \le \gamma] \tag{12}$$

where $E[W_j|\mathbf{W} \le \gamma],\ \ j = 1, 2$ are the conditional expected value of standardized normal variables.

At iteration t, after filling up the censored observed dataset, the complete dataset $\mathbf{Y}^{(t)}$ is then used to compute the expected log-likelihood function, conditional on $\hat{\boldsymbol{\theta}}^{(t-1)}$,

$$Q(\boldsymbol{\theta}|\hat{\boldsymbol{\theta}}^{(t-1)}) = E[logL(\boldsymbol{\theta}|\mathbf{W}, \boldsymbol{\theta}^{(t-1)})] \tag{13}$$

where $\boldsymbol{\theta} = (\boldsymbol{\beta}, \boldsymbol{\Sigma})$ and $L(\boldsymbol{\theta}|\mathbf{W})$ denotes the likelihood function given the complete data. The expected MLE estimates satisfy $\hat{\boldsymbol{\theta}}^{(t)} = argmax\ \ Q(\boldsymbol{\theta}|\hat{\boldsymbol{\theta}}^{(t-1)})$. The value of $\boldsymbol{\beta}$ which maximizes (13) is

$$\hat{\boldsymbol{\beta}}^{(t)} = (\mathbf{X}'\mathbf{X})^{-1}\mathbf{X}'\mathbf{W}^{(t)}. \tag{14}$$

Given an estimate of $\boldsymbol{\beta}$, an unbiased estimate for $\boldsymbol{\Sigma}$ is

$$\hat{\boldsymbol{\Sigma}}^{(t)} = \frac{1}{n-m-1}(\mathbf{W}^{(t)} - \mathbf{X}\hat{\boldsymbol{\beta}}^{(t)})'(\mathbf{W}^{(t)} - \mathbf{X}\hat{\boldsymbol{\beta}}^{(t)})'. \tag{15}$$

3.2 Data Augmentation Algorithm

The data augmentation (DA) algorithm as described here is based on successive updating of the censored observations, and the corresponding ordinary least squares (OLS) estimates are computed using the augmented data.

At each iteration of the DA algorithm, censored values of each response variable $\mathbf{W}_{(j)}$ are sampled from their univariate truncated distribution conditional on the values of the remaining response variables, corresponding to the same subject. This procedure results in a sequence of random $m-$variate variables which converge in probability to the joint distribution of the $m-$variate latent variable $\mathbf{W} = (W_1, \ldots, W_m)$ [17].

In multivariate distributions, the acceptance-rejection algorithms are feasible, but the rate of convergence may be too low to be practical. Thus, a more efficient algorithm is the data augmentation, in which incomplete data is reconstructed using a Gibbs sampler-type algorithm [17, 18].

3.3 *Gibbs Sampler with Data Augmentation Algorithm*

The Gibbs sampling with data augmentation (GDA) algorithm [8] allows the use of a Bayesian approach to estimate the CMLR model, where inferences about the model parameters are obtained from the posterior distribution, $\pi(\boldsymbol{\beta}, \boldsymbol{\Sigma}|\mathbf{W})$, defined by

$$\pi(\boldsymbol{\beta}, \boldsymbol{\Sigma}|\mathbf{W}) \propto L(\boldsymbol{\beta}, \boldsymbol{\Sigma}|\mathbf{W}) \times \pi(\mathbf{B}, \boldsymbol{\Sigma}), \tag{16}$$

where $L(\boldsymbol{\beta}, \boldsymbol{\Sigma}|\mathbf{W})$ is the likelihood function of the observed data and $\pi(\mathbf{B}, \boldsymbol{\Sigma})$ represents the joint prior distribution of the parameters.

The Likelihood Function. As in [19], model (2) may be rewritten equivalently as

$$\mathbf{W}^* = \mathbf{X}^*\mathbf{B} + \epsilon, \tag{17}$$

where $\mathbf{W}^* = (\mathbf{W}'_{(1)}, \ldots, \mathbf{W}'_{(m)})'$ is a $mn \times 1$ vector, $\mathbf{X}^* = diag(\mathbf{X}^{(1)}, \ldots, \mathbf{X}^{(m)})$ is a $mn \times (mk + m)$ block diagonal matrix, where $\mathbf{X}^{(1)} = \ldots = \mathbf{X}^{(m)} = \mathbf{X}$, $\mathbf{B} = (\boldsymbol{\beta}'_{(1)}, \ldots, \boldsymbol{\beta}'_{(m)})'$ is a $(mk + m) \times 1$ vector of the regression coefficients and $\epsilon = (\epsilon'_{(1)}, \ldots, \epsilon'_{(m)})'$ is a $mn \times 1$ vector of the disturbances, assumed to be normally distributed, with zero mean and covariance matrix $\boldsymbol{\Sigma} \otimes \mathbf{I}_n$. Then, the likelihood function for $\boldsymbol{\beta}$ and $\boldsymbol{\Sigma}$ may be rewritten as

$$\begin{aligned} L(\boldsymbol{\beta}, \boldsymbol{\Sigma}|\mathbf{W}^*) =& (2\pi)^{-nm/2}|\boldsymbol{\Sigma}|^{-n/2}\exp\Big\{-\frac{1}{2}\epsilon'\boldsymbol{\Sigma}^{-1} \otimes \mathbf{I}_n\epsilon\Big\}. \\ =& (2\pi)^{-nm/2}|\boldsymbol{\Sigma}|^{-n/2}\exp\Big\{-\frac{1}{2}(\mathbf{W}^* - \mathbf{X}^*\mathbf{B})'\boldsymbol{\Sigma}^{-1} \otimes \mathbf{I}_n(\mathbf{W}^* - \mathbf{X}^*\mathbf{B})\Big\} \end{aligned} \tag{18}$$

where $\otimes$ is the Kronecker product and $\mathbf{I}_n$ is the identity matrix of order n.

Using the properties of the *trace* of a matrix [14] and considering that $\hat{\boldsymbol{\beta}} = (\mathbf{X}'\mathbf{X})^{-1}\mathbf{X}'\mathbf{W}$ and $\mathbf{A} = (\mathbf{W} - \mathbf{X}\hat{\boldsymbol{\beta}})'(\mathbf{W} - \mathbf{X}\hat{\boldsymbol{\beta}})$ are jointly sufficient for $\boldsymbol{\beta}$ and $\boldsymbol{\Sigma}$ [19], the likelihood function (18) can be simplified to

$$\begin{aligned} L(\boldsymbol{\beta}, \boldsymbol{\Sigma}|\mathbf{W}) =& (2\pi)^{-nm/2}|\boldsymbol{\Sigma}|^{-n/2} \\ & \times \exp\Big\{-\frac{1}{2}tr\boldsymbol{\Sigma}^{-1}\mathbf{A} - \frac{1}{2}(\mathbf{B} - \hat{\mathbf{B}})'\boldsymbol{\Sigma}^{-1} \otimes \mathbf{X}'\mathbf{X}(\mathbf{B} - \hat{\mathbf{B}})\Big\}. \end{aligned} \tag{19}$$

The Prior Distribution. Now, let's assume that $\boldsymbol{\beta}$ and $\boldsymbol{\Sigma}$ are independent [19]. Then, a non-informative prior distribution for $\boldsymbol{\beta}$ and $\boldsymbol{\Sigma}$ can be written as

$$\pi(\boldsymbol{\beta}, \boldsymbol{\Sigma}) = \pi(\boldsymbol{\beta})\pi(\boldsymbol{\Sigma}). \tag{20}$$

Due to the invariance property [19], we have that

$$\begin{aligned} \pi(\boldsymbol{\beta}) &\propto C, \\ \pi(\boldsymbol{\Sigma}) &\propto |\boldsymbol{\Sigma}|^{-\frac{m+1}{2}}, \end{aligned} \tag{21}$$

where C is a constant. Then, $\pi(\boldsymbol{\beta}, \boldsymbol{\Sigma}) \propto |\boldsymbol{\Sigma}|^{-\frac{m+1}{2}}$.

The Posterior Distribution. Using the prior distribution in (21) in conjunction with the likelihood function (19), the posterior distribution of $\boldsymbol{\beta}$ and $\boldsymbol{\Sigma}$ is given by

$$\begin{aligned} \pi(\boldsymbol{\beta}, \boldsymbol{\Sigma}|\mathbf{W}) &\propto L(\boldsymbol{\beta}, \boldsymbol{\Sigma}|\mathbf{W}) \times \pi(\mathbf{B}, \boldsymbol{\Sigma}) \\ &\propto |\boldsymbol{\Sigma}|^{-\frac{n+m+1}{2}} \exp\Big\{ -\frac{1}{2} tr\, \boldsymbol{\Sigma}^{-1}\mathbf{A} - \frac{1}{2}(\mathbf{B}-\hat{\mathbf{B}})'\boldsymbol{\Sigma}^{-1} \otimes \mathbf{X}'\mathbf{X}(\mathbf{B}-\hat{\mathbf{B}})\Big\} \\ &\propto \exp\Big\{ -\frac{1}{2}(\mathbf{B}-\hat{\mathbf{B}})'\boldsymbol{\Sigma}^{-1} \otimes \mathbf{X}'\mathbf{X}(\mathbf{B}-\hat{\mathbf{B}})\Big\} \\ &\quad \times |\boldsymbol{\Sigma}|^{-\frac{n+m+1}{2}} \exp\Big\{ -\frac{1}{2} tr\big(\boldsymbol{\Sigma}^{-1}\mathbf{A}\big)\Big\}. \end{aligned} \tag{22}$$

From Eq. (22) and taking only the terms involving each model parameter, the conditional posterior distribution of $\mathbf{B}$ and $\boldsymbol{\Sigma}$ can be expressed as

$$\pi(\mathbf{B}, \boldsymbol{\Sigma}|\mathbf{W}) = \pi(\mathbf{B}|\boldsymbol{\Sigma}, \mathbf{W})\pi(\boldsymbol{\Sigma}|\mathbf{W}), \tag{23}$$

with

$$\pi(\mathbf{B}|\boldsymbol{\Sigma}, \mathbf{W}) \propto exp\Big\{ -\frac{1}{2}(\mathbf{B}-\hat{\mathbf{B}})'\boldsymbol{\Sigma}^{-1} \otimes \mathbf{X}'\mathbf{X}(\mathbf{B}-\hat{\mathbf{B}})\Big\} \tag{24}$$

and

$$\pi(\boldsymbol{\Sigma}|\mathbf{W}) \propto |\boldsymbol{\Sigma}|^{-\frac{n+m+1}{2}} \exp\Big\{ -\frac{1}{2} tr\big(\boldsymbol{\Sigma}^{-1}\mathbf{A}\big)\Big\}. \tag{25}$$

The functional form of (24) and (25) show that

$$\begin{aligned} \pi(\mathbf{B}|\boldsymbol{\Sigma}, \mathbf{W}) &\propto N_{(mk+m)}\Big(\hat{\mathbf{B}}, \boldsymbol{\Sigma} \otimes (\mathbf{X}'\mathbf{X})^{-1}\Big) \\ \pi(\boldsymbol{\Sigma}|\mathbf{W}) &\propto IW(n, \mathbf{A}), \end{aligned} \tag{26}$$

where $IW(.)$ stands for inverted Wishart distribution [20]. Thus, observations from the joint distribution $\pi(\mathbf{B}, \boldsymbol{\Sigma}|\mathbf{W})$ can be drawn, iteratively, through the GDA algorithm.

The GDA Algorithm. The GDA algorithm has two main steps: (1) update the parameters' values from the posterior distributions, based on the data from the previous iterations and (2) use data augmentation (DA) algorithm (see Sect. 3.2) to update the censored observations, based on the current parameters' values. The successive updating of the model parameters and censored observations will result in a sequence of random $m-$variate variables which converge to the joint posterior distribution of $\boldsymbol{\theta} = (\boldsymbol{\beta}, \boldsymbol{\Sigma})$ [7, 17].

4 Simulation Study

To analyse the performance of the above procedures, consider a bivariate censored LR model ($m = 2$) with one predictor.[1] The datasets, of size $n = 100, 500$ and 1000, are generated using two sets of regression coefficients $\boldsymbol{\beta}^{(1)}$ and $\boldsymbol{\beta}^{(2)}$, each one combined with three different covariance matrices (low $\boldsymbol{\Sigma}^{(1)}$, moderate $\boldsymbol{\Sigma}^{(2)}$ and high correlation $\boldsymbol{\Sigma}^{(3)}$), as follows:

$$\boldsymbol{\beta}^{(1)} = \begin{bmatrix} 2 & 1 \\ 0.6 & 0.89 \end{bmatrix} \text{ and } \boldsymbol{\beta}^{(2)} = \begin{bmatrix} 0.2 & 0.3 \\ 0.4 & 0.24 \end{bmatrix}, \tag{27}$$

$$\boldsymbol{\Sigma}^{(1)} = \begin{bmatrix} 2 & 0.1 \\ 0.1 & 1.5 \end{bmatrix}, \boldsymbol{\Sigma}^{(2)} = \begin{bmatrix} 2 & -0.4 \\ -0.4 & 1.5 \end{bmatrix} \boldsymbol{\Sigma}^{(3)} = \begin{bmatrix} 2 & 0.8 \\ 0.8 & 1.5 \end{bmatrix}. \tag{28}$$

Values of LOD (L_1 and L_2) were set so that the observed response variables $Y_{(1)}$ and $Y_{(2)}$ have five different pairwise levels of censorship: $A = (5\%, 5\%)$, $B = (5\%, 20\%)$, $C = (5\%, 40\%)$, $D = (20\%, 20\%)$ and $E = (40\%, 40\%)$. We generate 100 realizations of each of these 90 scenarios to assess the finite sample behaviour of the estimates.

To illustrate the comparison between the methods, boxplots of biases corresponding to the three scenarios of censorship (low, medium and high) are represented in Figs. 1, 2, 3 and 4.

The overall results, illustrated in Figs. 1 (weak correlation) and 2 (strong correlation), indicate that the proposed methods produce approximately unbiased estimates for the regression parameters, $\boldsymbol{\beta}$, with decreasing variance as the sample size increases. However, as the correlation increases, the estimates present slight bias especially for high censoring.

[1] The generalization of this study to more than one independent variable is trivial for DA and GDA. However, the computation of the EM estimates may be hindered by the need to obtain the moments of the truncated multivariate distributions.

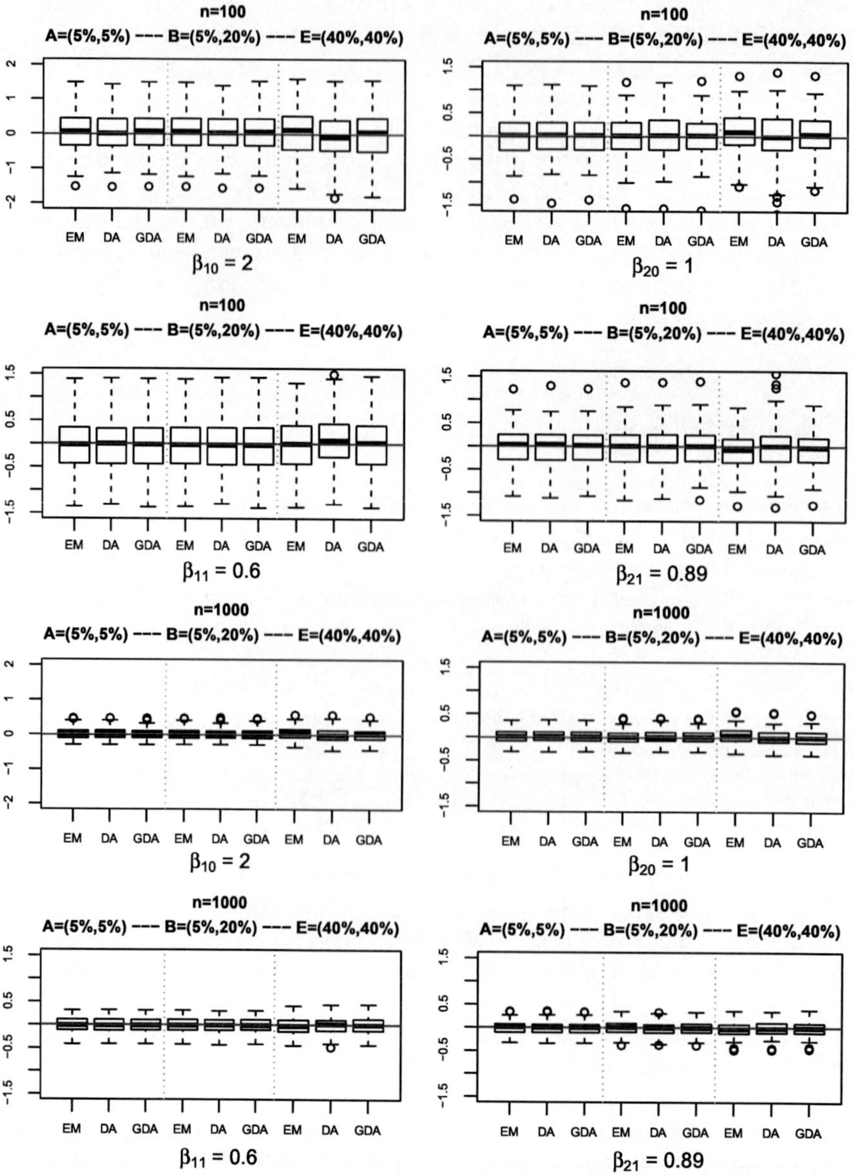

Fig. 1 Biases of $\hat{\beta}^{(1)}$ based on data generated from the model with $\boldsymbol{\Sigma}^{(1)}$, for $n = 100$ (*top*) and $n = 1000$ (*down*)

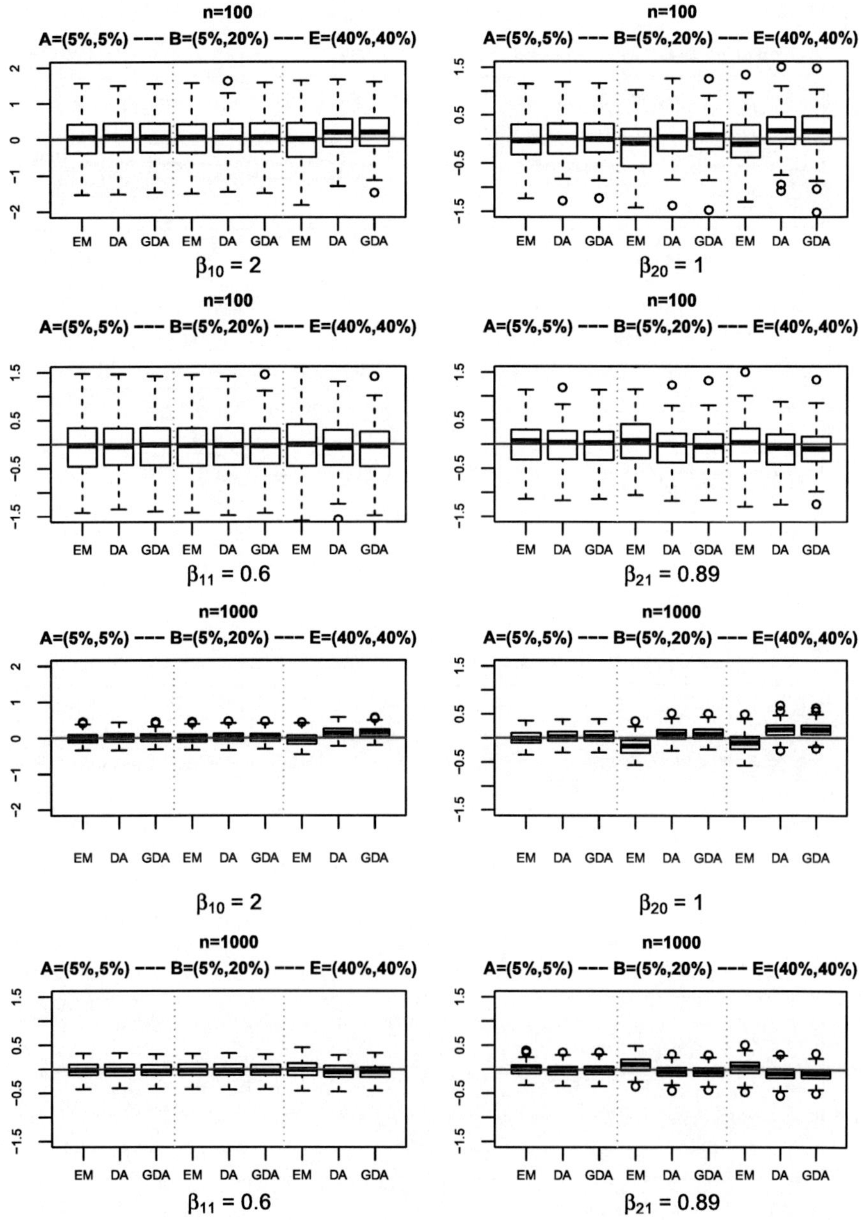

Fig. 2 Biases of $\hat{\beta}^{(1)}$ based on data generated from the model with $\boldsymbol{\Sigma}^{(3)}$, for $n = 100$ (*top*) and $n = 1000$ (*down*)

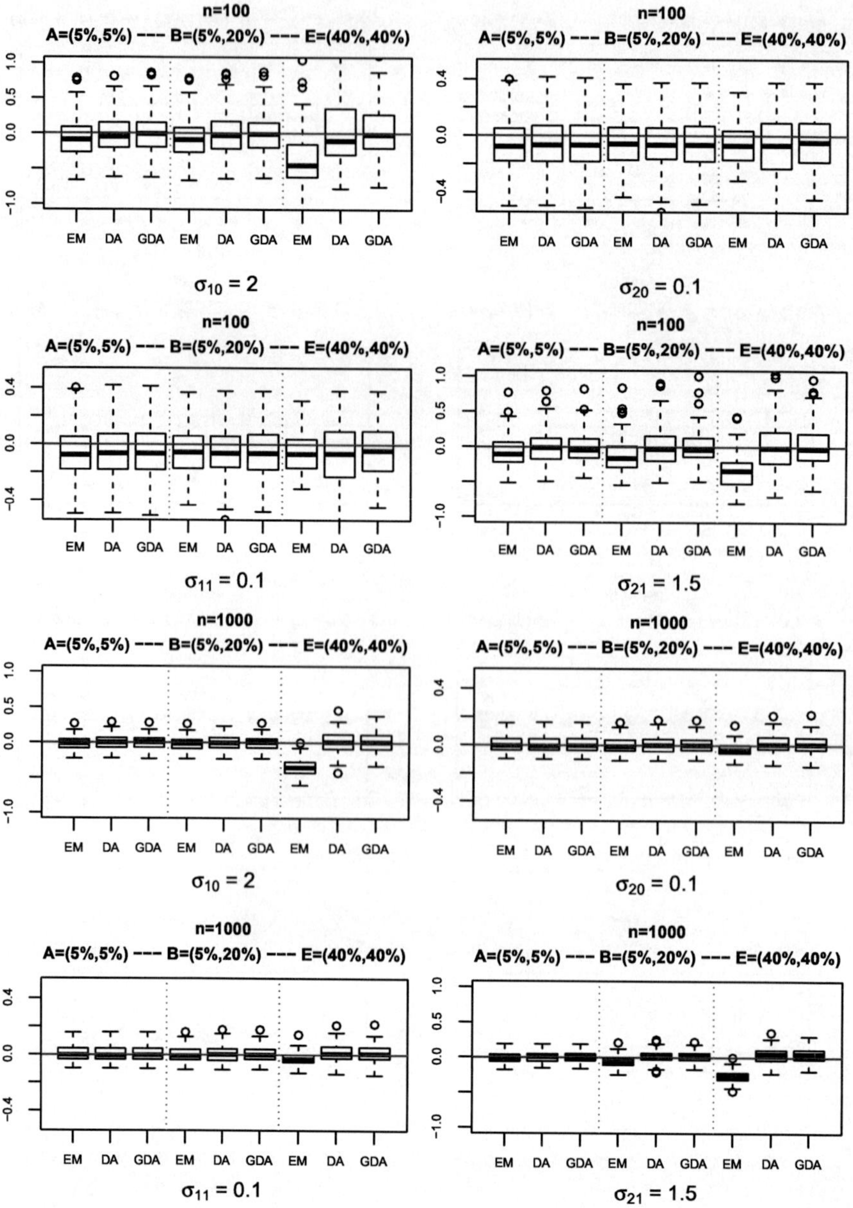

Fig. 3 Biases of $\hat{\boldsymbol{\Sigma}}^{(1)}$ based on data generated from the model with $\beta^{(1)}$, for $n = 100$ (*top*) and $n = 1000$ (*down*)

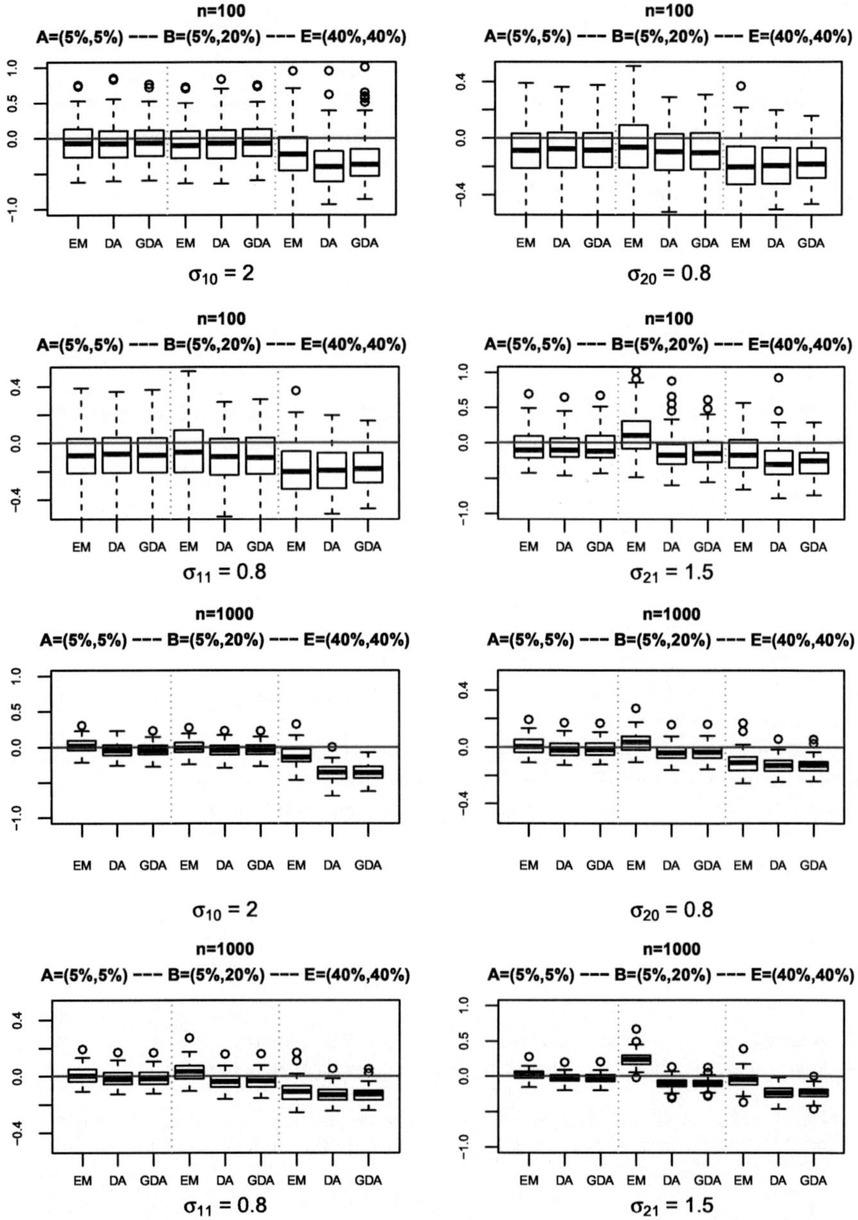

Fig. 4 Biases of $\hat{\boldsymbol{\Sigma}}^{(3)}$ based on data generated from the model with $\beta^{(1)}$, for $n = 100$ (*top*) and $n = 1000$ (*down*)

The DA and GDA approaches yield estimates for $\boldsymbol{\Sigma}$, illustrated in Figs. 3 and 4, approximately unbiased and with decreasing variance as the sample size increases under weak correlation $\boldsymbol{\Sigma}^{(1)}$. Under high correlation, $\boldsymbol{\Sigma}^{(3)}$, and high censoring rate, the bias increases for all the approaches, with EM showing lower bias. The results indicate that $\boldsymbol{\Sigma}$ is under-estimated in all scenarios but this does not affect the estimates of $\boldsymbol{\beta}$. This behaviour is expected since, in theory, the estimator of $\boldsymbol{\beta}$ is independent of the estimator of $\hat{\boldsymbol{\Sigma}}$ [14].

5 Final Remarks

One of the main features of multivariate LR is cross-correlation among the response variables. The censorship may distort the correlation pattern in multivariate data. Then, in this work, we propose three methods based on filling up data: EM, DA and GDA. Results from the simulation study show that both DA and GDA estimates are consistent for low and moderate correlation.

This study has been conducted for the bivariate case. The main issue when considering $m > 2$ is related to the computation of the conditional expected value of the multivariate censored variable, needed to compute the EM estimates. Since general expressions for this conditional mean are given in [16], it is our aim to implement higher order cases in the future. Furthermore, we aim to develop methods for censored multivariate time series data.

Acknowledgements This work is supported by Fundação Calouste Gulbenkian and the Center for Research and Development in Mathematics and Applications (CIDMA) through the Portuguese Foundation for Science and Technology (FCT—Fundação para a Ciência e a Tecnologia), reference UIDB/04106/2020.

References

1. Anderson: Multivariate Statistical Analy. Wiley, New York (2003)
2. Lee, G., Scott, C.: EM algorithms for multivariate gaussian mixture models with truncated and censored data. Comput. Stat. & Data Anal. **56**(9), 2816–2829 (2012)
3. Hopke, P.K., Liu, C., Rubin, D.B.: Multiple imputation for multivariate data with missing and below-threshold measurements: time-series concentrations of pollutants in the arctic. Biometrics **57**(1), 22–33 (2001)
4. Andersen, A., Benn, C.S., Jørgensen, M.J., Ravn, H.: Censored correlated cytokine concentrations: multivariate tobit regression using clustered variance estimation. Stat. Med. **32**(16), 2859–2874 (2012)
5. Alejo, J., Montes-Rojas, G.: Quantile regression under limited dependent variable (2021). arxiv:2112.06822
6. Li, S., Hu, T., Tong, T., Sun, J.: Semiparametric regression analysis of multivariate doubly censored data. Stat. Model. **20**(5), 502–526 (2019)

7. Chen, H., Quandt, S.A., Grzywacz, J.G., Arcury, T.A.: A Bayesian multiple imputation method for handling longitudinal pesticide data with values below the limit of detection. Environmetrics **24**(2), 132–142 (2012)
8. Tanner, M.A., Wong, W.H.: The calculation of posterior distributions by data augmentation. J. Amer. Stat. Assoc. **82**(398), 528–540 (1987)
9. Chib, S.: Bayes inference in the tobit censored regression model. J. Econ. **51**(1), 79–99 (1992)
10. Zeger, S.L., Brookmeyer, R.: Regression analysis with censored autocorrelated data. J. Amer. Stat. Assoc. **81**(395), 722–729 (1986)
11. Dempster, A.P., Laird, N.M., Rubin, D.B.: Maximum likelihood from incomplete data via the EM algorithm. J. R. Stat. Soc.: Ser. B **39**(1), 1–22 (1977)
12. Lockwood, J.R., Schervish, M.J.: MCMC strategies for computing Bayesian predictive densities for censored multivariate data. J. Comput. Graph. Stat. **14**(2), 395–414 (2005)
13. Muthén, B.: Moments of the censored and truncated bivariate normal distribution. Br. J. Math. Stat. Psychol. **43**(1), 131–143 (1990)
14. Johnson, D., Wichern, R.: Applied Multivariate Statistical Analysis. Pearson Prentice Hall, Upper Saddle River (2007)
15. Cohen, A.C.: Restriction and selection in samples from bivariate normal distributions. J. Amer. Stat. Assoc. **50**(271), 884–893 (1955)
16. Tallis, G.M.: The moment generating function of the truncated multi-normal distribution. J. Roy. Stat. Soc.: Ser. B (Methodol.) **23**(1), 223–229 (1961)
17. Breslaw, J.A.: Random sampling from a truncated multivariate normal distribution. Appl. Math. Lett. **7**, 1–6 (1994)
18. Horrace, W.C.: Some results on the multivariate truncated normal distribution. J. Multivar. Anal. **94**(1), 209–221 (2005)
19. Tiao, G.C., Zellner, A.: On the Bayesian estimation of multivariate regression. J. R. Stat. Soc.: Ser. B **26**(2), 277–285 (1964)
20. Wishart, J.: The generalised product moment distribution in samples from a normal multivariate population. Biometrika **20A**(1–2), 32–52 (1928)

A Methodology to Reveal Terrain Effects from Wind Farm SCADA Data Using a Wind Signature Concept

Alda Carvalho, Daniel C. Vaz, Tiago A. N. Silva, and Cláudia Casaca

Abstract Terrain features can deviate wind, causing heterogeneity in wind power distribution that varies with oncoming wind direction. An opportunity to review a wind farm layout, and improve its performance, arises with the need to replace end-of-life turbines. A methodology that adds value to wind data recorded over time by a supervisory control and data acquisition (SCADA) system is proposed. Time series portions, i.e., "time bands", with steady wind are identified and validated to compute a proposed index, S_B, that quantifies the significance of the directional distribution of these "time bands" number. S_B polar plots bring out terrain effects. Additionally, a wind signature concept is introduced, which is a convenient way of graphically displaying, over the topographic map of the wind farm, wind speed, direction, and turbulence at the location of a given turbine, providing an expeditious assessment of

A. Carvalho (✉)
CIMOSM, ISEL - Instituto Superior de Engenharia de Lisboa, Polytechnic Institute of Lisbon, Lisbon, Portugal
e-mail: alda.carvalho@isel.pt

CEMAPRE-REM, University of Lisbon, Lisbon, Portugal

D. C. Vaz
UNIDEMI, Department of Mechanical and Industrial Engineering, NOVA School of Science and Technology, Universidade Nova de Lisboa, Caparica, Portugal
e-mail: dv@fct.unl.pt

Laboratório Associado de Sistemas Inteligentes, LASI, Guimarães, Portugal

T. A. N. Silva
UNIDEMI, Department of Mechanical and Industrial Engineering, NOVA School of Science and Technology, Universidade Nova de Lisboa, Caparica, Portugal
e-mail: tan.silva@fct.unl.pt

Laboratório Associado de Sistemas Inteligentes, LASI, Guimarães, Portugal

CIMOSM, IPL-Polytechnic Institute of Lisbon, Lisbon, Portugal

C. Casaca
CIMOSM, ISEL - Instituto Superior de Engenharia de Lisboa, Polytechnic Institute of Lisbon, Lisbon, Portugal
e-mail: claudia.casaca@isel.pt

R. Bispo et al. (eds.), *Recent Developments in Statistics and Data Science*,
Springer Proceedings in Mathematics & Statistics 398,
https://doi.org/10.1007/978-3-031-12766-3_21

the wind pattern at a turbine-level scale. The proposed methodology is applied to the case study of four turbines in complex terrain in northern Portugal, revealing some effects of terrain features for various directions of oncoming wind.

Keywords Complex terrain · Micro-sitting · Wind turbine replacement · Applied statistics · Data mining · Flow pattern

1 Introduction

Energy production from renewable sources is increasingly playing a leading role in the development and implementation of sustainable energy and environmental policies to mitigate global warming [1, 2].

Worldwide, the rate of installation of modern horizontal axis wind turbines (HAWT) was rather moderate up to about 2004, with global annual installed capacities below 10 GW/yr, but after 2009 the values have been four times higher [3]. Since the life expectancy of wind turbines is around 18–25 years [3], around 2030, it is expected a significant increase in the number of turbines that reach their end of life and, therefore, need to be decommissioned and replaced.

Taking the example of Europe, the power per turbine doubled over about a decade [4]. In repowering a wind farm, after a lifetime of about two decades, a single new turbine can replace 4 old ones. Therefore, wind farms layout will need to be revised, creating an opportunity to improve the performance of the wind farm. The placement of new turbines will benefit from knowledge about local wind collected over the years. Indeed, wind farms continuously record operational data.

The positioning of turbines in a wind farm taking into consideration local effects of terrain, obstacles, or other turbines is referred to as micro-sitting. In micro-sitting, negative effects should be avoided, namely wind velocity deficit and/or increased turbulence when the wind from a predominant direction interacts with a terrain feature or when a turbine becomes immersed in the wake of another one, leading to reduced power production (up to 40%).

Considering the financial return of the investment in wind farms, the main challenge in applying wind-based knowledge is the improvement of wind turbine reliability to reduce its downtime. The performance and other operational parameters of wind turbines can be monitored through supervisory control and data acquisition systems (SCADA). SCADA data allows monitoring power production in the wind farm and, at the same time, gathers a large amount of information about wind flow and the functioning of various components, at a low cost [5–7]. The analysis of a SCADA dataset, by itself, can become challenging due to the constantly changing operating conditions of the turbine and the random nature of environmental conditions (wind speed and direction, air density, turbulence, etc.). A methodology for analysing this dynamic dataset can improve the understanding of wind farm operation, enhancing its performance, as well as the capability to anticipate equipment malfunctions [5, 8, 9]. Several methodologies can be used in forecasting or to extract useful information from SCADA data [5, 10–12].

With the aging of wind farms the propensity for the occurrence of failures increases and, when the turbines eventually reach their end of life, the need to replace them with newer turbines arises. Because of continuing technological advances, the new turbines are different from the previously installed ones, as they may be larger and more efficient, and this issue calls for rethinking the wind farm layout. Both failure prediction and wind farm layout benefit from information, and this has generated much interest in studying the large amount of data provided by the monitoring tools [13].

Monitoring how efficiency varies with wind direction is seen as a crucial task to assess the actual performance of wind farms, as this is affected by wake interactions and terrain complexity [14]. Indeed, wind characteristics can be significantly affected by surrounding terrains features [15–18]. The shape, orientation, and steepness of valleys and hills, result in hill shielding and valley channelling effects [19]. Upwind terrain or topographical conditions may affect both wind speed and wind direction.

While turbines in a wind farm located on a large flat terrain or offshore experience about the same wind regardless of oncoming direction, that is not the case with complex terrains. In [20], an analysis of a wind farm in a complex terrain reveals complex flow patterns at turbine-level scale. The results suggest a switch between at least two flow patterns. Thus, micro-sitting should not rely on wind assessment just at a single location in a wind farm, considered a representative location, but the flow pattern dependence on wind direction should be taken into consideration.

Dai et al. [21] have analysed SCADA data for a cluster of four turbines on a mountainous location in Chenzhou, China, to obtain the joint distribution surface of wind speed and direction. This surface exhibits peaks that characterize the specific turbine cluster studied. However, this analysis provides just a perception of the wind averaged over a year or a season.

In a recent work, Nai-Zhi et al. [22] have looked at extracting wake features from SCADA data to precisely account for the variation of wake expansion with local environment and inflow factors, for a specific wind farm. Such effects of topography on wake expansion had never been reflected in existing analytical wake models. Massive SCADA data has been analysed and processed to extract wake expansion features contained in it. Then, the relationship between the local inflow information and expansion features has been established by a machine learning algorithm. Wind speed and direction have been identified as the most important variables. That work, however, has been focused on the effects of wakes.

Castellani et al. [23] have proposed a very interesting methodology to derive from SCADA data knowledge useful for wind farm optimization. As the authors well put it, this "*is a challenging task, involving engineering, physics, statistics, and computer science skills*". In their approach, to automatically identify the dominant patterns of rotor orientations, a sub-cluster of turbines is selected, e.g., affected by wakes, and the properly discretized nacelles' orientations are post-processed through simple statistical methods. Castellani et al. have shown that non-trivial alignments with respect to the wind direction arise, as it is also found in the present work. Their study concerned a wind farm laying on a very gentle terrain in southern Italy and, thus, was more focused on the effect of wakes, although the authors mention that their methodology can be applied to address local effects associated with complex terrains.

Wind data gathered at each turbine may assist in producing a picture of the wind flow pattern. In principle, the comparison of wind speed and wind direction between the time series of data from neighbouring turbines can be used to infer the effects that the terrain, or obstacles around these turbines, have on local wind. However, it may not be possible to detect hidden changes if they are overwhelmed by the complexity of the signals collected by the anemometers, especially when wind direction and speed vary abruptly and frequently over time and small distances. To overcome this issue, in this paper, we propose a concept of using time bands, i.e., sufficiently long continuous portions of the time series for which wind is steady in direction and/or speed. Also, seeking combining orography with data, we propose the concept of local wind signature, i.e., a convenient way of graphically displaying over a map of the wind farm, wind direction, speed, and turbulence at each turbine. When used to display entries of different time bands, a dynamic representation results and small differences in wind characteristics between turbines can be seen, suggesting that the time band technique can indeed assist in the analysis of the effects of terrain, obstacles, and wakes.

2 Background

2.1 SCADA Data

SCADA systems are fully disseminated in different industrial applications to perform automated and synchronized data collection from numerous sensors. In a wind farm, environmental and operational related data is measured at an acquisition rate that depends on the situation, although the standard for wind-related data, e.g., wind speed and direction, is to acquire one data point at each second and then downsampling the dataset to store 10-minute statistics metrics, such as average, extreme or standard deviation values [24].

2.2 Data Pre-processing/Cleansing

The step of data pre-processing or preparation aims at ensuring that time series of different variables, and furthermore, of different wind turbines (T) are compatible, i.e., that the time-stamps indeed match. Thus, after loading the dataset and defining the time period of interest, all data vectors are stored in multidimensional arrays, as these vectors might contain different sizes. Then, one initializes all variables as arrays of `nan` with the exact size of the expected time-stamp vector and, for each variable of interest, one should compare the time-stamp vectors of different turbines:

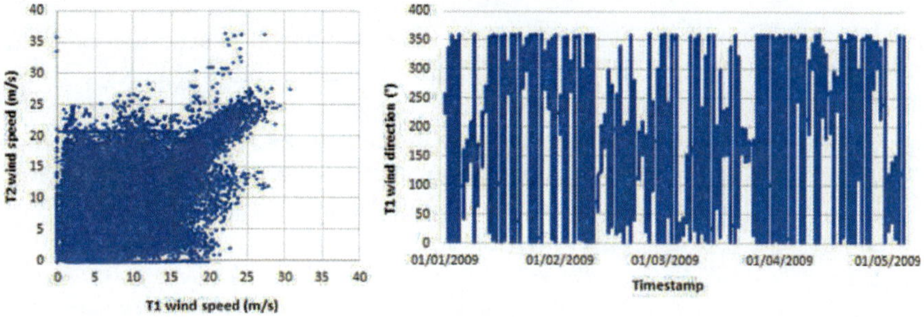

Fig. 1 Scatter plot comparing the raw wind speed dataset for two turbines over a period of four years (left). Line plot for raw wind direction dataset over 125 days (right)

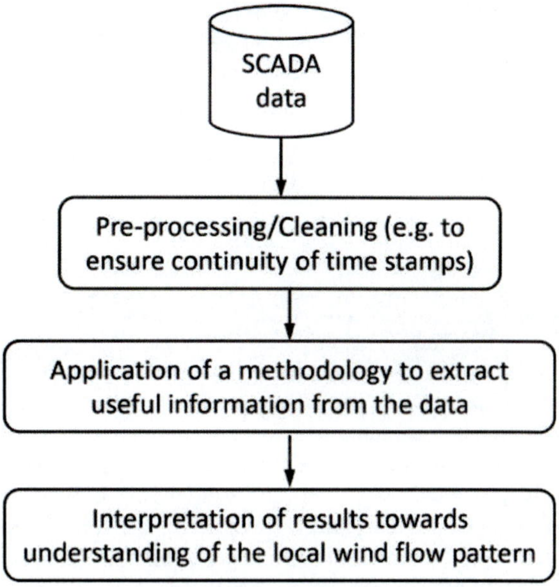

Fig. 2 A flowchart illustrating the main steps of the analysis of SCADA data towards the study of local wind flow

(i) if both time-stamp vectors match, one records the variable vectors as they are; (ii) otherwise, one identifies missing time-stamp entries and records the existing data at its registered time-stamps, leaving the non-matched data entries as `nan`. The compatible dataset is saved in a unique file, containing the synchronized data vectors. Note that the term synchronized here stands for compatible data entries, regarding their recording time-stamp. It is worthy to mention that this data preparation task is applied with a general purpose and thus one can treat the dataset using missing-data imputation techniques [25], before data cleansing and filtering.

In Fig. 1, on the left, it is possible to see a scatter plot of wind speed measured at two neighbouring turbines. Not all instances (here represented by the points) are aligned along the identity line, many samples have significant differences in wind speed. In Fig. 1, on the right, it is possible to see the temporal evolution of wind direction. Besides the natural variability of the time series, abrupt changes are seen between 0° and 360°: circular statistics can be used to deal with this problem.

The proposed methodology is illustrated in the flowchart of Fig. 2. It presents the main steps of the analysis to derive understanding of the local wind flow from SCADA raw data. Details on the various steps of the analysis are given in Sect. 3.

2.3 Variables of Interest

As mentioned before, SCADA data has a large set of variables. In order to study the terrain effect on local wind farm pattern, the main variables of interest are wind speed (U), wind direction (θ), and turbulence intensity (TI),

$$TI = \frac{\sigma_U}{\overline{U}} \tag{1}$$

where σ_U is the standard deviation of the wind speed time series and $\overline{U}$ is the wind speed time average [24].

2.4 Frequency Wind Roses

Useful information can be obtained from data by conveniently displaying parts of it graphically. An example is frequency wind roses, in which the frequency of winds, at a particular location and over a time period, is plotted by wind direction, producing a polar plot with spokes of a variety of lengths. Longer spokes correspond to directions of greater wind frequency. Most often, the spokes are subdivided in colour bands representing a selection of wind speed bins. Commonly called wind rose, it provides a view of how wind speed is distributed over all directions.

The set of the frequency wind roses of the wind measured at the various turbines in a farm (Fig. 3) is useful but not sufficient for the understanding of the wind pattern over the farm. They are useful because they give an indication of possible changes in wind direction as it flows between neighbouring turbines. On the other hand, they are insufficient since the results in wind frequency wind roses are integrated over time and, thus, do not provide an instantaneous picture of the wind direction at the various turbines. This means that associating directions of high (or low) frequencies between wind frequency wind roses of neighbouring turbines may point towards an erroneous flow pattern because this flow pattern may not coincide with any actual instantaneous flow pattern over the farm. For simple terrains, i.e., terrains for which a wind pattern is dominant throughout the period analysed, it may be easy to spot how wind is being deflected by some sole feature in the terrain. However, for complex terrain, the frequency wind roses result from the superposition of several wind patterns, and

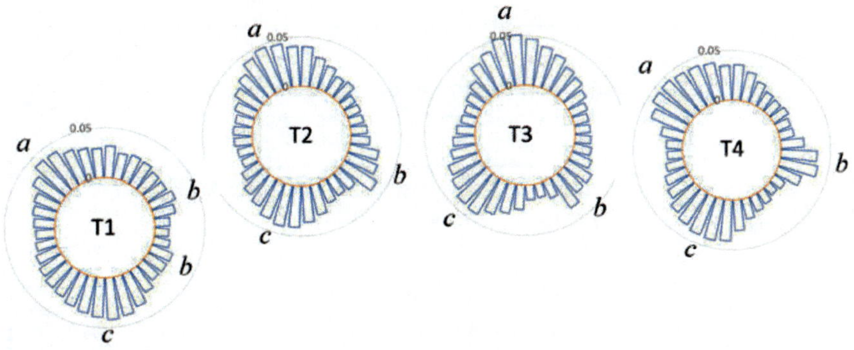

Fig. 3 Frequency wind roses for the 4 turbines of the wind farm discussed as case study

thus, it can be difficult do understand how exactly the wind is being deflected along the vicinity of a sequence of turbines.

2.5 Fluctuations in the Direction Signal

In principle, one expects to get an understanding of the flow pattern over the wind farm through observation of simultaneous wind directions at multiple turbines. However, it would be very difficult to use this approach to reach conclusions about the flow pattern because the fluctuations exhibited by direction signals (time series) are not exclusively due to the effects from terrain topology. While the terrain can introduce fluctuations in the signal, for example, as observed in the perturbed flow in the wake of a hill or another obstacle, the direction signals include additional effects from fluctuations of the oncoming wind itself, related with atmospheric instabilities, weather systems, amongst other causes. For the aforementioned approach to be useful, it is necessary to remove fluctuations in the signal that are not attributable to terrain effects. In this paper a procedure is proposed to identify portions of the time series where the wind is considered to be steady, as will be defined in Sect. 3.

3 The Proposed Methodology

3.1 Overview

In this section we detail the methodology that is being offered to uncover terrain effects from SCADA data collected by the various wind turbines in a wind farm. This corresponds to the step "*Application of a methodology to extract useful information*

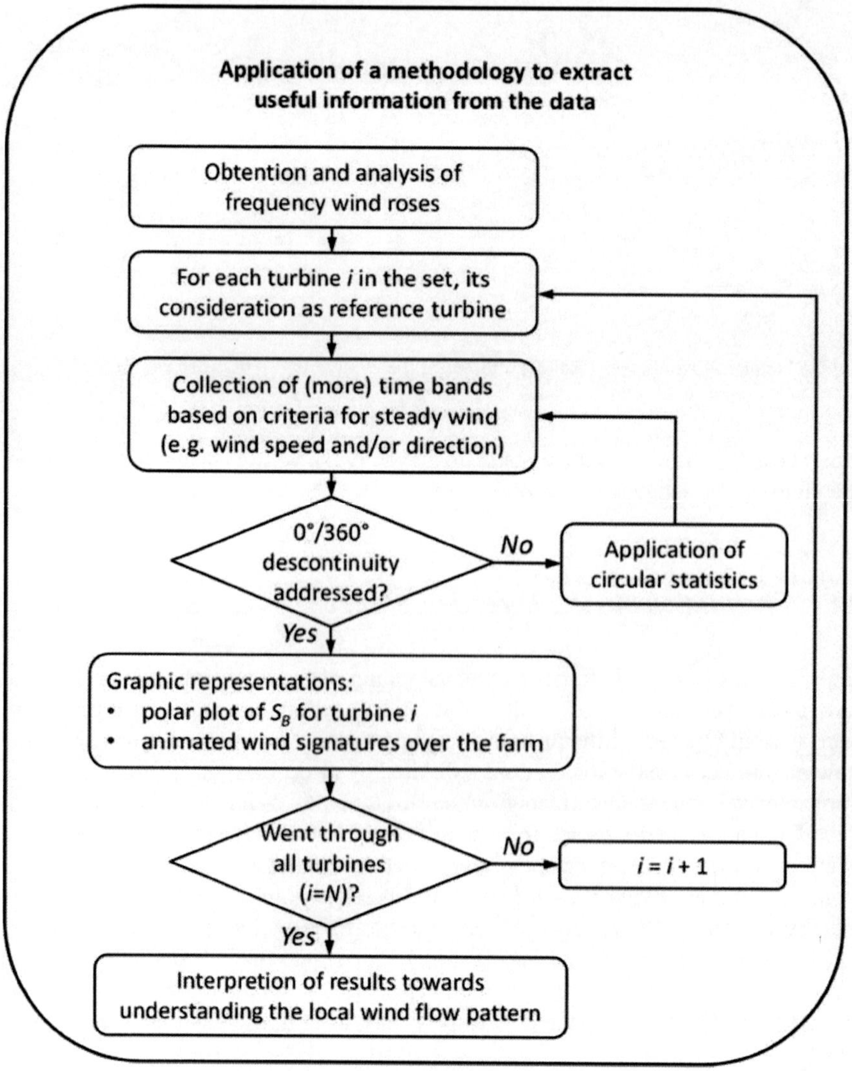

Fig. 4 Flowchart detailing the proposed methodology to uncover terrain effects from SCADA data

from the data" in the flowchart of Fig. 2. As a roadmap for the present section, that step has been expanded in Fig. 4.

3.2 Steady Wind

The main idea behind the analysis is to obtain time bands in which the wind can be considered constant, or steady. For clarity, herein, constant/steady wind, is that for which a given property, or combination of properties, remain(s) within a specified small interval(s). The more intuitive variables of interest related to wind are wind speed and wind direction, but it could also be any other recorded by the SCADA system, like air temperature or wind speed standard deviation. Filtering the time series with given criteria of constant wind will produce several portions, which are herein called time bands.

It must be noted that constant, or steady, wind should not be confused with stationary wind, since the later has a precise technical meaning. It is associated with decomposing the velocity of random wind as a sum of a constant mean wind velocity and three turbulence components (longitudinal, lateral, and vertical), modelled as stationary Gaussian random processes [26]. On the other hand, steady wind, as employed in the present study, is understood as wind for which over a period of time the instantaneous values of one or more variables of interest related to wind remain between a specified interval.

Denoting by T the variable of interest, this interval may be specified in absolute terms (especially for wind direction), $T_{(n)} - T_{(1)} < \delta_T$, or in relative terms, $\max\left(T_{(n)}/\overline{T} - 1,\ 1 - T_{(1)}/\overline{T}\right) < \varepsilon_T$, where $T_{(1)} \leq T_{(2)} \ldots \leq T_{(n)}$ are the ascending order statistics and $\overline{T}$ is the sample mean from a period of time, here represented by $(T_1, T_2, ..., T_n)$. Such steadiness criteria can be applied to more than one variable, with distinct intervals, and may concern the variables registered at a single reference turbine or at several turbines.

3.3 Harvesting and Selection of Time Bands

As pointed out in Sect. 2.5, the effects of terrain topology on the wind pattern may be masked by stronger fluctuations in wind direction due to other causes, originated far away, upwind of the wind farm. Hence, for the analysis of terrain effects on local wind direction to be feasible, it is of the most importantance to retain for analysis just the portions of the time series in which wind does not exhibit direction fluctuations as it approaches the wind farm. Since weather masts are not available around the whole periphery of a wind farm, it is necessary to resort to the wind measurements at the turbines themselves. However, one has to allow for fluctuations in wind direction caused by terrain features, that is to say, the time series should not be filtered for portions where the wind direction is steady for *all* turbines. Therefore, the filter is applied to the variable(s) of one turbine (or at most, a fraction of the total number of turbines) taken as reference.

Given the circular nature of wind direction, a second step involving circular statistics should desirably be included in the process of obtaining time bands, to ensure

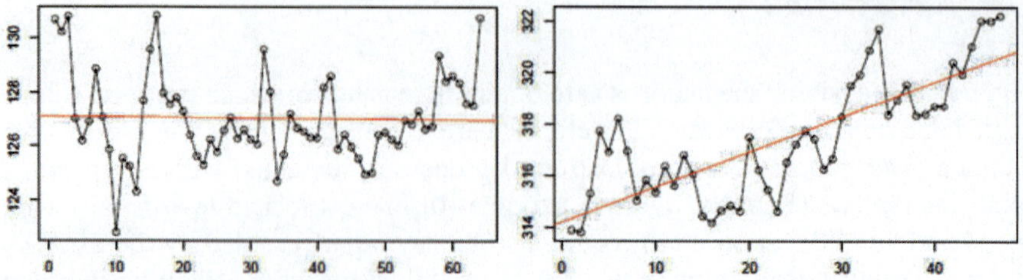

Fig. 5 Example of trends in the time bands: without trend (left); and with trend (right)

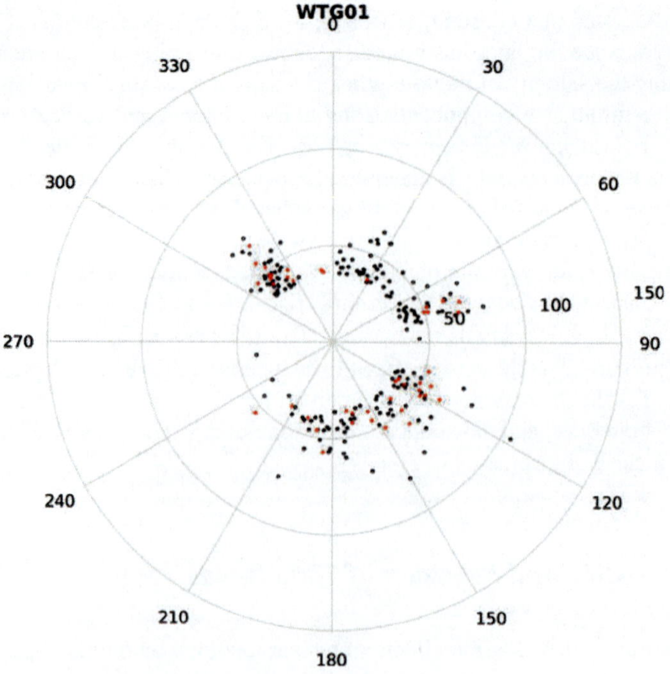

Fig. 6 Polar plot of time bands collected for T1 as reference turbine: time bands without trend (black) and rejected time bands for having trend (red)

that time bands associated with the north direction and of significance to the analysis are not missed because of the 0°/360° discontinuity.

After applying the first criterion, the resulting time bands may not be stationary. For the wind flow analysis, it is important to ensure that the time bands do not present a trend. Two examples of time bands can be seen in Fig. 5. The second part of this step is the Sieve-bootstrap Student's t-test [27]. The null hypothesis of no trend is tested against the alternative hypothesis of linear trend. The significance 1% is defined as threshold for rejection and time bands with p-value$<$ 1% are removed.

In Fig. 6 it is possible to see the polar plot of T1 of the case study. Each point represents a time band, where the radial distance represents the time band length and angular coordinate represents the time band mean direction. All the time bands are represented in Fig. 6 and the red dots correspond to the time bands rejected due to linear trend.

3.4 Time Band Significance Index

At this point of the analysis, polar plots such as that of Fig. 6 are available for each turbine. However, one should exercise care in giving significance to the number of time bands found in one direction. In fact, a large number of time bands in a given direction, relatively to the average number of time bands per direction, may stem from the wind blowing more frequently from that direction. And the opposite is also true.

So, to weigh the significance to attribute to the number of time bands along a directional sector, found when considering a given turbine as reference turbine, we put forward a non-dimensional index (significance of number of time bands along a directional sector):

$$S_B = \frac{N_B/N_{T,B}}{N/N_T} \tag{2}$$

where: N is the number of observations in the directional sector, for a given turbine, N_T is the number of total valid observations in the time series, for the same turbine, N_B is the number of time bands found in the directional sector and $N_{T,B}$ is the total number of time bands found in all directions.

Figure 7 shows polar plots of S_B, again, for the case study wind farm described later in Sect. 4. For clarity, what is actually plotted is $\log(S_B)$.

When $S_B < 1$, (the spokes in the polar charts point inwards) it means that the number of time bands found in that direction are relatively few, given the total

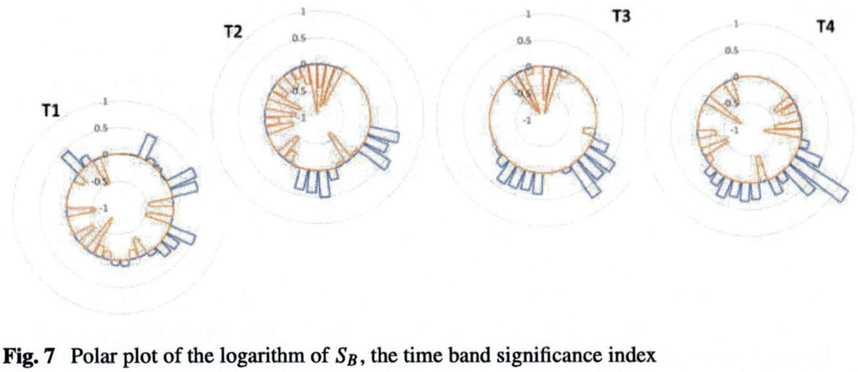

Fig. 7 Polar plot of the logarithm of S_B, the time band significance index

number of bands found in all directions, and the probability of wind blowing from that direction. Such directions with relatively few time bands should then be interpreted as despite having a number of periods of steady wind—sufficient to produce valid time bands—the number of these periods is not significant, and hence, over the whole time series, the more general situation along that direction is that the wind is in fact unsteady. As will be seen from the discussion of the case study presented in the next section (4. Case Study), the process of identifying time bands, of distributing them over directions, and of classifying the significance of the number of time bands along a direction based on the evaluation of the proposed figure of merit S_B, produces polar plots that when overlayed on a wind farm map can tell us which terrain features are having an influence on local wind direction and direction fluctuations. This adds clarity and confidence to any preliminary impression of the wind pattern obtained from the wind frequency roses. However, equally to these latter graphs, polar plots of S_B also do not provide an instantaneous view of the wind pattern over the farm. That is to say, one does not know which spokes on the polar plots of S_B of one turbine correspond, *at the same time instant*, to certain prominent spokes on another-turbine's plot. This lack of knowledge can lead to erroneous formulations of wind patterns over the farm, and do avoid them, it is necessary to look at mean values of wind directions at each turbine, calculated along the collected time bands. Since these values are taken over the same period of time, they can be assessed in ensemble to provide a coarse picture of the flow over the farm. Next, we propose a graphical representation that is very convenient at this point of the analysis. Besides just direction, other variables are added to the graphical representation and result in what we label instantaneous wind-signature at each turbine.

3.5 Instantaneous Wind Signatures

As mentioned before, a better understanding of the wind flow pattern is essential to improve the wind farm layout. By combining orography with wind statistical data, it is possible to bring forward some hidden correlations. In this section we propose a schematic representation of local *wind signature* using wind speed, direction and turbulence (see Fig. 8, left). Using an interactive dynamic geometry application such as Geogebra [28], it is possible quickly visualize (and animate) the wind signature overlapped with the wind farm map. In Fig. 8 (right) it is possible to see a particular frame (corresponding to one-time band) with its own signature, here represented by a triangle that summarizes the three wind measures of interest (speed, direction, and turbulence).

Stacking several frames (each corresponding to a valid time band), wind signature of the same time period (time band) can be inspected in a graphical and fast way. When several time bands exhibit a similar wind pattern, then the pattern can be identified as one possible stable pattern observed in the farm, again and again, like has been found in [23]. If not, then despite the fact wind remained sufficiently steady to yield a time band, the flow pattern registered is not a common one.

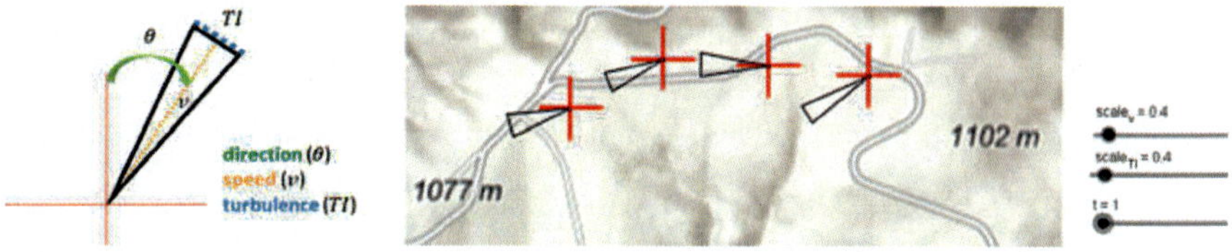

Fig. 8 Wind signature: schematic representation based on wind speed, direction, and turbulence intensity (left). Wind farm signature animation (right)

Wind signatures provide filtered information that is of good use for the aerodynamic specialists concerned with micro-sitting of turbines. A comprehensive and in-depth discussion of the last step of the procedure outlined in Fig. 4 is out of the scope of the present paper and its application to the wind farm under study will be the subject of a future publication.

4 Case Study

In this section we present the proposed methodology applied to a group of 4 turbines located in Freita, in northern Portugal (see Fig. 9). The variables of interest for this study are wind speed (m/s) and wind direction (°), measured by the wind turbines' anemometers. The four wind turbines are located at the border of a plateau raising 500 m above neighbouring terrain and their average is approximately 400 m. The dataset used in this study relates to the period 2009–2013 with a 10 min interval. The complete dataset has 262944 observations, although there are some missing or incorrect values.

After applying the criteria defined in Sect. 3.2, it is possible to see the number of resulting time bands after the 10° range criteria. The average number of the resulting time bands is approximately 200, with around 25% rejected due to linear trend (Sect. 3.3). The average length of the resulting time bands is approximately 8 h.

The situation of $S_B < 1$ can be seen for wind coming aligned with gullies 2 and 3 (labelled g2 and g3) in Fig. 9 and reaching turbines 2 and 3, respectively. Therefore, even though there may be situations in which the wind comes channelled by the gullies, and remains steady in direction (resulting in validated time bands), there are many more situations in which due to possible misalignment with the gullies, or due to some other causes (e.g., thermal effects), the wind comes perturbed, fluctuating in the direction in a such a way that the signal does not comply with the criteria set for steady wind.

Other situations with $S_B < 1$ can be seen in the polar plot of turbine T1, corresponding to perturbed flow in the wake of the hill SW of the turbine, and in the polar plot of turbine T4, for winds coming from NEE, off-aligned with gullies (g6) and ridges in that direction and thus exhibiting fluctuations in direction.

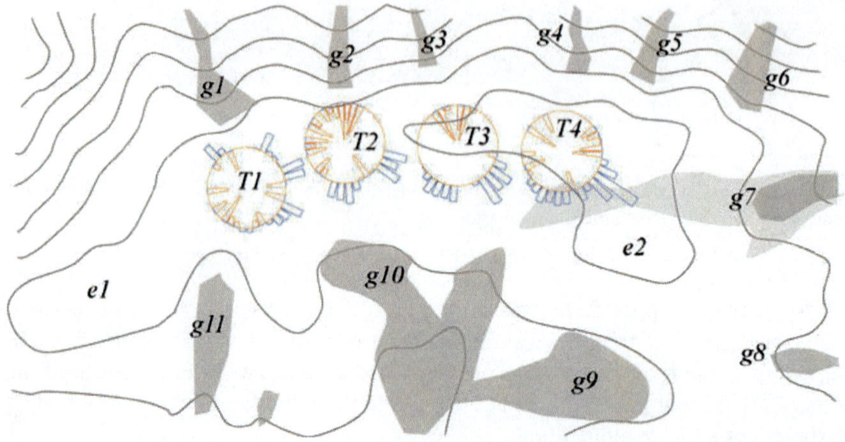

Fig. 9 Locations of turbines T1 to T4 over the topography of the wind farm: shaded areas are gullies (g1 to g11) and e1 and e2 are elevations

Moving on to the directions for which $S_B > 1$ (spokes in the polar charts pointing outwards), an interesting situation can be seen associated with the wide valley (g10) south of turbines T2 and T3. Wind approaching from south is possibly spread out, as a result of the uphill broadening of the valley, and reaches turbines T1 through T4 at somewhat different directions. The polar plots seem rotated in relation to one another, as an effect of the terrain feature causing deflection of the wind being relatively close to this group of turbines, so that each "sees" the feature from different angles.

Other situations can be seen in the results but to lack of space their discussion is left for another publication.

5 Conclusions

This work aims at presenting a methodology to reveal terrain effects on wind, from SCADA data, registered on a wind farm in the northern Portugal over a time period of 5 years, using a wind signature concept. By the use of the proposed methodology, it is shown that it is possible to process data in order to obtain useful information on wind patterns that are developed as the oncoming wind changes direction.

For the same direction of oncoming wind, a number of possible wind patterns may be observed, being overall similar, except for a given turbine. To explain the heterogeneity of wind patterns, it is necessary to look into the effect that other variables may have on local wind signatures. Future work may address other variables of interest apart from the wind speed and direction which have been the focus of the current work, e.g., ambient temperature, atmospheric stability, hour of day, season, or weather conditions.

Further improvements should involve numerical simulation to emphasize specific details on the analysis to establish in a systematic framework the capability of studying wind patterns in any given wind farm.

Acknowledgements This work was developed and financially supported under the framework of project MoDMaPE2 from the Polytechnic Institute of Lisbon (IDI&CA, 2020). Alda Carvalho acknowledge the support provided by the Portuguese Foundation for Science and Technology (FCT.IP/MCTES) for the work carried out in the framework of the research centre CEMAPRE/REM (ref. UIDB/05069/2020). Daniel Vaz and Tiago Silva acknowledge Fundação para a Ciência e a Tecnologia (FCT, IP) for its financial support via the project UIDB/00667/2020 (UNIDEMI).

References

1. E. E. Agency, E. T. C. for Air Pollution, C. C. Mitigation: Renewable Energy in Europe 2018: Recent Growth and Knock On Effects. Publications Office (2018)
2. Gielen, D., Boshell, F., Saygin, D., Bazilian, M.D., Wagner, N., et al.: The role of renewable energy in the global energy transformation. Energ. Strat. Rev. **24**, 38–50 (2019)
3. Liu, P., Barlow, C.Y.: Wind turbine blade waste in 2050. Waste Manage. **62**, 229–240 (2017)
4. Serrano-González, J., Lacal-Arántegui, R.: Technological evolution of onshore wind turbines—a market-based analysis. Wind Energy **19**(12), 2171–2187 (2016)
5. Lebranchu, A., Charbonnier, S., Bérenguer, C., Prévost, F.: A combined mono- and multi-turbine approach for fault indicator synthesis and wind turbine monitoring using SCADA data. ISA Trans. **87**, 272–281 (2019)
6. Yadav, G., Paul, K.: Architecture and security of SCADA systems: a review. Int. J. Crit. Infrastruct. Prot. **34**, 100433 (2021)
7. Yang, W., Court, R., Jiang, J.: Wind turbine condition monitoring by the approach of SCADA data analysis. Renew. Energy **53**, 365–376 (2013)
8. Astolfi, D., Castellani, F., Terzi, L.: Mathematical methods for SCADA data mining of onshore wind farms: performance evaluation and wake analysis. Wind Eng. **40**(1), 69–85 (2016)
9. Luo, L., Zhuang, Y., Duan, Q., Dong, L., Yu, Y., et al.: Local climatic and environmental effects of an onshore wind farm in North China. Agric. For. Meteorol. **308–309**, 108607 (2021)
10. Herbert, G.J., Iniyan, S., Sreevalsan, E., Rajapandian, S.: A review of wind energy technologies. Renew. Sustain. Energy Rev. **11**(6), 1117–1145 (2007)
11. Kusiak, A., Zhang, Z., Verma, A.: Prediction, operations, and condition monitoring in wind energy. Energy **60**, 1–12 (2013)
12. Liu, H., Tian, H.-Q., Chen, C., Fei Li, Y.: A hybrid statistical method to predict wind speed and wind power. Renew. Energy **35**(8), 1857–1861 (2010)
13. Cambron, P., Masson, C., Tahan, A., Pelletier, F.: Control chart monitoring of wind turbine generators using the statistical inertia of a wind farm average. Renew. Energy **116**, 88–98 (2018)
14. Castellani, F., Astolfi, D., Terzi, L., Hansen, K.S., Rodrigo, J.S.: Analysing wind farm efficiency on complex terrains. J. Phys: Conf. Ser. **524**, 012142 (2014)
15. Palomino, I., Martín, F.: A simple method for spatial interpolation of the wind in complex terrain. J. Appl. Meteorol. **34**(7), 1678–1693 (1995)
16. Bullard, J., Wiggs, G., Nash, D.: Experimental study of wind directional variability in the vicinity of a model valley. Geomorphology **35**(1–2), 127–143 (2000)
17. Hesp, P.A., Smyth, T.A., Nielsen, P., Walker, I.J., Bauer, B.O., et al.: Flow deflection over a foredune. Geomorphology **230**, 64–74 (2015)

18. Lange, J., Mann, J., Berg, J., Parvu, D., Kilpatrick, R., et al.: For wind turbines in complex terrain, the devil is in the detail. Environ. Res. Lett. **12**(9), 094020 (2017)
19. He, Y., Chan, P., Li, Q.: Wind characteristics over different terrains. J. Wind Eng. Ind. Aerodyn. **120**, 51–69 (2013)
20. Casaca, C., Vaz, D., Silva, T.A.N., Carvalho, A.: An analysis of wind farm data to evidence local wind pattern switches near a plateau. In: Loja, M. et al. (ed.) Proceedings of 4th International Conference on Numerical and Symbolic Computation: Developments and Applications (SYMCOMP2019), ISBN: 978-989-99410-5-2, @ECCOMAS (2019)
21. Dai, J., Tan, Y., Yang, W., Wen, L., Shen, X.: Investigation of wind resource characteristics in mountain wind farm using multiple-unit SCADA data in Chenzhou: a case study. Energy Convers. Manage. **148**, 378–393 (2017)
22. Nai-Zhi, G., Ming-Ming, Z., Bo, L.: A data-driven analytical model for wind turbine wakes using machine learning method. Energy Convers. Manage. **252**, 115130 (2022)
23. Castellani, F., Astolfi, D., Sdringola, P., Proietti, S., Terzi, L.: Analyzing wind turbine directional behavior: SCADA data mining techniques for efficiency and power assessment. Appl. Energy **185**, 1076–1086 (2017)
24. I. E. Commission: International standard iec 61400-12-1:2017—power performance measurements of electricity producing wind turbines (2017)
25. Sun, C., Chen, Y., Cheng, C.: Imputation of missing data from offshore wind farms using spatio-temporal correlation and feature correlation. Energy **229**, 120777 (2021)
26. Tubino, F., Solari, G.: Time varying mean extraction for stationary and nonstationary winds. J. Wind Eng. Ind. Aerodyn. **203**, 104187 (2020)
27. Chang, Y., Park, J.Y.: A sieve bootstrap for the test of a unit root. J. Time Ser. Anal. **24**(4), 379–400 (2003)
28. Hohenwarter, M., et al.: GeoGebra 5.0.507.0 (2018). http://www.geogebra.org

A Robust Version of the FGLS Estimator for Panel Data

Anabela Rocha and M. Cristina Miranda

Abstract Panel or longitudinal data sets are frequent in financial and economic studies. This type of data combines cross-sectional with time-series data, providing extra information and allowing to evaluate and measure the statistical effects that would otherwise keep unknown. Different degree of restrictions upon the structure of the data leads to different approaches with least squares methodology. This results in estimators that can be highly affected by a violation of those assumptions. The Feasible Generalized Least Squares estimator (FGLS) is an estimator that preserves good properties without requiring strong distribution requisites. In spite of this, it is highly affected by the presence of observations too much different from all the rest. These are known as atypical observations or outliers. Economical and financial real data often present this type of data and the FGLS estimator may be seriously affected by those observations. This might be avoided if a robust option is chosen. Although robustness is the main concern in recent econometric modelling, there is still much to do in this field. Recent studies in those fields point to the advantage of using robust estimators. With this work, we want to contribute to the use of robust methodologies in the estimation of panel data models and present a robust version of FGLS, the RFGLS (Robust Feasible Generalized Least Squares). In this paper, the performance of the proposed estimator is compared with the FGLS using real data previously analysed by some authors.

Keywords FGLS · Panel data · Robust estimation

A. Rocha (✉) · M. C. Miranda
ISCA and CIDMA, University of Aveiro, Aveiro, Portugal
e-mail: anabela.rocha@ua.pt

M. C. Miranda
e-mail: cristina.miranda@ua.pt

M. C. Miranda
CEAUL, University of Lisbon, Lisbon, Portugal

R. Bispo et al. (eds.), *Recent Developments in Statistics and Data Science*,
Springer Proceedings in Mathematics & Statistics 398,
https://doi.org/10.1007/978-3-031-12766-3_22

1 Introduction and Preliminaries

In econometric studies, it is very frequent to use data referring to records of a set of variables of interest, over some period of time. The units of study may be households, firms, countries, individuals, etc. This leads to a set of longitudinal data set or, as usually denoted by econometricians, a set of panel data. Following records from a set of variables for a period of time may reveal more information than the observation of those same variables in a single moment (cross-sectional data).

Longitudinal data or panel data (PD) studies may be found within a long range of areas of knowledge. This is a frequently used methodology in demographic and economic research areas, but also in biological [1], climate and environment [2]. Several national institutes conduct panel data studies following families, companies or individuals, keeping records of some variables of interest for a predefined period of time. As an example, Baltagi [3] refers to the National Longitudinal Surveys (NLS) of the U.S. Bureau of Labor Statistics. The NLSY97 consists of a sample of 8984 people with information on the labour market and educational experiences. Data were collected for 18 rounds, from 1997−98 to 2017−18.

Typically, a panel data set consists of a number of observations, concerning different units taken repeatedly for a number of times, usually small when compared to the number of units under study. The units may be companies, individuals, countries, families, etc., depending on the object of study—macro or microeconomics. One of the main motivations of this approach is the presence of heterogeneity among individuals. Panel data models allow the detection of effects that would be imperceptible with cross-sectional data or with time-series data.

Panel data model analysis requires data to satisfy several conditions. Only with such data, it is possible to obtain suitable estimators for the parameters of the models under consideration. Most of the time, however, real data don't behave as one would expect. So, it is important to look for estimators that can respond adequately, even when data don't fulfil the necessary conditions. The answer to this problem consists of looking for robust estimators. In this paper the authors present a new proposal for a robust version of the Feasible Generalized Least Square (FGLS) estimator.

This paper is organized as follows. After a brief introduction, we refer to the framework of panel data, as well as the main concepts of robust methodologies. Section 2 provides the main results for the FGLS estimator in panel data. In Sect. 3, a new version of a robust FGLS is presented. Then, in Sect. 4, Grunfeld data is used as presented in one of the recent versions, available in [4]. This paper is concluded in Sect. 5 with a brief discussion of the main results and conclusions.

1.1 Panel Data Model (PDM)

A panel data model may be defined by the following equation:

$$y_{it} = \beta_0 + \mathbf{X}'_{it}\beta + u_{it}, \qquad i = 1, ..., N; t = 1, ..., T, \tag{1}$$

where y_{it} denotes the observation of the dependent variable Y under study; the i subscript refers to the unit, (individual, country,...) and the t index is used for the time periods in which the observations are collected for each of the individuals i; $\beta_0 \in \mathbb{R}$, $\mathbf{X}'_{it}$ is the vector of observations of the K independent variables at time t for the individual i and β is a $K \times 1$ vector of coefficients of the model.

The simplest way of analyzing panel data is to treat it like a cross-sectional data set, ignoring eventual individual or time effects. This is known as the pooling model. Choosing the model depends on the nature of the study and/or the variables under consideration.

We will consider the usual approach of splitting the two components of the random error u_{it} so the existence of an unobservable individual effect, μ_i might be distinguishable from the rest of disturbance ν_{it},

$$u_{it} = \mu_i + \nu_{it}. \tag{2}$$

The fact that the term μ_i is time-invariant allows it to accommodate the existence of a specific individual effect, not expressed in the regression equation. Depending on the assumptions we can make about the terms μ_i, we consider different models for estimating the model parameters.

When we make an option for the fixed effects model, it does not necessarily mean that we are considering the μ_i as nonstochastic terms. It may possible to have some arbitrary correlations between the unobserved effect and the explainable variables [5]. Strict exogeneity is assumed, meaning that the independent variables X_{it} are independent from the error ν_{it}, for all i and t. The error term ν_{it} is assumed to be independent and identically distributed (i.i.d.) with constant variance, say, σ_ν^2. This approach is adequate if we aim to obtain inference results, only valid for the i individuals under study. The methodology used to obtain the estimators, in this case, is a consequence of the Frisch-Waugh-Lovell theorem and is similar to the one applied when dummy variables are present in the model. This approach is called the within estimation. For example, if the individuals are some banks in Portugal, this would be equivalent to define a set of dummy variables, one for each bank present in the study. In this case, the inference would be conditional to those same banks and the Ordinary Least Squares (OLS) methodology would be applied to obtain the estimators.

If we aim to extend the results to the population, then we go for the random effects (RE) model, in which μ_i are assumed to be random. In the RE model, in addition to the assumptions made for the FE model, it is also assumed that: μ_i are i.i.d. with constant variance σ_μ^2; μ_i are independent of ν_{it} and X_{it} are independent of ν_{it} and μ_i.

According to Baltagi [3], the model (1) can be written as $y = Z\delta + u$ and the error (2) can be written as

$$u = Z_\mu \mu + \nu, \tag{3}$$

with $u' = (u_{11}, ..., u_{1T}, u_{21}, ..., u_{2T}, ..., u_{N1}, ..., u_{NT})$, $\mu' = (\mu_1, ..., \mu_N)$ and $\nu = (\nu_{11}, ..., \nu_{1T}, ..., \nu_{N1}, ..., \nu_{NT})$.

The covariance matrix of these errors is Ω and its structure depends on the type of model considered—fixed or random effects.

1.2 Robust Methods for PDM

A panel data set contains observations of several variables for a period of years (or months for example) referring to a set of individuals (countries or firms). Real data sets often present atypical observations or outliers. Outliers can be interpreted as observations with a low probability of belonging to the same distribution as the one that characterizes the majority of the rest of the data. It is important to detect multivariate outliers in this type of data, but visual observation is not easy, because these observations can be masked by the complex structure of this type of data. Rousseeuw and Van Zomeren [6] proposed a detection robust methodology for identifying multivariate outliers.

The classical estimation of PDM parameters, namely FGLS, may be seriously affected by the presence of outliers in the sample which should not occur within Robust estimation. Some robust procedures for PDM have been proposed in the last years, in [7–15], for example. Some of these proposals are stated for fixed effects models, others are for random effects models; some of them are directed to dynamic models and others to static models. In these studies, the authors adapted robust regression methods [16] to PDM. Although there are already some proposals for robust methods in the case of PDM, there are still few papers with an application of robust methodologies. In the fields of economics and finance, the most commonly used estimators are those obtained from the application of the least squares method. In spite of the existence of numerous robust proposals for these estimators, we find them rarely applied in empirical studies. The authors of this paper suggest a most user-friendly version of a robust procedure, expecting to witness a more widespread use from the community of nonstatistical researchers.

2 The FGLS Estimator

For the RE model, the error covariance matrix is Ω is given by,

$$\Omega = E(\mathbf{u}\mathbf{u}') = \sigma_\mu^2(\mathbf{I}_N \otimes \mathbf{J}_T) + \sigma_\nu^2(\mathbf{I}_N \otimes \mathbf{I}_T), \tag{4}$$

with $\mathbf{J}_T$ being a matrix of ones of dimension T, $\mathbf{I}_N, \mathbf{I}_T$ identity matrices of order N, T, respectively.

In case of the FE model, this matrix is simplified and has the expression:

$$\Omega = E(\mathbf{u}\mathbf{u}') = \sigma_\nu^2(\mathbf{I}_N \otimes \mathbf{I}_T), \tag{5}$$

After obtaining the inverse Ω^{-1}, a Generalized Least Squares (GLS) estimator may be obtained as a weighted least squares estimator. The matrix Ω may be decomposed, but the problem is that the component variances are unknown. Several proposals were considered to overcome this difficulty and the framework of Feasible Generalized Least Squares (FGLS) was developed. The methodology involved consists of using an estimated matrix $\hat{\Omega}$.

One of the most frequent approaches considers the process of estimation in two steps: first using an Ordinary Least Square (OLS) methodology, and in the second step, the residuals of the first fitted values are used to estimate Ω. With the estimated matrix Ω under suitable conditions, we obtain the FGLS estimator:

$$\hat{\delta}_{FGLS} = (\mathbf{X}'\hat{\Omega}^{-1}\mathbf{X})^{-1}\mathbf{X}'\hat{\Omega}^{-1}\mathbf{Y}. \tag{6}$$

Asymptotic results provide good properties for the FGLS estimator when applied with large samples, see [3] and [5].

3 A Robust FGLS Estimator

The presented proposal consists of robustifying the FGLS estimator, recalling that its implementation includes three steps:

(i) estimate the parameters by the PLS (Pooled Least Squares) and collect the residuals, considering them as error estimates; (ii) estimate the covariance matrix of the errors Ω with the residuals of the former step, using the sample covariance matrix; (iii) estimate the model parameters by FGLS with the estimated covariance matrix obtained in the former step.

The RFGLS (Robust Feasible Generalized Least Squares) estimator proposed in this work results from applying a robust method in the second step of FGLS. The correspondent algorithm is as follows:

1. estimate the parameters by PLS and compute the residuals,
2. estimate the covariance matrix of the errors using the robust estimator CovOGK,

3. estimate the model parameters with FGLS using the robust estimated of covariance matrix obtained at the previous step.

The robust covariance matrix estimator OGK (Orthogonalized Gnanadesikan-Kettenring) was proposed by Maronna and Zamar [17]. It allows to get robust location and scale estimators. The OGK estimator results from a transformation of a previously proposed estimator by Gnanadesikan and Kettenring [18]. This original proposal allows to obtain a robust estimate of the covariance matrix, but the resulting matrix may not be positive definite. To overcome this problem, Maronna and Zamar [17] performed a geometric transformation (orthogonalization). This transformation is based on the fact that the eigenvalues of the covariance matrix are the variances along the directions defined by the respective eigenvectors; this ensures that the obtained matrix is positive definite [16]. To calculate the OGK estimator, it is necessary to consider robust and efficient location and scale functions. In [17], Maronna and Zamar used a weighted mean and τ-scale estimator. The OGK estimator does not have an explicit form, but it can be obtained by applying a set of computational steps, which can be seen in detail in [16].

4 Illustration with the Grunfeld Data

Grunfeld data [4] is a set of data widely used in econometric literature and teaching econometrics activity. It consists of a set of annual records from the American firms: General Motors, US Steel, General Electric, Chrysler, Atlantic Refining, IBM, Union Oil, Westinghouse, Goodyear, Diamond Match and American Steel. Data refer to the period between 1935 and 1954.

There is a total of 220 observations, corresponding to twenty years and eleven firms for five variables:

- the dependent variable—*invest*, representing the firm investments in dollars;
- two independent variables—*value* referring to the market value, and *capital* regarding the firm capital;
- the variable *firm* identifying the different firms recorded;
- the variable *year*, a year identifier.

There are multiple versions of these data in the literature. The version used in this study is the latest version, available at https://eeecon.uibk.ac.at/~zeileis/grunfeld/Grunfeld.csv.

The original Grunfeld data were first analysed in the frame of Grunfeld's PhD in Economics, where he studied *"The Determinants of Corporate Investment"* [19]. This set of data continues to be widely used in order to illustrate different panel data studies for research and educational purposes.

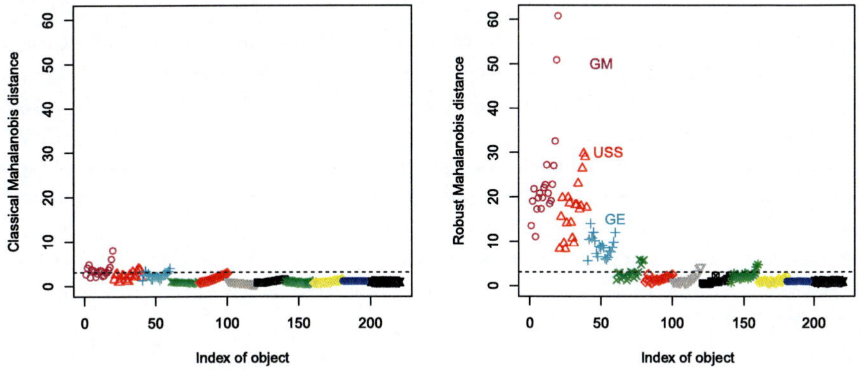

Fig. 1 Detection of multivariate outliers with Mahalanobis distance

Grunfeld formulated a model that describes the dependence of the investment, (y), from the value (x_1) and the capital (x_2) [20], translated by the investment equation:

$$invest_{it} = \beta_0 + \beta_1 value_{it} + \beta_2 capital_{it} + u_{it}, \tag{7}$$

with $i = 1, ..., 11$ e $t = 1, ..., 20$.

A preliminary analysis is important to detect the main characteristics of data. Panel data analysis requires suitable conditions that should be present, otherwise, we compromise the validity of the results. As in multiple fields of research, econometric data sets often exhibit atypical observations that demand particular attention. It is important to investigate the existence of outliers before proceeding to the statistical analysis. Due to the nature of data, a simple boxplot might not do the task, i.e., without convenient multivariate tools, one might miss the detection of an outlier.

Outliers detection of Grunfeld data was made in accordance with the proposed methodology for multivariate outliers detection, in [6], with classic and robust Mahalanobis distance and assuming the normality of the error terms. To support the computations, R language [21] was used, in particular, the *Moutlier* function from *chemometrics package* [22]. The pertinence of the use of this methodology is illustrated in Fig. 1.

As shown in Fig. 1, the robust method highlights three outliers, i.e., firms that are associated with variable values that are far away from those observed for the remaining firms: these are the firms General Motors (GM), US Steel (USS) and General Electrics (GE).

In this paper, we applied both classic and robust methods to obtain parameter estimates of the Grunfeld model. The presence of outliers within Grunfeld data justifies the use of robust estimation methods. The parameters estimation process was made considering the fixed effects model and the random effects model, using FGLS and RFGLS, respectively. To compare the performance of the two estimators, we performed a residual analysis, according to [12].

To estimate the model parameters, we used two R packages: for the FGLS estimates we used the function *pggls* from the package *plm* (a package for panel data analysis) [23]; for the RFGLS estimates, we used the function *covOGK* from *robustbase* (package with robust methods) [24].

We initially considered the *pggls* function and then modified it, so we could obtain an adapted version of the function that includes the robust covariance matrix. During the FGLS estimator calculation process, we replaced the required matrix with a new, robustified version, computed with the *covOGK* function. The result is a modified robust version of the FGLS estimator, i.e., we obtained new RFGLS estimates of the parameters.

4.1 Model Parameters Estimates

Table 1 contains the values of the parameters estimates, found for the hypotheses and methods considered. We can observe some differences between the model parameters estimates obtained with the two different estimators, FGLS e RFGLS.

In order to evaluate the performance of the two estimators considered, the multivariate residuals were calculated for each of the fitted models and a residual analysis was carried out, comparing the mean and standard deviation values obtained.

Figure 2 shows that, for the fixed effects model, the robust method performs better. The residuals of the fixed effects model obtained after applying the robust method RFGLS present smaller mean values (at the left) and standard deviation (right) for almost every company.

Figure 3 shows that, for the random effects model, the robust method performs better too. The residuals of the fitted random effects model produced, after applying the robust method RFGLS, present smaller mean and standard deviations values for almost every firm.

Note that both the mean and standard deviation of the residuals obtained were lower for the robust method. For both type of models, random or fixed effects, the residuals obtained with the robust method presented lower mean and standard deviation. It is clear that the robust estimated model is less affected by the identified outliers (for the three firms, GM, USS, GE) than the classical estimated model.

Table 1 Model parameters estimates

	FE		RE	
	$\hat{\beta}_1$	$\hat{\beta}_2$	$\hat{\beta}_1$	$\hat{\beta}_2$
FGLS	0.110	0.309	0.114	0.228
RFGLS	0.113	0.295	0.124	0.191

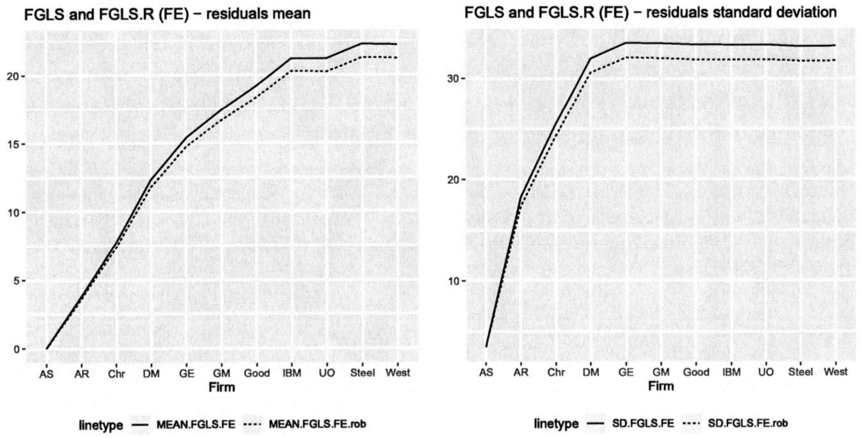

Fig. 2 FGLS and RFGLS mean and MSE—fixed effects model

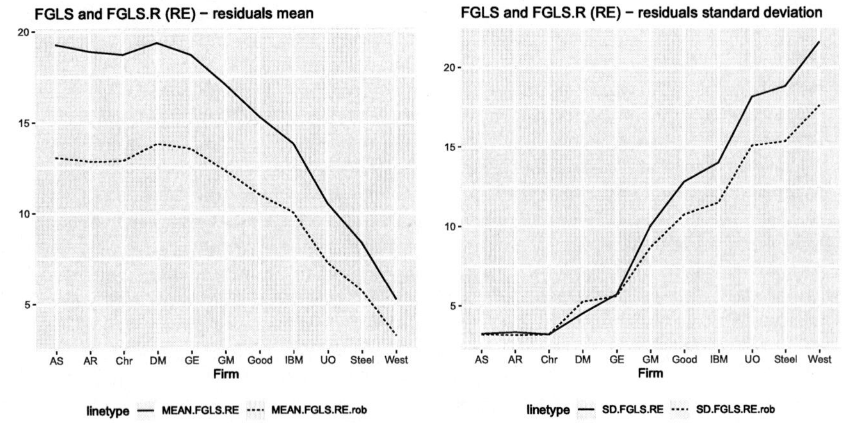

Fig. 3 FGLS and RFGLS mean and MSE—random effects model

5 Concluding Remarks and Future Work

The panel data approach is a frequent way to represent Economical and Financial data. In these areas of study, real data often contain outliers. Robust methods are recommended for this type of data analysis. Robust Mahalanobis distance turned possible to detect outliers that were present in the Grunfeld data set. The robust estimator was the one with better performance as this estimator produced residuals with less mean and less standard deviation. To continue this research, the authors intend to do a simulation study in order to evaluate the RFGLS estimator properties. A Monte Carlo study could be used to evaluate the estimated bias of the new estimators. Assumptions on the idiosyncratic component ν_{it} might fail having to face with autocorrelation and heteroskedasticity, so common in economics and finance. It is important to study the behaviour of this new estimator in those adverse scenarios. Furthermore, the authors seek to improve the RFGLS estimator, inserting robust procedures in the remaining steps of FGLS estimator.

Acknowledgements This work is supported by The Center for Research and Development in Mathematics and Applications (CIDMA) through the Portuguese Foundation for Science and Technology (FCT - Fundaç a para a Ciência e a Tecnologia), references UIDB/04106/2020 and UIDP/04106/2020.

References

1. Morita, M., Ohtsuki, H., Hiraiwa-Hasegawa, M.: A panel data analysis of the probability of childbirth in a Japanese sample: new evidence of the two-child norm. Am. J. Hum. Biol. **28**(2), 220–225 (2016)
2. Kalkuhl, M., Wenz, L.: The impact of climate conditions on economic production. Evidence from a global panel of regions. J. Environ. Econ. Manag. **103**, 102–360 (2020)
3. Baltagi, B.H.: Econometric Analysis of Panel Data . Springer (2021)
4. Kleiber C, Z.A.: The Grunfeld Data at 50. German Econ. Rev. **11**(4), 404–417 (2010)
5. Wooldridge, J.M.: Econometric Analysis of Cross Section and Panel Data 2e. MIT Press (2010)
6. Rousseeuw, P.J., van Zomeren, B.C.: Unmasking multivariate outliers and leverage points: rejoinder. J. Am. Stat. Assoc. **85**(411), 633–639 (1990)
7. Koenker, R.: Quantile regression for longitudinal data. J. Multivar. Anal. **91**(1), 74–89 (2004)
8. Bramati, M.C., Croux, C.: Robust estimators for the fixed effects panel data model. Economet. J. **10**(3), 521–540 (2007)
9. Aquaro, M., Cizek, P., Aquaro, M., Cizek, P.: One-step robust estimation of fixed-effects panel data models. Comput. Stat. Data Anal. **57**(1), 536–548 (2013)
10. Dhaene, G., Zhu, Y., Dhaene, G., Zhu, Y.: Median-based estimation of dynamic panel models with fixed effects. Comput. Stat Data Anal. **113**(C), 398–423 (2017)
11. Cízek, P., Aquaro, M.: Robust estimation and moment selection in dynamic fixed-effects panel data models. Comput. Stat. **33**(2), 675–708 (2018)
12. Mazlina, N., Bakar, A., Midi, H.: The Applications of Robust Estimation in Fixed Effect Panel Data Model, pp. 341–346. Atlantis Press (2019)
13. Midi, H., Muhammad, S.: Robust estimation for fixed and random effects panel data models with different centering methods. J. Eng. Appl. Sci. **13**, 7156–7161 (2018)
14. Bakar, N.M.A., Midi, H.: Robust weights of generalized m-estimator for panel data. AIP Conf. Proc. **1905**, 5–10 (2017)
15. Beyaztas, B.H., Bandyopadhyay, S.: Data driven robust estimation methods for fixed effects panel data models. J. Stat. Comput. Simul. **0**(0), 1–25 (2021)
16. Maronna, R.A., Martin, R.D., Yohai, V.J.: Robust Statistics: Theory and Methods. Wiley, New York (2006)
17. Maronna, R.A., Zamar, R.H.: Robust estimates of location and dispersion for high-dimensional datasets. Technometrics **44**(4), 307–317 (2002)
18. Gnanadesikan, R., Kettenring, J.R.: Robust estimates, residuals, and outlier detection with multiresponse data. Biometrics **28**(1), 81–124 (1972)
19. Grunfeld, Y.: Determinants of Corporate Investment, Demand for Durable Goods. Ph.D. thesis, Chicago: University of Chicago Press (1960)
20. Gujarati, D.N., Porter, D.C.: Basic Econometrics, 5 edn. McGraw-Hill, Irwin (2011)
21. R Core Team: R: A Language and Environment for Statistical Computing. R Foundation for Statistical Computing, Vienna, Austria (2021)

22. Varmuza, K., Filzmoser, P.: Introduction to Multivariate Statistical Analysis in Chemometrics. Chapman & Hall/CRC Press, Boca Raton, FL (2016)
23. Croissant, Y., Millo, G.: Panel data econometrics in R: The `plm` package. J. Stat. Softw. **27**(2), 1–43 (2008)
24. Maechler, M., Rousseeuw, P., Croux, C., Todorov, V., Ruckstuhl, A. et al.: `robustbase`: Basic Robust Statistics (2021). R package version 0.93-9

The Extended Chen–Poisson Marginal Rate Model for Recurrent Gap Time Data

Ivo Sousa-Ferreira, Cristina Rocha, and Ana Maria Abreu

Abstract A new parametric model for recurrent gap time data based on the extended Chen–Poisson distribution is proposed. The model is characterized by a marginal rate function derived from a non-homogeneous Poisson process, which allows us to deduce the conditional distribution of each gap time given the previous recurrence time. The proposed model is quite flexible since it accommodates several shapes of the marginal rate function. Moreover, it is shown that this model has the Chen marginal rate model as a limiting case. The maximum likelihood method is applied for parameter estimation in the presence of right-censoring. A simulation study is conducted to evaluate the properties of the maximum likelihood estimators in various scenarios. The likelihood ratio test is also investigated for model selection between the proposed model and its limiting case. An application to small bowel motility data is considered to illustrate the potential of the new model in comparison with other competing models.

Keywords Extended Chen–Poisson distribution · Gap times · Non-homogeneous Poisson process · Parametric model · Recurrent events

---

I. Sousa-Ferreira (✉) · C. Rocha
Department of Statistics and Operational Research, Faculty of Sciences, University of Lisbon, Lisbon, Portugal
e-mail: ivo.ferreira@staff.uma.pt

C. Rocha
e-mail: cmrocha@fc.ul.pt

I. Sousa-Ferreira · A. M. Abreu
Department of Mathematics, Faculty of Exact Sciences and Engineering, University of Madeira, Funchal, Portugal
e-mail: abreu@staff.uma.pt

I. Sousa-Ferreira · C. Rocha
CEAUL, Faculty of Sciences, University of Lisbon, Lisbon, Portugal

A. M. Abreu
CIMA, University of Madeira, Funchal, Portugal

R. Bispo et al. (eds.), *Recent Developments in Statistics and Data Science*,
Springer Proceedings in Mathematics & Statistics 398,
https://doi.org/10.1007/978-3-031-12766-3_23

1 Introduction

In longitudinal studies, it is common for subjects to experience several episodes of a certain event of interest during the observation period. Such outcomes have been termed *recurrent events* and are often encountered in medical studies on disease relapses, reliability studies on repeated machine breakdowns, financial studies on successive defaults on bank loans, among others. In many settings, researchers have more interest in the time between consecutive events (i.e., gap times) than in the time-to-events (e.g., Gail et al. [1]). For instance, in medical studies it is often intended to model the time elapsed since the last event when subjects can recover after the occurrence of each event, such as in asthma attacks, epileptic seizures and re-hospitalizations.

The canonical models to analyse gap times are based on renewal processes [2, 3]. These models are formulated under the assumption that gap times can be directly modelled without specifying a dependence structure within subjects. Since the independence assumption is untenable in most situations, more general models have been formulated over the years through conditional distributions, including a variety of regression models to evaluate covariate effects (e.g., [4–8]), gap time models with frailty terms (e.g., [9, 10]) and joint distribution of the gap times via copula functions (e.g., [11, 12]). For a comprehensive understanding on the existing methods to analyse recurrent gap time data, the reader is referred to Cook and Lawless [3] and Aalen et al. [13].

Another approach in gap time modelling consists in deducing the conditional distribution of the gap times under the classical assumption that the number of recurrent events up to a given time follows a non-homogeneous Poisson process (NHPP), for which the gap times are generally not independent [3]. In this context, Zhao and Zhou [14] proposed an additive semiparametric model based on a marginal rate function (mrf) that is derived from a NHPP. This model has the advantage of allowing estimation of the covariate effects without specifying the form of the baseline rate function. Nonetheless, when the research interest is also to study how the recurrence rate evolves over time, an adequate parametric model would be more convenient. With this motivation, Macera et al. [15] and Louzada et al. [16, 17] suggested a parametric form for the baseline rate function based on the exponential-Poisson (EP), Poisson-exponential (PE) and Weibull distributions, respectively. However, these parametric models only allow monotonic rates. Hence, alternative distributions should be considered to provide more flexibility to model gap times between recurrent events.

For complex phenomena associated with a subject's lifetime, it is admissible to consider non-monotonic hazard shapes. In this sense, Sousa-Ferreira et al. [18] recently proposed a new flexible generalization of the Chen distribution [19] by compounding it with a zero-truncated Poisson (ZTP) distribution, which is called extended Chen–Poisson (ECP) distribution. For this distribution, the hazard and survival functions at time t are defined, respectively, as

$$h_0(t; \lambda, \gamma, \phi) = \frac{\lambda\gamma\phi t^{\gamma-1} e^{t^{\gamma}+\lambda\left(1-e^{t^{\gamma}}\right)}}{e^{\phi e^{\lambda\left(1-e^{t^{\gamma}}\right)}} - 1}, \qquad t > 0, \tag{1}$$

and

$$S_0(t; \lambda, \gamma, \phi) = \frac{1 - e^{-\phi e^{\lambda\left(1-e^{t^{\gamma}}\right)}}}{1 - e^{-\phi}}, \qquad t > 0 \tag{2}$$

where $\lambda, \gamma > 0$ and $\phi \in \mathbb{R}\backslash\{0\}$ are the parameters of the distribution. A graphical analysis showed that the hazard function (1) can be monotonic increasing, monotonic decreasing, unimodal, bathtub, increasing-decreasing-increasing (IDI) or decreasing-increasing-decreasing-increasing (DIDI), so it has the potential to cover a wide variety of situations. Therefore, the ECP distribution is a promising candidate for the development of a new model for recurrent events.

The ECP distribution arises in the context of competitive and complementary risks (CCR) settings for single event analysis, wherein it is only possible to observe the minimum or maximum lifetime among all causes that could trigger the occurrence of the event, instead of observing the lifetime associated with a particular cause. In these circumstances, the cause responsible for the occurrence of the event is often unknown, as well as the number of existing causes. As discussed by Ramos et al. [20], when it is assumed that the number of causes follows a ZTP distribution, both the minimum and maximum distributions can be unified in a simple form, by extending the parameter space of the ZTP distribution into $\mathbb{R}\backslash\{0\}$, giving rise to the extended Poisson family of distributions. Since the ECP distribution [18] belongs to this family, it has two special cases when $\phi < 0$ (distribution of the minimum) and $\phi > 0$ (distribution of the maximum), which refer to the Chen–Poisson and Poisson-Chen distributions, respectively. In recurrent events analysis, it is also plausible that the nature of the recurrence process involves a CCR scenario. The EP and PE marginal rate models proposed by Macera et al. [15] and Louzada et al. [16], respectively, are able to deal with these kind of problems. According to Ramos et al. [20], since the EP and PE distributions belong to the unified Poisson family, the resulting models for recurrent events can be merged into a single model, named extended exponential-Poisson (EEP) marginal rate model.

In the light of the above context, we propose a new parametric model for recurrent gap time data, considering the ECP form (1) to specify the baseline rate function. The remainder of the paper is organized as follows. Section 2 begins with the formulation of the proposed model and with the study of its properties. The maximum likelihood (ML) method is applied for parameter estimation, in the presence of a right censoring mechanism, in Sect. 3. A simulation study is performed to assess the frequentist properties of the ML estimators in Sect. 4, while in Sect. 5 the proposed model is applied in the analysis of the small bowel motility data in [2]. Some concluding remarks are presented in Sect. 6.

2 Formulation of the ECP Marginal Rate Model

Suppose that there are n independent subjects in study and that each one can experience a maximum of K_i $(i = 1, \ldots, n)$ recurrences of an event. For the ith subject, let T_{ik} be the time from the beginning of study until the occurrence of the kth event $(k = 1, \ldots, K_i)$ and $W_{ik} = T_{ik} - T_{i,k-1}$ be the gap time between the $(k-1)$th and kth events, where $0 \equiv T_{i0} < T_{i1} < \ldots < T_{iK_i}$. Let $N_i(t)$ denote the number of recurrences of an event up to time $t \geq 0$. The recurrence process $N_i(\cdot)$ of the ith subject is assumed to be a NHPP with independent increments. In order to simplify the notation, an arbitrary subject is considered and the subscript i is dropped.

Zhao and Zhou [14] proposed a model wherein the general form of the mrf[1] of $N(t_{k-1} + w)$ is characterized by

$$h(w|t_{k-1}) = h_0(t_{k-1} + w), \qquad w > 0, \tag{3}$$

where $h_0(\cdot) \geq 0$ is a baseline rate function. Under the assumptions of a NHPP [3], the average number of recurrences over the interval $(t_{k-1},\ t_{k-1} + w]$ is given by

$$\begin{aligned} E[N(t_{k-1} + w) - N(t_{k-1})] &= \int_{t_{k-1}}^{t_{k-1}+w} h_0(u)du = \int_0^w h_0(t_{k-1} + u)du \\ &= H_0(t_{k-1} + w) - H_0(t_{k-1}) = H(w|t_{k-1}) \end{aligned}$$

and the survival function of the kth gap time, W_k, conditional on $T_{k-1} = t_{k-1}$ is

$$S(w|t_{k-1}) = \exp\big\{ - H(w|t_{k-1})\big\} = \frac{S_0(t_{k-1} + w)}{S_0(t_{k-1})}, \tag{4}$$

where $H_0(t) = \int_0^t h_0(u)du$ and $S_0(t) = \exp\big\{ - H_0(t)\big\}$ are the baseline cumulative rate and baseline survival functions, respectively, and $H(w|t_{k-1})$ is the cumulative rate function of the recurrence process. So, the dependence structure among gap times within a subject is expressed by the conditional survival function (4), which represents the probability of not suffering any event during a gap time of length w, given that the subject survived beyond the time t_{k-1}. Note that, since $W_1 = T_1 - T_0 = T_1$, it follows that $S(w|t_0) = S_0(w)$.

To estimate $h_0(\cdot)$, Zhao and Zhou [14] considered a non-parametric method based on kernel estimation, while other researchers assumed a specific parametric form for the baseline rate function, by considering an EEP [15, 16] or a Weibull [17] form. Since the exponential distribution is a particular case of the EEP and Weibull distributions, the exponential marginal rate model will in turn be a sub-model of a marginal rate model (3) based on those distributions. This leads to an important special case of the Poisson process, corresponding to the classical homogenous Poisson process

[1] It represents the marginal (i.e. unconditional on the complete process history) instantaneous probability of occurring an event at time $t_{k-1} + w$.

(HPP). This is the only case where it is assumed that the gap times between recurrent events are independent and identically distributed exponential random variables.

To the best of our knowledge, all fully parametric marginal rate models proposed so far only have monotonic rate functions. This drawback motivated the development of a more flexible model. Specifically, conditional on $T_{k-1} = t_{k-1}$, we assume that the baseline rate function has an ECP form (1). Then, it follows from (3) that the mrf of the recurrence process is

$$h(w|t_{k-1}) = \frac{\lambda\gamma\phi(t_{k-1}+w)^{\gamma-1}\mathrm{e}^{(t_{k-1}+w)^{\gamma}+\lambda\left(1-\mathrm{e}^{(t_{k-1}+w)^{\gamma}}\right)}}{\mathrm{e}^{\phi\mathrm{e}^{\lambda\left(1-\mathrm{e}^{(t_{k-1}+w)^{\gamma}}\right)}}-1}, \qquad w > 0, \qquad (5)$$

and, together with (2) and (4), the survival function of the kth gap time, W_k, conditional on the previous recurrence time is

$$S(w|t_{k-1}) = \frac{1-\mathrm{e}^{-\phi\mathrm{e}^{\lambda\left(1-\mathrm{e}^{(t_{k-1}+w)^{\gamma}}\right)}}}{1-\mathrm{e}^{-\phi\mathrm{e}^{\lambda\left(1-\mathrm{e}^{t_{k-1}^{\gamma}}\right)}}}, \qquad w > 0, \qquad (6)$$

where $\lambda, \gamma > 0$ and $\phi \in \mathbb{R}\backslash\{0\}$. Hereafter, the distribution of $W_k|T_{k-1} = t_{k-1}$ will be called ECP marginal rate model. In the same line of the EEP marginal rate model [15, 16, 20], the proposed model provides a practical interpretation in CCR settings. When $\phi < 0$ (or $\phi > 0$), $W_k|T_{k-1} = t_{k-1}$ represents the minimum (or maximum) time among all causes responsible for the event occurrence. Moreover, it should be noted that the Chen marginal rate model is a limiting case of the proposed model, since when ϕ approaches 0 it follows that the mrf (5) reduces to $\lim_{\phi\to 0} h(w|t_{k-1}) = \lambda\gamma\left(t_{k-1}+w\right)^{\gamma-1}\exp\{\left(t_{k-1}+w\right)^{\gamma}\}$, which is the form of the hazard function of the Chen distribution [19] at time $t_{k-1}+w$.

The mrf (5) is able to take the same flexible shapes reported for the hazard function (1) of the ECP distribution [18]. Figure 1 depicts some possible rate shapes for different sets of parameter values. Although the mrf (5) presents an expression similar to the hazard function (1) of the ECP distribution, the survival functions (2) and (6) are clearly distinct. Actually, considering that $W_1 = T_1 - T_0 = T_1$, the ECP marginal rate model is equal to the ECP distribution only for $k = 1$. In other words, the first gap time follows an ECP distribution, while the subsequent gap times follow the conditional distribution given by (6).

The cumulative distribution function (cdf), $F(w|t_{k-1}) = 1 - S(w|t_{k-1})$, can be directly obtained from (6). Applying the inverse transformation method [21] to the cdf, a pseudo-random sample from the ECP marginal rate model can be generated considering the expression

$$W_k = \left\{\log\left[1-\lambda^{-1}\log\left(-\phi^{-1}\log\left(U_k-(U_k-1)\mathrm{e}^{-\phi e^{\lambda\left(1-\mathrm{e}^{t_{k-1}^{\gamma}}\right)}}\right)\right)\right]\right\}^{1/\gamma} - t_{k-1}, \qquad (7)$$

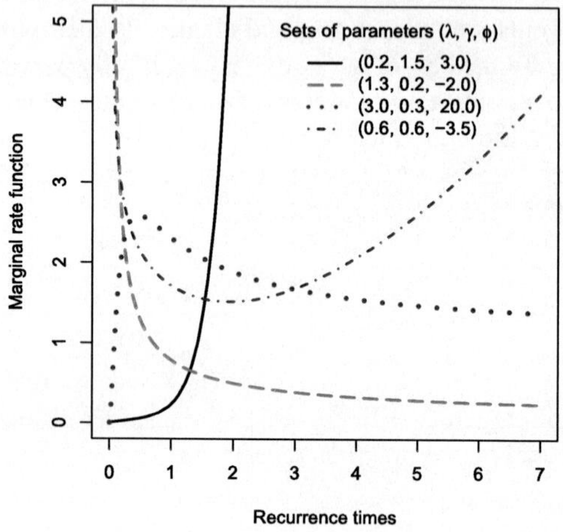

Fig. 1 Some ECP marginal rate functions of the recurrence process $N(t_{k-1}+w)$ for an arbitrary subject, considering the sets of parameter values $(\lambda, \gamma, \phi) = (0.2, 1.5, 3.0)$, $(1.3, 0.2, -2.0)$, $(3.0, 0.3, 20.0)$ and $(0.6, 0.6, -3.5)$ that correspond to an increasing, decreasing, unimodal and bathtub shapes, respectively

where U_k is a random variable with standard uniform distribution. Thus, for an arbitrary subject, the realizations of T_k can be recursively obtained for $k = 1, \ldots, K$ by $t_k = t_{k-1} + w_k$, with $t_0 = 0$.

Based on the raw moments of the ECP distribution [18], the general expression of the rth raw moment of $W_k | T_{k-1} = t_{k-1}$ can be straightforwardly deduced by making the change of variable $v = \exp\{\lambda(1 - \mathrm{e}^{w^\gamma})\}$, resulting in

$$E(W_k^r | t_{k-1}) = A \int_0^B \mathrm{e}^{-\phi v} \left[\log\left(1 - \frac{\log(v)}{\lambda}\right)\right]^{r/\gamma} dv - t_{k-1}, \quad r \in \mathbb{N},$$

with $A = \phi/(1 - \mathrm{e}^{-\phi B})$ and $B = \exp\{\lambda\big(1 - \mathrm{e}^{t_{k-1}^\gamma}\big)\}$. Hence, the mean and variance of $W_k | T_{k-1} = t_{k-1}$ are given, respectively, by

$$E(W_k | t_{k-1}) = A \int_0^B \mathrm{e}^{-\phi v} \left[\log\left(1 - \frac{\log(v)}{\lambda}\right)\right]^{1/\gamma} dv - t_{k-1}$$

and

$$\mathrm{Var}(W_k | t_{k-1}) = A \int_0^B \mathrm{e}^{-\phi v} \left[\log\left(1 - \frac{\log(v)}{\lambda}\right)\right]^{2/\gamma} dv - t_{k-1} - [E(W_k | t_{k-1})]^2.$$

Interestingly, it can be shown that $E(W_k | t_{k-1})$ corresponds to the mean residual life function of the ECP distribution at time t_{k-1}, studied in [18].

3 Statistical Inference

The inferential procedures are based on the well-known ML method and its large sample properties. Suppose that data are available from n independent subjects, that to each subject i corresponds a vector (w_{ik}, δ_{ik}), $i = 1, \ldots, n$ and $k = 1, \ldots, K_i$, where $w_{ik} = t_{ik} - t_{i,k-1}$ is the observed gap time, $0 < t_{i1} < \ldots < t_{iK_i}$ are the observed time-to-events corresponding to the K_i recurrences and δ_{ik} is a censoring indicator variable that equals 0 or 1 when w_{ik} is right-censored or completely observed, respectively.

Let $\boldsymbol{\vartheta} = (\lambda, \gamma, \phi)'$ be the vector of parameters of the ECP marginal rate model. Assuming that the censoring mechanism is non-informative, the ML estimate of $\boldsymbol{\vartheta}$ can be obtained by direct maximization of the log-likelihood function given by

$$\ell(\boldsymbol{\vartheta}) = \sum_{i=1}^{n}\sum_{k=1}^{K_i}\Bigg\{\lambda\delta_{ik} + \log(\lambda\gamma)\delta_{ik} + \delta_{ik}(t_{i,k-1} + w_{ik})^{\gamma} - \lambda\delta_{ik}\mathrm{e}^{(t_{i,k-1}+w_{ik})^{\gamma}}$$
$$+ (\gamma - 1)\delta_{ik}\log(t_{i,k-1} + w_{ik}) + \delta_{ik}\log\left(\frac{\phi}{\mathrm{e}^{\phi\mathrm{e}^{\lambda\left(1-\mathrm{e}^{(t_{i,k-1}+w_{ik})^{\gamma}}\right)}} - 1}\right) \quad (8)$$
$$+ \log\left(\frac{1 - \mathrm{e}^{-\phi\mathrm{e}^{\lambda\left(1-\mathrm{e}^{(t_{i,k-1}+w_{ik})^{\gamma}}\right)}}}{1 - \mathrm{e}^{-\phi\mathrm{e}^{\lambda\left(1-\mathrm{e}^{t_{i,k-1}^{\gamma}}\right)}}}\right)\Bigg\}.$$

Care is needed when $\phi < 0$, since the values of $\log\{1 - \exp[-\phi\exp(\lambda(1 - \mathrm{e}^{t^{\gamma}}))]\}$, $t > 0$, and $\log(\phi)$, cannot be computed. This problem is easily overcome by considering that $\log\{\phi/[\exp[\phi\exp(\lambda(1 - \mathrm{e}^{(t_{i,k-1}+w_{ik})^{\gamma}}))] - 1]\} \in \mathbb{R}$ and $\log\left\{\{1 - \exp[-\phi\exp(\lambda(1 - \mathrm{e}^{(t_{i,k-1}+w_{ik})^{\gamma}}))]\}/\{1 - \exp[-\phi\exp(\lambda(1 - \mathrm{e}^{t_{i,k-1}^{\gamma}}))]\}\right\} \in \mathbb{R}_0^-$, $\forall\lambda, \gamma > 0$ and $\phi \in \mathbb{R}\backslash\{0\}$.

For large samples, the inference for λ, γ and ϕ can be based on the corresponding ML estimates and their estimated standard errors, evaluated in standard fashion from the observed information matrix. For computational implementation, the `optim` function available in `R` [22] statistical software (version 4.1.3) is applied to maximize the log-likelihood function (8) through the Broyden–Fletcher–Goldfarb–Shanno optimization method.

The likelihood ratio (LR) test is used for model selection between the ECP and Chen marginal rate models, considering the hypotheses $H_0 : \phi = 0$ versus $H_1 : \phi \neq 0$. The LR statistic is given by $-2\{\ell(\hat{\boldsymbol{\vartheta}}_0) - \ell(\hat{\boldsymbol{\vartheta}})\}$, where $\ell(\hat{\boldsymbol{\vartheta}}_0)$ and $\ell(\hat{\boldsymbol{\vartheta}})$ are the log-likelihoods under the null and alternative hypotheses, respectively, with $\hat{\boldsymbol{\vartheta}}_0 = \arg\max_{(\lambda,\gamma,0)} \ell(\boldsymbol{\vartheta})$ and $\hat{\boldsymbol{\vartheta}} = \arg\max_{(\lambda,\gamma,\phi)} \ell(\boldsymbol{\vartheta})$. Note that, since the baseline distribution unifies the Poisson-Chen ($\phi > 0$) and Chen–Poisson ($\phi < 0$) distributions, the true parameter $\phi = 0$ lies on the boundary of the parameter space in these sub-models. Following Zhou and Maller [23], in this case the asymptotic distribution of the LR test is a 50-50 mixture of a chi-square distribution with 1 degree of freedom (χ_1^2) and a point mass at 0. This result was also considered for model selection between the EEP and exponential marginal rate models [15, 16].

4 Simulation Study

A simulation study is performed to assess the adequacy of the inferential procedures described previously. The pseudo-random samples in the presence of random censoring are generated from (7), assuming that the event times follow an ECP marginal rate model and the censoring times are uniformly distributed. The percentage of pseudo-random censoring is specified as 5, 15 and 30%, following the procedures discussed in [21]. Different sample sizes, $n = 20$, 100 and 500, and number of recurrences, $k = 2$, 5 and 10, are considered. For simplicity, it is assumed that all subjects experience at least $k - 1$ recurrences, which means that only the kth gap time can be censored. The sets of parameter values $\boldsymbol{\vartheta} = (\lambda, \gamma, \phi) = (0.2, 1.5, 3.0)$, $(1.3, 0.2, -2.0)$, $(3.0, 0.3, 20.0)$ and $(0.6, 0.6, -3.5)$ were selected in order to yield increasing, decreasing, unimodal and bathtub shapes of the mrf, respectively, as shown in Fig. 1. Thus, 108 scenarios are investigated. For each one, 1000 pseudo-random samples are generated.

The results reported in Table 1 refer to scenarios with 30% of censoring. However, similar results hold for smaller censoring percentages and also for other sets of parameter values. From Table 1, it is seen that the averages of the ML estimates of λ, γ and ϕ tend to the true value of the parameter and their standard errors tend to zero, as the sample size and number of recurrences increase. These results suggest that the ML estimators are asymptotically unbiased. However, it appears that ϕ has poor average estimates and high standard errors for small sample sizes. This aspect is more visible for the set of parameter values corresponding to a unimodal mrf, but then it fades for large sample sizes and large number of recurrences. The coverage probabilities (CP) of the 95% confidence interval (CI) were also calculated for each parameter, representing the proportion of the 1000 generated 95% CIs that include the actual value of the parameter. The results show that, in general, the CP are close to the nominal level of 95%.

Additionally, the performance of the LR test is analysed in two different situations, depending on whether the parameter ϕ is positive or negative. In the first, the hypotheses $H_0 : \phi = 0$ versus $H_1 : \phi > 0$ are tested considering the parameters $\lambda = 0.2$ and $\gamma = 1.5$, while in the second situation the hypotheses $H_0 : \phi = 0$ versus $H_1 : \phi < 0$ are tested considering the parameters $\lambda = 0.6$ and $\gamma = 0.6$. Under H_0, the first and second sets of parameter values lead to the Chen marginal rate model with increasing and bathtub shapes of the mrf, respectively. The results for these two situations are compiled in Tables 2 and 3, respectively, which contain the empirical proportions of type I error under the null hypothesis, as well as the empirical power of the test to detect different alternative hypothesis, at the 5% nominal significance level. In both cases, as the sample size and number of recurrences increase, the empirical significance levels are closer to the nominal level and the empirical power

Table 1 The averages (Av) of the 1000 ML estimates for $\boldsymbol{\vartheta} = (\lambda, \gamma, \phi)'$, their standard errors (SE) and coverage probabilities (CP) of the 95% CIs

$\boldsymbol{\vartheta}$	k	n	Av($\hat{\boldsymbol{\vartheta}}$)	SE($\hat{\boldsymbol{\vartheta}}$)	CP ($\hat{\boldsymbol{\vartheta}}$)
(0.2, 1.5, 3.0)	2	20	(0.262, 1.520, 5.254)	(0.201, 0.325, 5.853)	(0.870, 0.941, 0.995)
		100	(0.205, 1.516, 3.099)	(0.079, 0.145, 1.442)	(0.936, 0.949, 0.983)
		500	(0.199, 1.506, 2.989)	(0.034, 0.059, 0.566)	(0.966, 0.965, 0.968)
	5	20	(0.215, 1.510, 3.672)	(0.105, 0.152, 2.644)	(0.952, 0.962, 0.996)
		100	(0.200, 1.505, 3.038)	(0.043, 0.061, 0.894)	(0.956, 0.972, 0.984)
		500	(0.200, 1.502, 2.996)	(0.019, 0.026, 0.382)	(0.959, 0.964, 0.960)
	10	20	(0.204, 1.507, 3.297)	(0.067, 0.079, 1.807)	(0.944, 0.966, 0.987)
		100	(0.200, 1.502, 3.035)	(0.028, 0.033, 0.698)	(0.952, 0.958, 0.964)
		500	(0.200, 1.500, 3.001)	(0.013, 0.015, 0.306)	(0.963, 0.960, 0.953)
(1.3, 0.2, −2.0)	2	20	(1.372, 0.205, −2.195)	(0.807, 0.044, 2.632)	(0.971, 0.979, 1.000)
		100	(1.311, 0.200, −2.119)	(0.487, 0.022, 1.568)	(0.959, 0.970, 0.996)
		500	(1.300, 0.200, −2.036)	(0.236, 0.010, 0.718)	(0.960, 0.956, 0.972)
	5	20	(1.234, 0.207, −2.438)	(0.448, 0.031, 1.704)	(0.883, 0.928, 0.949)
		100	(1.290, 0.201, −2.073)	(0.260, 0.017, 0.906)	(0.940, 0.934, 0.956)
		500	(1.308, 0.200, −1.987)	(0.126, 0.008, 0.430)	(0.942, 0.942, 0.953)
	10	20	(1.261, 0.205, −2.274)	(0.369, 0.022, 1.383)	(0.873, 0.898, 0.923)
		100	(1.294, 0.201, −2.045)	(0.193, 0.011, 0.693)	(0.921, 0.925, 0.929)
		500	(1.301, 0.200, −2.000)	(0.087, 0.005, 0.309)	(0.956, 0.949, 0.957)
(3.0, 0.3, 20.0)	2	20	(3.220, 0.333, 64.973)	(0.704, 0.127, 31.372)	(0.773, 0.797, 0.653)
		100	(3.107, 0.298, 31.026)	(0.350, 0.051, 16.260)	(0.926, 0.927, 0.876)
		500	(3.013, 0.301, 20.991)	(0.153, 0.023, 5.394)	(0.961, 0.961, 0.948)
	5	20	(3.161, 0.299, 42.324)	(0.564, 0.052, 25.113)	(0.879, 0.888, 0.813)
		100	(3.028, 0.300, 22.412)	(0.254, 0.023, 8.557)	(0.953, 0.958, 0.942)
		500	(3.005, 0.300, 20.383)	(0.111, 0.010, 3.202)	(0.956, 0.959, 0.951)
	10	20	(3.088, 0.299, 30.078)	(0.453, 0.028, 17.191)	(0.934, 0.941, 0.884)
		100	(3.012, 0.300, 21.196)	(0.198, 0.012, 5.692)	(0.959, 0.951, 0.942)
		500	(3.000, 0.300, 20.144)	(0.087, 0.006, 2.332)	(0.947, 0.943, 0.952)
(0.6, 0.6, −3.5)	2	20	(0.814, 0.604, −3.350)	(0.537, 0.122, 3.862)	(0.956, 0.978, 0.972)
		100	(0.692, 0.592, −3.463)	(0.308, 0.054, 2.008)	(0.926, 0.972, 0.956)
		500	(0.627, 0.596, −3.534)	(0.162, 0.022, 1.047)	(0.896, 0.962, 0.922)
	5	20	(0.653, 0.595, −3.586)	(0.285, 0.069, 1.797)	(0.903, 0.959, 0.968)
		100	(0.624, 0.596, −3.449)	(0.143, 0.032, 0.856)	(0.939, 0.954, 0.964)
		500	(0.606, 0.599, −3.486)	(0.061, 0.014, 0.374)	(0.944, 0.951, 0.954)
	10	20	(0.623, 0.602, −3.592)	(0.210, 0.048, 1.309)	(0.861, 0.881, 0.908)
		100	(0.610, 0.600, −3.492)	(0.109, 0.025, 0.672)	(0.918, 0.925, 0.919)
		500	(0.603, 0.600, −3.490)	(0.048, 0.011, 0.301)	(0.946, 0.944, 0.957)

Table 2 Empirical proportions of type I error and power of the LR test at the 5% nominal significance level, considering $\lambda = 0.2$ and $\gamma = 1.5$

	Empirical type I error			Empirical power								
				$\phi = 0.5$			$\phi = 2.0$			$\phi = 3.5$		
n	$k = 2$	$k = 5$	$k = 10$	$k = 2$	$k = 5$	$k = 10$	$k = 2$	$k = 5$	$k = 10$	$k = 2$	$k = 5$	$k = 10$
20	0.056	0.045	0.040	0.050	0.075	0.073	0.119	0.243	0.411	0.220	0.504	0.716
100	0.049	0.048	0.050	0.076	0.095	0.202	0.263	0.656	0.912	0.647	0.977	1.000
500	0.043	0.056	0.055	0.077	0.255	0.573	0.717	0.996	0.999	0.992	1.000	1.000

Table 3 Empirical proportions of type I error and power of the LR test at the 5% nominal significance level, considering $\lambda = 0.6$ and $\gamma = 0.6$

	Empirical type I error			Empirical power								
				$\phi = -0.5$			$\phi = -2.0$			$\phi = -3.5$		
n	$k = 2$	$k = 5$	$k = 10$	$k = 2$	$k = 5$	$k = 10$	$k = 2$	$k = 5$	$k = 10$	$k = 2$	$k = 5$	$k = 10$
20	0.054	0.045	0.041	0.008	0.026	0.134	0.038	0.176	0.456	0.091	0.412	0.730
100	0.054	0.052	0.046	0.059	0.111	0.217	0.292	0.591	0.882	0.579	0.867	0.982
500	0.041	0.041	0.044	0.117	0.272	0.566	0.792	0.957	1.000	0.968	0.999	1.000

increases, as expected. Nevertheless, some care is needed since there is a remarkable drop of the empirical power when the LR test is performed closer to the boundary of the parameter space of ϕ, which is worsened by small sample sizes and small number of recurrences.

5 Application to Bowel Motility Data

In this section, the ECP marginal rate model is illustrated through a data set concerning the cyclical motility pattern of the small bowel during a fasting state, available in Aalen and Husebye [2]. The bowel motility data was also used by Louzada et al. [16] as an application example for the PE marginal rate model. The study involved 19 healthy subjects, for whom the intraluminal pressure in the small bowel were monitored continuously for 13 h and 40 min. In order to induce a fed state, a standardized mixed meal was served. The fed state is characterized by irregular contractions, lasting from 4 to 7 h. Afterwards, the fasting state starts with a cyclical bowel motility pattern. The aim of this study is to analyse the gap times between successive cycles during the fasting state, also known as migrating motor complex periods. The recurrent events are associated with the initial time of the consecutive cycles. For all subjects, the last gap time is censored due to the end of the study.

Table 4 Marginal rate models for recurrent events fitted to bowel motility data

Marginal rate model, [ref.]	Marginal rate function, $h(w\|t_{k-1})$, $w > 0$
Exponential (HPP), [3]	$\lambda_1, \quad \lambda_1 > 0$
Weibull, [17]	$\lambda_2\gamma_2(t_{k-1}+w)^{\gamma_2-1}, \quad \lambda_2, \gamma_2 > 0$
EEP, [15, 16, 20]	$\dfrac{\lambda_3\phi_3 e^{-\lambda_3(t_{k-1}+w)}}{e^{\phi_3 e^{-\lambda_3(t_{k-1}+w)}}-1}, \quad \lambda_3 > 0, \ \phi_3 \in \mathbb{R}\backslash\{0\}$
Chen	$\lambda_4\gamma_4(t_{k-1}+w)^{\gamma_4-1}e^{(t_{k-1}+w)^{\gamma_4}}, \quad \lambda_4, \gamma_4 > 0$
ECP	$\dfrac{\lambda_5\gamma_5\phi_5(t_{k-1}+w)^{\gamma_5-1}e^{(t_{k-1}+w)^{\gamma_5}+\lambda_5\left(1-e^{(t_{k-1}+w)^{\gamma_5}}\right)}}{e^{\phi e^{\lambda_5\left(1-e^{(t_{k-1}+w)^{\gamma_5}}\right)}}-1},$ $\lambda_5, \gamma_5 > 0, \ \phi_5 \in \mathbb{R}\backslash\{0\}$

Table 5 ML estimates and their 95% CI, −log-likelihood and AIC of the marginal rate models fitted to bowel motility data

Marginal rate model	Parameter	ML estimate	95% CI	$-\hat{\ell}$	AIC
Exponential (HPP)	λ_1	0.532	(0.416, 0.649)	130.457	262.915
Weibull	λ_2	0.208	(0.067, 0.348)	125.246	254.492
	γ_2	1.447	(1.144, 1.750)		
EEP	λ_3	0.727	(0.579, 0.875)	124.101	252.201
	ϕ_3	4.119	(1.734, 6.503)		
Chen	λ_4	0.229	(0.117, 0.341)	130.323	264.646
	γ_4	0.519	(0.455, 0.583)		
ECP	λ_5	1.665	(1.417, 1.912)	122.235	250.470
	γ_5	0.276	(0.239, 0.314)		
	ϕ_5	47.421	(38.479, 56.363)		

For comparison purposes, the marginal rate models listed in Table 4 were fitted to bowel motility data. Table 5 presents the ML estimates and the corresponding 95% CIs for the parameters of the fitted models, as well as the −log-likelihood and observed values of the Akaike information criterion (AIC). Note that the HPP model is a special case of the Weibull and EEP marginal rate models when $\gamma_2 = 1$ and $\phi_3 \to 0$, respectively. Thus, for these models, the LR test can be used to check the independence assumption between the gap times by considering the null hypotheses H_0: $\gamma_2 = 1$ and H_0: $\gamma_3 = 0$, as referred in [15–17]. The first situation involves testing inside the parameter space of γ_2, while the second involves testing at the boundary of the parameter space of ϕ_3. Thus, the 95% percentiles, $a_{0.95}$ and $b_{0.95}$, of the asymptotic distributions of the LR statistic under H_0: $\gamma_2 = 1$ and H_0: $\phi_3 = 0$, respectively, can be calculated from $P(\chi_1^2 \geq a_{0.95}) = 0.95 \Rightarrow a_{0.95} = 3.841$ and $1/2 + 1/2P(\chi_1^2 \geq b_{0.95}) = 0.95 \Rightarrow b_{0.95} = 2.706$. Since the corresponding observed values of LR statistic are equal to 10.423 and 12.713 (both with a p-value < 0.001), there is evidence against the null hypotheses, indicating that a model that takes into account the correlation between the gap times is preferred. The

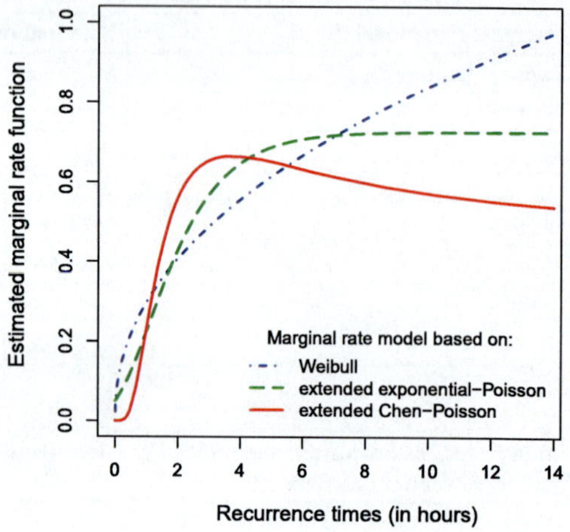

Fig. 2 Estimated marginal rate functions of the Weibull, EEP and ECP marginal rate models fitted to bowel motility data

Chen and ECP marginal rate models are also able to handle the lack of independence between gap times, since they are derived from a NHPP. Once again, the LR test can be used for model selection between these two models, by testing $H_0 : \phi_5 = 0$. In this case, given that the LR test yields an observed value of 16.176 (with a p-value < 0.0001), there is evidence in favour of the ECP marginal rate model.

The Weibull, EEP and ECP model-based estimates of the mrf are depicted in Fig. 2. Both Weibull and EPE marginal rate models provide an increasing rate, with the latter stabilizing from a certain time onwards. In contrast to these monotonic rate shapes, the model based on the ECP distribution exhibits an unimodal shape. The ECP marginal rate model has the lowest AIC value, which means that it is the preferred among all the models that were fitted to the bowel motility data. Additionally, the Cox-Snell residuals were used to informally assess the overall goodness-of-fit of the models. The residuals are defined as $\hat{r}_{ik} = \hat{H}(w_{ik}|t_{i,k-1})$, $i = 1, \ldots, n$ and $k = 1, \ldots, K_i$, where $\hat{H}(w_{ik}|t_{i,k-1})$ is the estimated cumulative rate function of the fitted model [3]. When the model is appropriate, the graphical representation of the pairs $\left(\hat{r}_{ik}, \hat{H}_{NA}(\hat{r}_{ik})\right)$, where $\hat{H}_{NA}(\hat{r}_{ik})$ is the Nelson–Aalen estimate of the cumulative rate function based on the residuals, yields a straight line through the origin with slope 1. Figure 3 displays the Cox-Snell residuals plots of the EEP and ECP marginal rate models (which have the lowest AIC values) on the log scale, in order to easily identify departures from linearity. Although both models show close agreement, the proposed model provides a better fit to the data. This improvement in the goodness-of-fit is potentially due to its ability to capture a non-monotonic shape of the mrf.

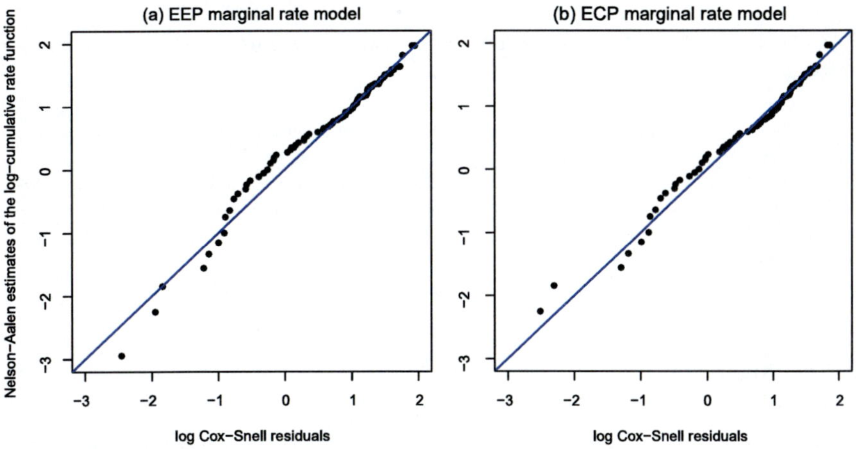

Fig. 3 Cox-Snell residuals to informally evaluate the goodness-of-fit of the (**a**) EEP and (**b**) ECP marginal rate models fitted to bowel motility data

6 Concluding Remarks

In this work, the applicability of the ECP lifetime distribution [18] is expanded for modelling gap times between recurrent events by proposing a new marginal rate model based on this distribution. Since the ECP marginal rate model is derived from a NHPP, the conditional distribution of the gap times given the previous recurrence time is deduced. Under this formulation, the gap times are treated equally and so the relationship between events of the same subject is no longer a problem [14]. Several features of the new model were studied, such as the expressions of its mrf, survival function and rth raw moments of the gap times (in particular, for the mean and variance). The proposed model is innovative in the sense that it is able to take on non-monotonic rates. In fact, it turns out to be quite flexible, as its mrf can be monotonic increasing, monotonic decreasing, unimodal, bathtub, IDI or DIDI. Moreover, it was shown that the proposed model has the Chen marginal rate model as a limiting case. The ML method was applied for parameter estimation in the presence of right-censoring. The results of the simulation study allowed to check the efficiency of the ML estimators, as well as the performance of the LR test, in various scenarios with different sample sizes, number of recurrences, censoring percentages and shapes of the mrf.

In the application to the bowel motility data, the proposed ECP marginal rate model revealed a superior fit to the data in comparison with other competing models. Furthermore, the new model offers an important interpretation in CCR scenarios, considering that it is based on the ECP distribution. For the bowel motility data, the ML estimate of parameter ϕ of the ECP marginal rate model (as well as the EEP marginal rate model) was positive. This fact points out that, if there are unobservable causes contributing to the event occurrence, they emerge necessarily from a complementary risk setting.

Acknowledgements This work is partially financed by national funds through FCT—Fundação para a Ciência e a Tecnologia, under the projects UIDB/00006/2020 (CEAUL—Centro de Estatística e Aplicações) and UIDB/04674/2020 (Center for Research in Mathematics and Applications (CIMA) related with the Statistics, Stochastic Processes and Applications (SSPA) group). I. Sousa-Ferreira also acknowledges financial support to FCT for the Ph.D. grant DFA/BD/6459/2020.

References

1. Gail, M.H., Santner, T.J., Brown, C.C.: An analysis of comparative carcinogenesis experiments based on multiple times to tumor. Biometrics **36**(2), 255 (1980)
2. Aalen, O.O., Husebye, E.: Statistical analysis of repeated events forming renewal processes. Stat. Med. **10**(8), 1227–1240 (1991)
3. Jerald Lawless, R.J.C.: The Statistical Analysis of Recurrent Events. Springer, New York (2007)
4. Chang, S.-H.: Estimating marginal effects in accelerated failure time models for serial sojourn times among repeated events. Lifetime Data Anal. **10**(2), 175–190 (2004)
5. Ghosh, D.: Accelerated rates regression models for recurrent failure time data. Lifetime Data Anal. **10**(3), 247–261 (2004)
6. Huang, Y., Chen, Y.Q.: Marginal regression of gaps between recurrent events. Lifetime Data Anal. **9**(3), 293–303 (2003)
7. Luo, X., Huang, C.-Y., Wang, L.: Quantile regression for recurrent gap time data. Biometrics **69**(2), 375–385 (2013)
8. Sun, L., Park, D.-H., Sun, J.: The additive hazards model for recurrent gap times. Stat. Sin. **16**(3), 919–932 (2006)
9. Box-Steffensmeier, J.M., Boef, S.D.: Repeated events survival models: the conditional frailty model. Stat. Med. **25**(20), 3518–3533 (2006)
10. Duchateau, L., Janssen, P., Kezic, I., Fortpied, C.: Evolution of recurrent asthma event rate over time in frailty models. J. R. Stat. Soc.: Ser. C **52**(3), 355–363 (2003)
11. Barthel, N., Geerdens, C., Czado, C., Janssen, P.: Dependence modeling for recurrent event times subject to right-censoring with d-vine copulas. Biometrics **75**(2), 439–451 (2019)
12. Meyer, R., Romeo, J.S.: Bayesian semiparametric analysis of recurrent failure time data using copulas. Biom. J. **57**(6), 982–1001 (2015)
13. Aalen, O., Borgan, O., Gjessing, H.: Survival and Event History Analysis. Springer, New York (2008)
14. Zhao, X., Zhou, X.: Modeling gap times between recurrent events by marginal rate function. Comput. Stat. & Data Anal. **56**(2), 370–383 (2012)
15. Macera, M.A.C., Louzada, F., Cancho, V.G., Fontes, C.J.F.: The exponential-poisson model for recurrent event data: an application to a set of data on malaria in brazil. Biom. J. **57**(2), 201–214 (2014)
16. Louzada, F., Macera, M.A., Cancho, V.G.: The poisson-exponential model for recurrent event data: an application to bowel motility data. J. Appl. Stat. **42**(11), 2353–2366 (2015)
17. Louzada, F., Macera, M.A., Cancho, V.G.: A gap time model based on a multiplicative marginal rate function that accounts for zero-recurrence units. Stat. Methods Med. Res. **26**(5), 2000–2010 (2017)
18. Sousa-Ferreira, I., Abreu, A.M., Rocha, C.: The extended Chen-Poisson lifetime distribution: Accepted - November 2021. REVSTAT—Statistical Journal (2021)
19. Chen, Z.: A new two-parameter lifetime distribution with bathtub shape or increasing failure rate function. Stat. & Probab. Lett. **49**(2), 155–161 (2000)

20. Ramos, P.L., Dey, D.K., Louzada, F., Lachos, V.H.: An extended poisson family of life distribution: a unified approach in competitive and complementary risks. J. Appl. Stat. **47**(2), 306–322 (2019)
21. Ramos, P.L., Guzman, D.C.F., Mota, A.L., Rodrigues, F.A., Louzada, F.: Sampling with censored data: a practical guide (2020)
22. R Core Team: R: A Language and Environment for Statistical Computing. R Foundation for Statistical Computing, Vienna, Austria (2022)
23. Zhou, S., Maller, R.A.: The likelihood ratio test for the presence of immunes in a censored sample. Statistics **27**(1–2), 181–201 (1995)

On Classical Measurement Error within a Bayesian Nonparametric Framework

Emmanuel Bernieri and Miguel de Carvalho

Abstract This paper studies the impact of classical measurement error on a Dependent Dirichlet Process (DDP). Specifically, we study a Simulation-Extrapolation (SIMEX) algorithm, adapted to a nonparametric Bayesian framework, that assesses the impact of measurement error by inducing even further error in the covariate. We illustrate the algorithm via a battery of numerical experiments.

Keywords Classical measurement error · Dependent Dirichlet process · Nonparametric Bayes · Simulation-extrapolation

1 Introduction

Measurement error is a well-known statistical problem that occurs in regression applications, when covariates cannot be observed directly but are rather observed with error. See [1–5].

In this paper, we will devise an algorithm for accounting for classical measurement error on an infinite mixture of regression lines; such mixture model is known in nonparametric Bayesian parlance as dependent Dirichlet process [6–10].

The dependent Dirichlet process, developed by MacEachern in [9, 10] is a generalization of the Dirichlet process as a prior for a collection of covariate dependent random distribution. The focus of this paper is to examine the effect of the classical measurement error in a dependent Dirichlet process. With this aim in mind, we resort to a SIMEX algorithm, as proposed in [11], so to correct the effect of measurement error. While The nonparametric Bayesian framework has already been employed in a measurement error context [12–15], the inclusion of measurement error in the dependent Dirichlet process has not been explored yet in the literature to the best of our knowledge.

E. Bernieri · M. de Carvalho (✉)
School of Mathematics, University of Edinburgh, Edinburgh, Scotland
e-mail: Miguel.deCarvalho@ed.ac.uk

R. Bispo et al. (eds.), *Recent Developments in Statistics and Data Science*,
Springer Proceedings in Mathematics & Statistics 398,
https://doi.org/10.1007/978-3-031-12766-3_24

The remainder of the article is organized as follows. Section 2 presents the SIMEX-DDP algorithm. Then in Sect. 3, we present some numerical experiments to assess the performance of the algorithm in a controlled environment. Then we will discuss the results of our research and conclude.

2 Simulation Extrapolation for a Conditional Dirichlet Process

2.1 Background

When data are too complex to be described by a single distribution, statisticians typically use mixture models that consist of weighted sums of distributions. A well-known example is the K-normal mixture model whose density is given by:

$$f(y \mid \boldsymbol{\omega}, \boldsymbol{\theta}) = \sum_{k=1}^{K} \omega_k \phi(y \mid \mu_k, \sigma_k^2), \tag{1}$$

where $\boldsymbol{\omega} = (\omega_1, \ldots, \omega_K)$ is a set of positive weights adding up to one, and $\boldsymbol{\theta} = (\mu_1, \ldots, \mu_K, \sigma_1^2, \ldots, \sigma_K^2)$ is a parameter containing the mean and variance of each component in the mixture.

Dirichlet process mixtures are a well-known nonparametric Bayesian approach that extends (1) by allowing for an infinite number of components. This is achieved by resorting to a prior on the space of probability measures, known as the Dirichlet Process (DP) [16, 17]. For example, the density of a Dirichlet process mixture of Normal distributions is given by:

$$f(y) = \int \phi(y, \mu, \sigma^2) \mathrm{d}G(\mu, \sigma^2), \quad G \sim \mathrm{DP}(\alpha, G_0). \tag{2}$$

Here G_0 is the centering distribution and $\alpha > 0$ is the so-called precision parameter. Note that $\mathrm{E}(G) = G_0$ and $\mathrm{var}(G) = G_0(1 - G_0)/(\alpha + 1)$.

Sethuraman gives a definition of the Dirichlet process in [18] as a constructive representation according to which $G \sim \mathrm{DP}(\alpha, G_0)$ has an almost sure representation of the form

$$G(\cdot) = \sum_{k=1}^{\infty} \omega_k \delta_{\boldsymbol{\theta}_k}(\cdot) \tag{3}$$

where $\boldsymbol{\theta}_k \overset{\text{iid}}{\sim} G_0$, $k = 1, 2, \ldots$, and $\omega_1 = v_1$, and for $k \geq 2$, $\omega_k = v_k \prod_{l<k}(1 - v_l)$, with $v_k \overset{\text{iid}}{\sim} \mathrm{Beta}(1, \alpha)$.

Now that we have introduced preparations on the Bayesian nonparametric framework of interest, we are ready to discuss a conditional error-contaminated version of (2).

2.2 Error-Contaminated Dependent Dirichlet Process

The dependent Dirichlet process proposed by MacEachern in [10] was built on top of the stick-breaking representation of Sethuraman [18]. A common approach to extend the Dirichlet process mixture in (2) to a conditional setting is to define the conditional density of a dependent nonparametric process in a very general manner as follows:

$$f(y \mid \mathbf{x}) = \int_{\Theta} K(\boldsymbol{\theta} \mid y) G_{\mathbf{x}}(d\boldsymbol{\theta}), \quad (y, \mathbf{x}) \in \mathbb{R} \times \mathcal{X}. \tag{4}$$

Here, $\boldsymbol{\theta} \subset \boldsymbol{\Theta} = \mathbb{R}^p$, K a kernel, and $\mathcal{X} \subset \mathbb{R}^q$ is the covariate space. In this paper we will choose a dependent Dirichlet process developed in [10] as a prior:

$$G_{\mathbf{X}} = \sum_{k=1}^{\infty} \omega_{k,\mathbf{x}} \delta_{\theta_{k,\mathbf{x}}}, \quad \omega_{1,\mathbf{x}} = v_{1,\mathbf{x}}, \quad \omega_{k,\mathbf{x}} = v_{k,\mathbf{x}} \prod_{l<k} (1 - v_{l,\mathbf{x}}), \tag{5}$$

where $\theta_{1,\mathbf{x}}, \ldots$ and $v_{1,\mathbf{x}}, \ldots$ are realizations of stochastic processes over $\mathcal{X}$, with $v_{k,\mathbf{x}} \sim \text{Beta}(1, \alpha_{\mathbf{x}})$, $\alpha_{\mathbf{x}} > 0$ is the precision parameter, and $\delta_{\theta_{k,\mathbf{x}}}$ denotes a point mass at $\theta_{k,\mathbf{x}}$. For example, assuming a Normal kernel and focusing on the single weight version of [10] (that sets $\omega_h = \omega_{h,\mathbf{x}}$), the DDP conditional density can be expressed as an infinite mixture of linear regression models that is:

$$f(y \mid \mathbf{x}) = \sum_{k=1}^{\infty} \omega_k \phi(y, \mathbf{x}^T \boldsymbol{\beta}_k, \sigma_k^2), \tag{6}$$

where the ω_k are similarly defined as in (3), and the $\boldsymbol{\beta}_k \in \mathbb{R}^p$ are regression parameters.

The current practice in the community is to learn about (6) from an error-free random sample $\{\mathbf{x}_i, y_i\}_{i=1}^n$. Yet, in practice, covariates may be subject to measurement error [19, 20], and it will be a goal of this paper to address this problem in the context of (4).

The classical measurement error type in the case of a single contaminated covariate has the following form:

$$W_i = X_i + U_i, \quad i = 1, \ldots, n, \tag{7}$$

where X_i and W_i are, respectively, the true and observed covariate, U_i is the measurement error, and n is the sample size. We assume $E[U_i \mid X_i] = 0$, and thus it follows that $E[U_i] = E[E[U_i \mid X_i]] = 0$ and:

$$\begin{aligned} \text{cov}(X_i, U_i) &= E[(X_i - \mu_X)(U_i - 0)] \\ &= E[X_i U_i] - \mu_X E[U_i] = E[E[X_i Ui \mid X_i]] \\ &= E[X_i E[U_i \mid X_i]] \\ &= 0, \end{aligned}$$

where $\mu_X = E[X_i]$, since X_i and U_i are uncorrelated we have:

$$\text{var}(W_i) = \sigma_X^2 + \sigma_U^2, \tag{8}$$

where σ_X^2 and σ_U^2 are the variance of X and U. A common metric to quantify the relative magnitude of the measurement error is the so-called reliability ratio:

$$\lambda = \frac{\sigma_X^2}{\sigma_X^2 + \sigma_U^2}. \tag{9}$$

Equation (9) warrants some remarks. The reliability ratio is important in measurement error because the ordinary least squares regression of $\mathbf{y}$ on $\mathbf{W}$ is a consistent estimator of $\beta_{x*} = \lambda \beta_x$ (see Chap. 1 of [20], or Chap. 3 of [19]). We can notice that the OLS regression of $\mathbf{y}$ on $\mathbf{W}$ will produce an estimator that is attenuated to zero. The more variance is induced by measurement error, the more the estimator will tend to zero.

The error-contaminated DDP conditional density is simply the conditional density in (6) contaminated with classical measurement error:

$$f(y \mid \mathbf{w}) = \sum_{k=1}^{\infty} \omega_k \phi(y; \mathbf{w}^T \boldsymbol{\beta}_k^*, \sigma_k^2), \tag{10}$$

where the $\boldsymbol{\beta}_k^* \in \mathbb{R}^p$ are the regression parameter of the DDP contaminated with measurement error.

So the question of interest is now the following: Given a sample with classical measurement error $\{\mathbf{w}_i, y_i\}_{i=1}^n$, how do we learn about (6)?

2.3 The SIMEX-DDP Algorithm

Before we are ready to introduce our SIMEX-DDP algorithm, we first review some background on SIMEX-based approaches. The SIMEX was developed in 1994 by Cook and Stefanski in [11]. It is a simulation-based method of estimating and reducing bias due to measurement error. The SIMEX methodology consists in adding measurement error to the data, studying the trend of measurement error induced bias against the variance of the added measurement error. To put differently, the underlying idea behind SIMEX is that we can estimate the effect of measurement error experimentally thanks to the simulation framework.

Suppose that we have our original dataset with additive measurement error, and we also have $M - 1$ additional datasets each with successively larger measurement error variance $(1 + \zeta_m)\sigma_u^2$, where $0 < \zeta_1 < \cdots < \zeta_M$ are known. Then thanks to (9) we can write that the parameter estimates for the mth dataset are consistently estimated by:

$$\hat{\beta}_{x,m} = \frac{\beta_x \sigma_x^2}{\sigma_x^2 + (1 + \zeta_m)\sigma_u^2}. \tag{11}$$

For each of the m dataset, we will have an estimate $\hat{\beta}_{x,m}$. If we consider the following dataset $\{\zeta_m, \hat{\beta}_{x,m}\}_{m=1}^{M}$ we can write the mean function of this regression as follows:

$$E(\hat{\beta}_{x,m} \mid \zeta) = \frac{\beta_x \sigma_x^2}{\sigma_x^2 + (1 + \zeta)\sigma_u^2}. \tag{12}$$

If we set $\zeta = -1$ in (12) we end up with β_x which is the value of interest.

We can write the SIMEX algorithm as follows:

- **Simulating**: Add independent measurement error with variance $\zeta_m \sigma_u^2$ are generated and added to the original data **W**. The total variance for the mth dataset is $(1 + \zeta_m)\sigma_u^2$.
- **Learning**: Parameter estimates are obtained for each of the generated datasets.
- **Averaging**: The first two steps are repeated a large number of times and the average value of the estimates for each level of contamination is calculated.
- **Extrapolating**: We have an average estimate for each of the mth dataset with known level of ζ; we use regression technique to find the estimate for $\zeta = -1$.

The SIMEX-DDP algorithm to be presented below is a straightforward extension of the standard SIMEX algorithm. The SIMEX-DDP procedure can be divided into four steps:

- **Simulating**: Add independent measurement error with variance $\zeta_m \sigma_u^2$ to the original data **W**. Simulate m datasets with increasing measurement error variance.
- **Learning**: Estimate (10) for each of the generated datasets.
- **Averaging**: After repeating the simulation and estimation steps a large number of times we average the estimates.
- **Extrapolating** to the ideal case of no measurement error ($\zeta = -1$) yields the SIMEX-DDP estimates of the conditional density.

The SIMEX-DDP consists in getting successive conditional expectation by fitting an increasing independent measurement error with variance $\zeta_m \sigma_u^2$ to the original **W** data. Then we use the same logic as the original SIMEX and we get end by extrapolating the true conditional expectation without measurement error.

Now that we have explicated the mechanics governing the proposed SIMEX-DDP algorithm, we will conduct a battery of numerical experiments so to evaluate its potential.

3 Numerical Experiments on Artificial Data

To evaluate the performance of the SIMEX algorithm from Sect. 2 we analyzed simulated data under the following four scenarios: linear mean, a mixture of linear means, nonlinear mean with constant variance, and another nonlinear mean with constant variance. We use the same dataset for each of the four scenarios, the sample size is $n = 200$. Covariates were independently generated from a standard Normal distribution, and the responses were generated as follows:

$$\begin{aligned}
\textbf{Scenario I:} \quad & y_i \mid x_i \sim N(2 + 4x_i, 2^2), \\
\textbf{Scenario II:} \quad & y_i \mid x_i \sim 0.5\, N(2 + 3x_i, 1^2) + 0.5\, N(6 + 2.5x_i, 1^2), \\
\textbf{Scenario III:} \quad & y_i \mid x_i \sim N(9 + 1.15x_i^2, 2.5^2), \\
\textbf{Scenario IV:} \quad & y_i \mid x_i \sim N(5 + 1.5x + 1.5 \times \sin(x), 1.5)).
\end{aligned}$$

In Scenario 1, we consider different homoscedastic linear mean regression models. Data for Scenario 2 are governed by the following mixtures of homoscedastic linear mean regression models. Scenarios 3 and 4 involve homoscedastic nonlinear mean regression models. For each of these scenarios, we consider three level of classical measurement error, $(0.1, 0.3, 0.5)$, and our SIMEX-DDP algorithm will be based on 10 iterations for each scenario and measurement error level. We use the same model specification as in [8].

On our numerical inquiry, we set $m = 10$ and $\zeta = 0.05$. Each blocked Gibbs sampler scans for 1500 draws for the posterior distribution after a burn-in of 500 samples. After fitting our models, we test them on an out-of-sample dataset of size $m = 100$ generated from a standard Normal distribution.

We can clearly see in Fig. 1 the effect of measurement error on the regression lines. The larger the variance of the contaminated data is the closer the slope of the regression line is of 0. Now that we have presented the artificial data for the numerical experiments let's see how SIMEX algorithm is working.

As it can be seen in Fig. 2, the SIMEX-DDP algorithm recovers the true from the contaminate dataset in this example with a high level of accuracy. To illustrate the accuracy of the algorithm under study, Fig. 3 depicts the boxplot of the distance between the estimated yield by our algorithm and the true value, and the distance between the estimate without using the SIMEX-DDP and the true value. As we

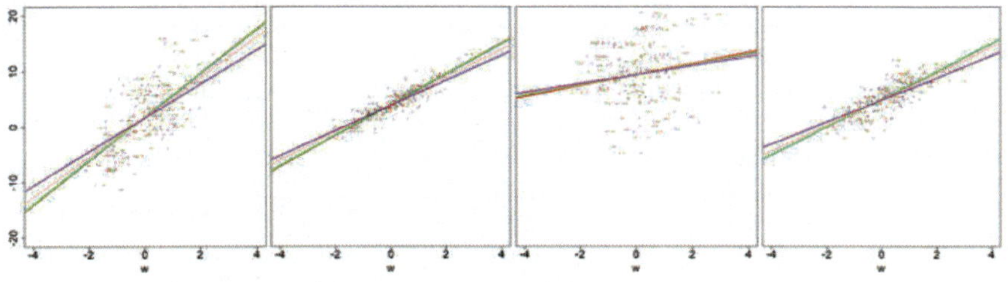

Fig. 1 Simulated datasets over different levels of measurement error (red point are observed without measurement error, green are observed with $\sigma_u^2 = 0.1$, pink with $\sigma_u^2 = 0.3$, and purple with $\sigma_u^2 = 0.5$), and their respective regression lines for each of the four scenarios. We use the same dataset for all the four scenarios

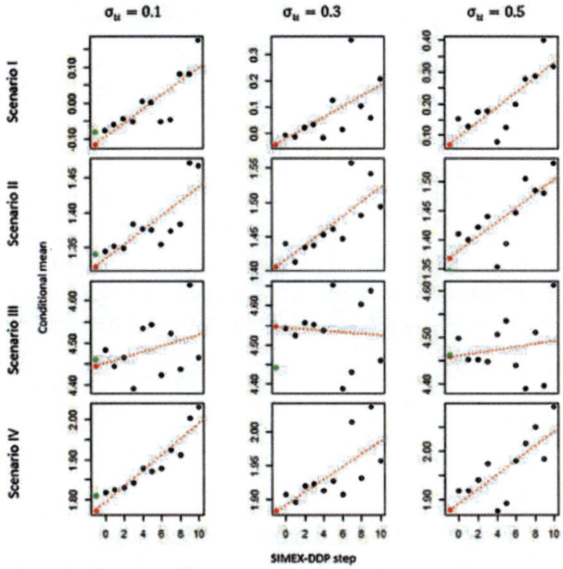

Fig. 2 Fitting of our first testing point for Scenario I to IV (rows) and for classical measurement error level of (0.1, 0.3, 0.5) (columns). On each graph, we can find the true value (green), the extrapolated value of our SIMEX algorithm (red) along with the regression line over the 10 iterations of the SIMEX-DDP algorithm that allowed us to estimate this value, and 10 iterations of the SIMEX algorithm (black)

can see on Fig. 3, the SIMEX-DDP algorithm consistently outperforms the naive approach that does not take into account measurement error. The only case (Scenario IV with level of measurement error of $\sigma_u = 0.1$) where the naive approach performs better, the difference in performance is negligible.

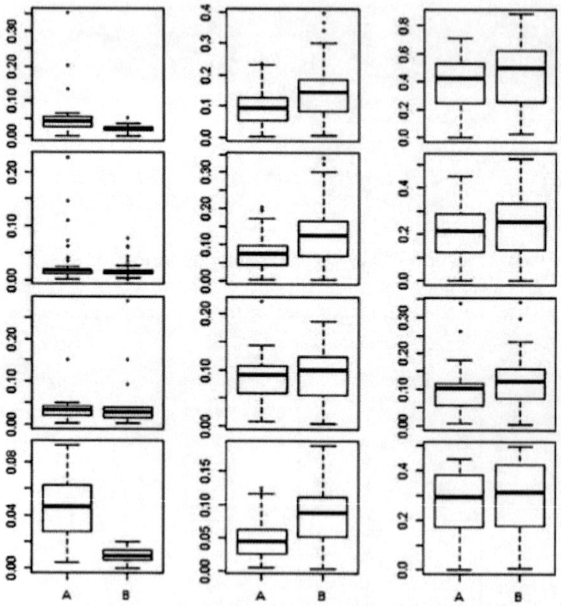

Fig. 3 Boxplot A corresponds to the distance between to true and estimated values thanks to the SIMEX-DDP algorithm for each of the 100 data points of our test set. Boxplot B corresponds to the distance between the true and estimated values without taking into account the presence of classical measurement error

4 Final Remarks

In this paper, we conduct a pilot study on a new approach to take care of classical measurement error within a Bayesian nonparametric context based on the famous Simulation-Extrapolation algorithm of Cook and Stenfaski. Specifically, we develop a SIMEX algorithm with the dependent Dirichlet process framework and test its performance on a numerical workout with various scenarios and measurement error level.

The preliminary results that we report in this paper suggest an interesting performance of the SIMEX-DDP algorithm. However, a Monte Carlo simulation is needed to examine the performance of the algorithm and confirm its potential. The algorithm that we develop here can be improved by adding extra flexibility to the regression line that we are using to estimate our (measurement) 'error-free' conditional density. For example, we could use B-spline basis functions to improve the performance of the algorithm. We can also acknowledge that the SIMEX-DDP is performant under all the four scenarios that we present, though at this stage, it remains unclear whether performance over Scenario IV could be improved.

Finally, it is important to consider that the SIMEX-DDP is highly computer intensive. Indeed, because we need to fit a dependent Dirichlet process at each simulation step of the SIMEX-DDP, the calculation cost is expensive and its regular use calls for a need of parallel computing or cloud-based computing. In our case, for each combination of scenarios-level of measurement error, we had to fit 12 times our data, one for the error-free dataset, one for the contaminated dataset, and then one time for each of the 10 steps of the algorithm. With our configuration of a test set of 200 observations, and with 1500 posterior draws for our blocked Gibbs sampler, it takes about 4 min on a machine with 64 cores with speed 3.20 Ghz.

References

1. Buonaccorsi, J.P., Lin, C.-D.: Berkson measurement error in designed repeated measures studies with random coefficients. J. Stat. Plan. Infer. **104**(1), 53–72 (2002)
2. Jones, D.Y., Schatzkin, A., Green, S.B., Block, G., Brinton, L.A., Ziegler, R.G., Hoover, R., Taylor, P.R.: Dietary fat and breast cancer in the national health and nutrition examination survey i epidemiologic follow-up study. J. Natl. Cancer Inst. **79**(3), 465–471 (1987)
3. Lerner, D.J., Kannel, W.B.: Patterns of coronary heart disease morbidity and mortality in the sexes: a 26-year follow-up of the framingham population. Amer. Heart J. **111**(2), 383–390 (1986)
4. Pierce, D.A., Stram, D.O., Vaeth, M., Schafer, D.W.: The errors-in-variables problem: considerations provided by radiation dose-response analyses of the a-bomb survivor data. J. Amer. Stat. Assoc. **87**(418), 351–359 (1992)
5. Rosner, B., Spiegelman, D., Willett, W.C.: Correction of logistic regression relative risk estimates and confidence intervals for measurement error: the case of multiple covariates measured with error. Amer. J. Epidemiol. **132**(4), 734–745 (1990)
6. de Carvalho, M., Barney, B., Page, G.: Affinity-based measures of biomarker performance evaluation. Stat. Methods Med. Res. **29**(3), 837–853 (2019)
7. De Iorio, M., Müller, P., Rosner, G.L., MacEachern, S.N.: An anova model for dependent random measures. J. Amer. Stat. Assoc. **99**(465), 205–215 (2004)
8. Inácio de Carvalho, V., de Carvalho, M., Branscum, A.J.: Nonparametric Bayesian regression analysis of the Youden index. Biometrics **73**, 1279–1288 (2017)
9. MacEachern, S.N.: Dependent nonparametric processes. In: ASA Proceedings of the Section on Bayesian Statistical Science, vol. 1, pp. 50–55. American Statistical Association, Alexandria, Virginia (1999)
10. MacEachern, S.N.: Dependent Dirichlet processes. Unpublished manuscript, Department of Statistics, The Ohio State University, pp. 1–40 (2000)
11. Cook, J.R., Stefanski, L.A.: Simulation-extrapolation estimation in parametric measurement error models. J. Amer. Stat. Assoc. **89**(428), 1314–1328 (1994)
12. Lee, Y., Jeong, T., Kim, H.: A Bayesian nonparametric mixture measurement error model with application to spatial density estimation using mobile positioning data with multi-accuracy and multi-coverage. Technometrics **62**(2), 173–183 (2020)
13. Ryu, D., Li, E., Mallick, B.K.: Bayesian nonparametric regression analysis of data with random effects covariates from longitudinal measurements. Biometrics **67**(2), 454–466 (2011)
14. Trippa, L., Waldron, L., Huttenhower, C., Parmigiani, G.: Bayesian nonparametric cross-study validation of prediction methods. Ann. Appl. Stat. **9**(1), 402–428 (2015)
15. Walker, S.G., Damien, P., Laud, P.W., Smith, A.F.: Bayesian nonparametric inference for random distributions and related functions. J. R. Stat. Soc.: Ser. B (Stat. Methodol.) **61**(3), 485–527 (1999)
16. Ferguson, T.S.: A Bayesian analysis of some nonparametric problems. Ann. Stat. 209–230 (1973)

17. Ferguson, T.S.: Prior distributions on spaces of probability measures. Ann. Stat. **2**(4), 615–629 (1974)
18. Sethuraman, J.: A constructive definition of Dirichlet priors. Stat. Sinica 639–650 (1994)
19. Carroll, R.J., Ruppert, D., Crainiceanu, C.M., Stefanski, L.A.: Measurement error in nonlinear models: a modern perspective. Chapman and Hall/CRC (2006)
20. Fuller, W.A.: Measurement Error Models, vol. 305. Wiley, New York (1987)

Author Index

R. Bispo et al. (eds.), *Recent Developments in Statistics and Data Science*, Springer Proceedings in Mathematics & Statistics 398,
https://doi.org/10.1007/978-3-031-12766-3